Nutritional Aspects
of
Osteoporosis

Second Edition

Second Edition

Nutritional Aspects of Osteoporosis

Edited by

Peter Burckhardt

Department of Medicine
CHUV
Lausanne, Switzerland

Bess Dawson-Hughes

Bone Metabolism Laboratory
Jean Mayer U.S.D.A. Human
Research Center on Aging
Tufts University
Boston, Massachusetts

Robert P. Heaney

University Chair
Creighton University
Omaha, Nebraska

ELSEVIER
ACADEMIC
PRESS

Amsterdam   Boston   Heidelberg   London   New York   Oxford
Paris   San Diego   San Francisco   Singapore   Sydney   Tokyo

Elsevier Academic Press
200 Wheeler Road, 6th Floor, Burlington, MA 01803, USA
525 B Street, Suite 1900, San Diego, California 92101-4495, USA
84 Theobald's Road, London WC1X 8RR, UK

This book is printed on acid-free paper. ∞

Library of Congress Cataloging-in-Publication Data
Application submitted

British Library Cataloguing in Publication Data
A catalogue record for this book is available from the British Library

ISBN: 0-12-141704-2

For all information on all Academic Press publications
visit our Web site at www.academicpress.com

Printed in the United States of America
04   05   06   07   08   09   9   8   7   6   5   4   3   2   1

SPONSORS

MAIN SPONSORS
Glaxo Smith Kline
National Diary Council USA
Nycomed
Novartis Consumer Health

SPONSORS
Eli Lilly
IOF
Minute Maid Company
MSD Switzerland
Nestlé
Nestlé Foundation
Novartis Pharma Switzerland
Organon
Procter & Gamble
Rhodia Pharma Solutions
Roche Vitamins
Serono Foundation for the Advancement of Medical Science

FURTHER CONTRIBUTORS
Robapharm
Servier

This symposium is endorsed by

IOF (International Osteoporosis Foundation – President P. Delmas)
NOF (National Osteoporosis Foundation, U.S. – President B. Dawson-Hughes)

CONTENTS

Sponsors   v

Contributors   xxi

Preface   xxvii

PART **I**

Calcium in Childhood

1. Bone Mineral Density of the Skull and Lower Extremities During Growth and Calcium Supplementation

Velimir Matkovic, John D. Landoll, Prem Goel, Nancy Badenhop-Stevens, Eun-Jeong Ha, Bin Li, and Zeljka Crncevic-Orlic

Abstract   3
Introduction   4
Methods   5
Results   6
Discussion   10
Acknowledgments   14
References   14

2. Calcium Retention in Adolescence as a Function of Calcium Intake: Influence of Race and Gender

Connie M. Weaver

Abstract   17

Introduction   17
Methods for Determining Calcium Retention and Metabolism   18
Racial Differences in Calcium Metabolism   19
Gender Differences in Calcium Metabolism   21
Further Directions   22
References   22

3. **Longitudinal Study of Diet and Lifestyle Intervention on
   Bone Mineral Gain in School Children and Adolescents:
   Effects of Asian Traditional Diet and Sitting Style on Bone
   Mineral**

   Takako Hirota, Tomoko Kusu, Mizuho Hara, and Kenji Hirota

   Abstract   25
   Introduction   26
   Subjects and Methods   26
   Results   27
   Discussion   30
   Acknowledgment   32
   References   32

4. **A Co-Twin Calcium Intervention Trial in Premenarcheal
   Girls: Cortical Bone Effects by Hip Structural Analysis**

   *Lynda Paton, Thomas Beck, Caryl Nowson, Melissa Cameron, Susan Kantor,
   Heather McKay, Mark Forwood and John D. Wark*

   Abstract   35
   Introduction   36
   Methods   37
   Statistical Analyses   39
   Results   39
   Discussion   41
   References   42

5. **Calcium Carbonate Supplementation is Associated
   with Higher Plasma IGF-1 in 16- to 18-Year-Old
   Boys and Girls**

   *Fiona Ginty, A. Prentice, A. Laidlaw, L. McKenna, S. Jones, S. Stear,
   and T.J. Cole*

   Abstract   45
   Introduction   46

Methods   47
Results   51
Discussion   54
Conclusions   55
Acknowledgments   56
References   56

PART II
Dairy Products, Calcium Metabolism

6. Nutrients, Interactions, and Foods: The Importance of Source
Robert P. Heaney

Introduction   61
Calcium and Diet Quality   62
Calcium and Protein   65
Phosphorus and Calcium   67
Conclusion   74
References   74

PART III
Vitamins, Flavonoids

7. Vitamin K and Bone Health
Cees Vermeer

Abstract   79
Introduction   80
Sites of Vitamin K Action   81
Similarities Between Calcium Metabolism in
    Bone and Arteries   82
Vitamin K Status and Bone Health   84
Vitamin K Status and Cardiovascular Health   85
Vitamin K Intervention Studies   86
Dietary Vitamin K Requirements for Bone and
    Vascular Health   87

Safety and Potential Adverse Side Effects of
  Vitamin K Supplements   88
References   89

8. **Dietary Vitamin A is Negatively Related to Bone Mineral
   Density in Postmenopausal Woment**

*Jasminka Z. Ilich, Rhonda A. Brownbill, Harold C. Furr,
and Neal E. Craft*

Abstract   93
Introduction   94
Methods   95
Results   98
Discussion   102
Summary and Conclusions   106
Acknowledgments   106
References   106

9. **Hesperidin, a Citrus Flavanone, Improves Bone
   Acquisition and Prevents Skeletal Impairment
   in Rats**

Marie-Noëlle Horcajada and Véronique Coxam

Abstract   109
Introduction   110
Methods   112
Results   115
Discussion   119
References   123

10. **Vitamin B-Complex, Methylenetetrahydrofolate
    Reductase Polymorphism and Bone: Potential
    for Gene-Nutrient Interaction**

H.M. Macdonal and D.M. Reid

Abstract   127
Introduction   128
What is the Role of Methylene Tetrahydrofolate Reductase
  (MTHFR) Enzyme?   128
MTHFR Polymorphism   129
Vitamin B-Complex   132
Conclusions   135
References   135

PART **IV**

Nutrition and Bone Health Miscellaneous

11. A Placebo Controlled Randomized Trial of Chromium
    Picolinate Supplementation on Indices of Bone and
    Calcium Metabolism in Healthy Women
    *Monica Adhikari, Brian W. Morris, Richard Eastell,
    and Aubrey Blumsohn*

    Abstract   141
    Subjects   144
    Methods   144
    Result   146
    Discussion   147
    Acknowledgments   150
    References   150

12. Nutrition and Teeth
    Elizabeth A. Krall

    Abstract   153
    Introduction   154
    Oral Bone Loss and Systemic Bone Mineral Density   154
    Nutrition, Periodontal Disease and Tooth Loss   156
    Relationship of Calcium, Vitamin D, and Phosphorus
      to Periodontal Disease and Tooth Loss   158
    Conclusions   161
    Summary   162
    References   162

13. Cognitive Dietary Restraint, Cortisol and Bone Density
    in Normal-Weight Women: Is There a Relationship?
    Susan I. Barr

    Abstract   165
    Introduction   166
    Possible Mechanism   167
    Assessment of Dietary Restraint   167
    Associations Between Dietary Restraint and
      Menstrual Disturbances   168

Associations Between Subclinical Menstrual Disturbances
and Bone Loss   172
Associations Between Dietary Restraint and Cortisol   172
Association Between Dietary Restraint and Bone   173
Summary   175
Acknowledgments   175
References   175

PART **V**

Vitamin D—First Part

14. **Functions of Vitamin D: Importance for Prevention of
Common Cancers, Type 1 Diabetes and Heart Disease**
Michael F. Holick

Evolution of Vitamin D   181
Photosynthesis and Regulation of Previtamin D_3 182
Vitamin D and Bone Health   183
Metabolism and Biologic Functions of Vitamin D   183
Prevalence and Consequences of Vitamin D Deficiency
on Bone Health   186
Other Health Consequences of Vitamin D Deficiency:
Increased Risk of Autoimmune Diseases, Solid
Tumors, and Cardiovascular Heart Disease   189
Clinical Applications for the Antiproliferative Activity
of $1,25(OH)_2D_3$ and its Analogs   193
Prevention and Treatment of Vitamin D Deficiency   194
Conclusion   197
Acknowledgment   198
References   198

15. **Evidence for the Breakpoint of Normal Serum
25-Hydroxyvitamin D: Which Level Is Required
in the Elderly?**
Paul Lips

Introduction   203
Assessing the Required Serum 25(OH)D Concentration   204
Evidence from Epidemiological and Intervention Studies   205

The Influence of Calcium Intake on Serum PTH
  and Vitamin D Metabolism   206
Staging of Vitamin D Deficiency   207
Conclusion   207
References   208

16. What is the Optimal Amount of Vitamin D for
    Osteoporosis?
Reinhold Vieth

Introduction   211
Vitamin D and Osteoporosis   213
Dosage Considerations   215
Hormonal 1,25(OH)$_2$D is not an Alternative to
  Nutritional Vitamin D   217
Summary   219
References   220

PART **VI**

Vitamin D—Second Part

17. Serum 25-Hydroxyvitamin D and the Health of the
    Calcium Economy
Robert P. Heaney

Introduction   227
Studies of Calcium Absorption   228
Osteoporotic Fractures   231
Comment   232
References   232

18. Defining Optimal 25-Hydroxyvitamin D Levels in
    Younger and Older Adults Based on Hip Bone Mineral
    Density
Heike A. Bischoff-Ferrari and Bess Dawson-Hughes

Abstract   235
PTH Versus BMD in Threshold Assessment for
  Optimal 25-OHD Levels   236

Rationale for Assessment of Optimal 25-OHD in the
Non-White Population   237
Methods Applied to Study the Association Between 25-OHD
and BMD in a Population-Based Sample   237
Results   238
Discussion   240
References   242

19. Vitamin D Supplementation in Postmenopausal Black
Women Improves Calcium Homeostasis and Bone
Turnover in Three Months
*Jeri W. Nieves, Barbara Ambrose, Elizabeth Vasquez, Marsha Zion,
Felicia Cosman, and Robert Lindsay*

Abstract   245
Introduction   246
Methods   247
Results   248
Discussion   250
Acknowledgment   251
References   251

20. Adherence to Vitamin D Supplementation in Elderly
Patients After Hip Fracture
Elena Segal, H. Zinnman, B. Raz, A. Tamir, and S. Ish-Shalom

Abstract   253
Introduction   254
Patients and Methods   254
Results   256
Discussion   256
Conclusion   258
References   259

21. Vitamin D Round Table
*Bess Dawson-Hughes, Robert P. Heaney, Michael Holick, Paul Lips,
Pierre J. Meunier, and Reinhold Vieth*

Introduction   263
What is the Optimal Level of 25(OH)D for the
Skeleton and Why?   264

How Much Vitamin D_3 is Needed to Reach the Optimal
Level of 25(OH)D?   266
References   268

PART **VII**

Acid Load From Food—First Part

22. **Effects of Diet Acid Load on Bone Health**
Lynda A. Frassetto, R. Curtis Morris, Jr, and Anthony Sebastian

Abstract   273
Determinants of the Setpoint at which Blood Acidity
and Plasma Bicarbonate Concentration are
Regulated in Normal Subjects   274
Chronic Metabolic Acidosis and Bone Wasting   279
Plasma Acid-Base Balance and Diet Acid Load in Humans   281
Crossing the Neutral Zone   288
Implications for Further Research   290
Acknowledgments   290
References   290

23. **Effect of Various Classes of Foodstuffs and Beverages
of Vegetable Origin on Bone Metabolism in the Rat**
Roman C. Mühlbauer

Abstract   297
Introduction   298
Materials and Methods   299
Results and Discussion   302
What Should We Eat?   309
References   311

24. **A Role for Fruit and Vegetables in Osteoporosis
Prevention?**
Susan A. New

Abstract   315
Introduction   316
Importance of Acid-Base Homeostasis to Optimum Health   316

A Link Between Acid-Base Maintenance and Skeletal Integrity?   317
Acidity of Foods and Skeletal Health: Concept of
    Potential Renal Acid Loads   318
Positive Link Between Fruit and Vegetables, Alkali, and
    Bone Health: A Review of Current Evidence   319
Concept of NEAP and its Potential Impact on the Skeleton   321
Calcium/Alkali Supplements and Optimum Bone Health   324
Fruit and Vegetables and Bone: Exploring Other
    Important Factors   324
Concluding Remarks   324
Acknowledgments   325
References   325

PART **VIII**

Acid Load From Food—Second Part

25. **The Ovine Model for the Study of Dietary Acid Base,
    Estrogen Depletion and Bone Health**

Jennifer M. Macleay, D.L. Wheeler, and A.S. Turner

Abstract   331
Introduction   332
Background and Significance   332
The Influence of Dietary Strong Ions   333
Determination of Dietary Acid Load   336
The Dairy Connection   338
Preliminary Studies   338
Effect of a Diet Low in Cation-Anion Balance on Bone
    Mineral Density in Mature Ovariectomized Ewes   339
Conclusion   345
Acknowledgments   345
References   346

26. **The Natural Dietary Potassium Intake of Humans:
    The Effect of Diet-Induced Potassium-Replete,
    Chloride-Sufficient, Chronic Low-Grade Metabolic
    Alkalosis, or Stone Age Diets for the 21st Century**

Lynda A. Frassetto, R. Curtis Morris, Jr, and Anthony Sebastian

Abstract   349

Ancestral Dietary Patterns   350
Ancestral Potassium Intakes   358
Acid-Base Relationship to Bone Health and Bone
  Mineral Density   360
Conclusions   361
Implications for Further Research   361
Acknowledgments   362
References   362

PART IX

Protein

27. N-Acetyl Cysteine Supplementation of Growing Mice: Effects on Skeletal Size, Bone Mineral Density, and Serum IGF-I

*Cheryl L. Ackert-Bicknell, Wesley G. Beamer, and
Clifford J. Rosen*

Abstract   369
Introduction   370
Materials and Methods   371
Results   372
Discussion   375
References   376

28. Dietary Protein Intakes and Bone Strength

*René Rizzoli, Patrick Ammann, Thierry Chevalley, and
Jean-Philippe Bonjour*

Introduction   379
Dietary Protein and Bone Mass Gain   380
Dietary Protein and Bone Mineral Mass   381
Dietary Protein and Bone Homeostasis   384
Effects of Correcting Protein Insufficiency   388
Dietary Protein and Fracture Risk   389
Conclusions   390
Acknowledgments   391
References   391

29. Dietary Protein and the Skeleton

Bess Dawson-Hughes

Abstract   399
Dietary Protein and Serum IGF-1   400
Protein and Acid-Base Balance   401
Protein and Urine Calcium Excretion   402
Protein and Calcium Absorption   402
Dietary Protein and Bone Turnover   403
Protein, Bone Loss, and Fractures   403
Potential Impact of Calcium Intake on Link Between
  Protein and Bone   405
References   406

PART **X**

Protein—Mineral Water

30. Milk Basic Protein Increases Bone Mineral Density and
    Improves Bone Metabolism in Humans

Yukihiro Takada, Seiichiro Aoe, Yasuhiro Toba, Kazuhiro Uenishi, Akira Takeuchi, Akira Itabashi

Abstract   413
Introduction   414
Human Study 1   416
Human Study 2   423
Conclusion   426
References   427

31. Dietary Balance in Physically Active and Inactive Girls

Jaana A. Nurmi-Lawton, Adam Baxter-Jones, Pat Taylor, Cyrus Cooper, Jacki Bishop, and Susan New

Abstract   431
Introduction   432
AIMS   433
Subjects and Methods   433
Results   433
Discussion   435
References   437

32. Mineral Waters: Effects on Bone and Bone Metabolism

Peter Burckhardt

Introduction   439
Calcium   440
Sodium   441
Sulfates   442
Carbonated Beverages   442
Fluoride   442
Acid Load   443
Alkaline Load   444
Potassium   445
Conclusions   445
References   445

Index   449

CONTRIBUTORS

Numbers in parentheses indicate the pages on which the authors' contributions begin.

CHERYL L. ACKERT-BICKNELL (369) The Jackson Laboratory, Bar Harbor, Maine

MONICA ADHIKARI (141) Human Nutrition Unit, University of Sheffield, Northern General Hospital, Sheffield, United Kingdom

BARBARA AMBROSE (245) Clinical Research, Helen Hayes Hospital, West Haverstraw, New York

PATRICK AMMANN (279) Division of Bone Diseases, WHO Collaborating Center for Osteoporosis Prevention, Department of Rehabilitation and Geriatrics, University Hospital, Geneva, Switzerland

SEIICHIRO AOE (413) Department of Home Economics, Otsuma Women's University, Chiyoda-ku, Tokyo, Japan

NANCY BADENHOP-STEVENS (3) Osteoporosis Prevention and Treatment Center, Bone and Mineral Metabolism Laboratory, and Department of Statistics, Columbus, Ohio

SUSAN I. BARR (165) Department of Agricultural Sciences, University of British Columbia, Vancouver, British Columbia, Canada

ADAM BAXTER-JONES (431) College of Kinesiology, University of Saskatchewan, Saskatoon, Canada

WESLEY G. BEAMER (369) The Jackson Laboratory, Bar Harbor, Maine

THOMAS BECK (35) Department of Radiology, Johns Hopkins University School of Medicine, Baltimore, Maryland

HEIKE A. BISCHOFF-FERRARI (235) Division of Aging and Robert B. Brigham Arthritis and Musculoskeletal Diseases Clinical Research Center, Brigham and Women's Hospital, Boston, Massachusetts

JACKIE BISHOP (431) Centre for Nutrition and Food Safety, School of Biomedical and Life Sciences, University of Surrey, Guildford, United Kingdom

AUBREY BLUMSOHN (141) Bone Metabolism Group, University of Sheffield, Northern General Hospital, Sheffield, United Kingdom

JEAN-PHILIPPE BONJOUR (279) Division of Bone Diseases, WHO Collaborating Center for Osteoporosis Prevention, Department of Rehabilitation and Geriatrics, University Hospital, Geneva, Switzerland

RHONDA A. BROWNBILL (93) School of Allied Health, University of Connecticut, Storrs, Connecticut

PETER BURCKHARDT (439) Department of Medicine, CHUV, Lausanne, Switzerland

MELISSA CAMERON (35) Cancer Council, Victoria, Australia

THIERRY CHEVALLEY (279) Division of Bone Diseases, WHO Collaborating Center for Osteoporosis Prevention, Department of Rehabilitation and Geriatrics, University Hospital, Geneva, Switzerland

T.J. COLE (45) Centre for Paediatric Epidemiology and Biostatistics, Institute of Child Health, London, United Kingdom

CYRUS COOPER (431) MRC Environmental Epidemiology Unit, Southampton General Hospital, Southampton, United Kingdom

FELICIA COSMAN (245) Clinical Research, Helen Hayes Hospital, West Haverstraw, New York

VÉRONIQUE COXAM (109) Unité des Maladies Métaboliques et Micronutriments, Groupe Ostéoporose, INRA de Theix, France

NEAL E. CRAFT (93) Craft Technologies, Inc., Wilson, North Carolina

ZELJKA CRNCEVIC-ORLIC (3) Department of Endocrinology, University of Rijeka, Rijeka, Croatia

BESS DAWSON-HUGHES (235, 263, 399) Bone Metabolism Laboratory, Jean Mayer U.S.D.A. Human Nutrition Research Center on Aging, Tufts University, Boston, Massachusetts

RICHARD EASTELL (141) Bone Metabolism Group, University of Sheffield, Northern General Hospital, Sheffield, United Kingdom

MARK FORWOOD (35) Anatomy and Developmental Biology, The University of Queensland, Brisbane, Australia

LYNDA A. FRASSETTO (273, 349) Department of Medicine and General Clinical Research Center, University of California, San Francisco, California

HAROLD C. FURR (93) Craft Technologies, Inc., Wilson, North Carolina

FIONA GINTY (45) Elsie Widdowson Laboratory, MRC Human Nutrition Research, Cambridge, United Kingdom

PREM GOEL (3) Osteoporosis Prevention and Treatment Center, Bone and Mineral Metabolism Laboratory, and Department of Statistics, Columbus, Ohio

EUN-JEONG HA (3) Osteoporosis Prevention and Treatment Center, Bone and Mineral Metabolism Laboratory, and Department of Statistics, Columbus, Ohio

MIZUHO HARA (25) Research Laboratory, Tsuji Academy of Nutrition, Osaka, Japan

ROBERT P. HEANEY (61, 227, 263) University Chair, Creighton University, Omaha, Nebraska

KENJI HIROTA (25) Department of Obstetrics and Gynecology, Nissei Hospital, Osaka, Japan

TAKAKO HIROTA (25) Research Laboratory, Tsuji Academy of Nutrition, Osaka, Japan

MICHAEL F. HOLICK (181, 263) Department of Endocrinology, Boston University School of Medicine, Boston, Massachusetts

MARIE-NOËLLE HORCAJADA (109) Unité des Maladies Métaboliques et Micronutriments, Groupe Ostéoporose, INRA de Theix, France

JASMINKA Z. ILICH (93) School of Allied Health, University of Connecticut, Storrs, Connecticut

S. ISH-SHALOM (253) Metabolic Bone Diseases Unit, Rambam Medical Center and The Bruce Rappaport Faculty of Medicine, Technion-Israel Institute of Technology, Haifa, Israel

AKIRA ITABASHI (413) Department of Clinical Laboratory Medicine, Saitama Medical School, Saitama, Japan

S. JONES (45) Elsie Widdowson Laboratory, MRC Human Nutrition Research, Cambridge, United Kingdom

SUSAN KANTOR (35) Department of Medicine, Royal Melbourne Hospital, University of Melborne, Victoria, Australia

ELIZABETH A. KRALL (153) Department of Health Policy and Health Services Research, Boston University School of Dental Medicine, Boston, Massachusetts

TOMOKO KUSU (25) Research Laboratory, Tsuji Academy of Nutrition, Osaka, Japan

A. LAIDLAW (45) Elsie Widdowson Laboratory, MRC Human Nutrition Research, Cambridge, United Kingdom

JOHN D. LANDOLL (3) Osteoporosis Prevention and Treatment Center, Bone and Mineral Metabolism Laboratory, and Department of Statistics, Columbus, Ohio

BIN LI (3) Osteoporosis Prevention and Treatment Center, Bone and Mineral Metabolism Laboratory, and Department of Statistics, Columbus, Ohio

ROBERT LINDSAY (245) Clinical Research, Helen Hayes Hospital, West Haverstraw, New York

PAUL LIPS (203, 263) Department of Endocrinology, Vrije Universiteit Medical Center, Amsterdam, The Netherlands

H.M. MACDONALD (127) Osteoporosis Research Unit, Department of Medicine and Therapeutics, University of Aberdeen, Aberdeen, United Kingdom

JENNIFER M. MACLEAY (331) College of Veterinary Medicine and Biomedical Sciences, Colorado State University, Fort Collins, Colorado

VELIMIR MATKOVIC (3) Osteoporosis Prevention and Treatment Center, Bone and Mineral Metabolism Laboratory, and Department of Statistics, Columbus, Ohio

HEATHER MCKAY (35) School of Human Kinetics, University of British Columbia, Vancouver, British Columbia, Canada

L. MCKENNA (45) Elsie Widdowson Laboratory, MRC Human Nutrition Research, Cambridge, United Kingdom

PIERRE J. MEUNIER (263) Rheumatology and Bone Disease, Edouard Herriot Hopital, Lyon, France

BRIAN W. MORRIS (141) Clinical Biochemistry, University of Sheffield, Northern General Hospital, Sheffield, United Kingdom

R. CURTIS MORRIS, JR. (273, 349) Department of Medicine and General Clinical Research Center, University of California, San Francisco, California

ROMAN C. MÜHLBAUER (297) Bone Biology Group, Clinical Research, University of Bern, Bern, Switzerland

SUSAN A. NEW (315, 431) Centre for Nutrition and Food Safety, School of Biomedical and Molecular Sciences, University of Surrey, Guildford, Surrey, United Kingdom

JERI W. NIEVES (245) Clinical Research, Helen Hayes Hospital, West Haverstraw, New York

CARYL NOWSON (35) School of Health Sciences, Deakin University, Burwood, Victoria, Australia

JAANA A. NURMI-LAWTON (431) Centre for Nutrition and Food Safety, School of Biomedical and Life Sciences, University of Surrey, Guildford, United Kingdom

LYNDA PATON (35) Department of Medicine, Royal Melbourne Hospital, University of Melborne, Victoria, Australia

A. PRENTICE (45) Elsie Widdowson Laboratory, MRC Human Nutrition Research, Cambridge, United Kingdom

B. RAZ (253) Endocrine Laboratory, Rambam Medical Center, Haifa, Israel

D.M. REID (127) Osteoporosis Research Unit, Department of Medicine and Therapeutics, University of Aberdeen, Aberdeen, United Kingdom

RENÉ RIZZOLI (279) Division of Bone Diseases, WHO Collaborating Center for Osteoporosis Prevention, Department of Rehabilitation and Geriatrics, University Hospital, Geneva, Switzerland

CLIFFORD J. ROSEN (369) The Jackson Laboratory, Bar Harbor, Maine and The Maine Center for Osteoporosis Research and Education, St. Joseph Hospital, Bangor, Maine

ANTHONY SEBASTIAN (273, 349) Department of Medicine and General Clinical Research Center, University of California, San Francisco, California

ELENA SEGAL (253) Metabolic Bone Diseases Unit, Rambam Medical Center, Haifa, Israel

S. STEAR (45) Elsie Widdowson Laboratory, MRC Human Nutrition Research, Cambridge, United Kingdom

YUKIHIRO TAKADA (413) Technology & Research Institute, Snow Brand Milk Products Co., Ltd., Saitama, Japan

AKIRA TAKEUCHI (413) Luke Hospital, Nakano, Tokyo, Japan

A. TAMIR (253) The Bruce Rappaport Faculty of Medicine, Technion-Israel Institute of Technology and the Department of Community Medicine and Epidemiology, Carmel Medical Center, Haifa, Israel

PAT TAYLOR (431) MRC Environmental Epidemiology Unit, Southampton General Hospital, Southampton, United Kingdom

YASUHIRO TOBA (413) Technology & Research Institute, Snow Brand Milk Products Co., Ltd., Saitama, Japan

A.S. TURNER (331) College of Veterinary Medicine and Biomedical Sciences, Colorado State University, Fort Collins, Colorado

KAZUHIRO UENISHI (413) Laboratory of Physiological Nutrition, Kagawa Nutrition University, Tokyo, Japan

ELIZABETH VASQUEZ (245) Clinical Research, Helen Hayes Hospital, West Haverstraw, New York

CEES VERMEER (79) Department of Biochemistry, University of Maastricht, The Netherlands

REINHOLD VIETH (211, 263) Department of Laboratory Medicine and Pathobiology, University of Toronto, and Pathology and Laboratory Medicine, Mount Sinai Hospital, Toronto, Canada

JOHN D. WARK (35) Bone and Mineral Service, Department of Medicine, Royal Melbourne Hospital, University of Melbourne, Victoria, Australia

CONNIE M. WEAVER (17) Department of Foods and Nutrition, Purdue University, West Lafayette, Indiana

D.L. WHEELER (331) College of Engineering, Colorado State University, Fort Collins, Colorado

H. ZINNMAN (253) Orthopedic Surgery Department, Rambam Medical Center, Haifa, Israel

MARSHA ZION (245) Clinical Research, Helen Hayes Hospital, West Haverstraw, New York

PREFACE

In the field of nutrition, clinical research, unlike research in animals, progresses with a rhythm that seems to correspond to the 3-year intervals that separate the International Symposia on Nutritional Aspects of Osteoporosis. The Proceedings of the 5th Symposium describe the progress over the last 3 years in research on nutrition and bone health. The Symposium reviews topics that are of ongoing interest to the scientific community, such as the effects of vitamin D, calcium, and protein intake on bone health. It also provides ample occasion to discuss less well-established topics, such as the influence of the acid-base balance of the diet on calcium metabolism. In addition, this Symposium included presentations of uncommon topics and original scientific papers. The Proceedings reflect this mixture of systematic reviews and presentations of specific experimental work that characterizes the meeting. The editors hope that the Proceedings make a contribution to this field.

Peter Burckhardt
Bess Dawson-Hughes
Robert P. Heaney

PART I

Calcium in Childhood

Bone Mineral Density of the Skull and Lower Extremities During Growth and Calcium Supplementation

VELIMIR MATKOVIC,[1] JOHN D. LANDOLL,[1] PREM GOEL,[1] NANCY BADENHOP-STEVENS,[1] EUN-JEONG HA,[1] BIN LI,[1] and ZELJKA CRNCEVIC-ORLIC[2]

[1]Osteoporosis Prevention and Treatment Center, Bone and Mineral Metabolism Laboratory, and Department of Statistics, The Ohio State University, Columbus, Ohio, USA; [2]Department of Endocrinology, University of Rijeka, Croatia

ABSTRACT

The skull occupies a higher proportion of the total skeletal mass during growth than later in life. The bone mineral areal density of the skull is the highest among the other skeletal regions of interest due to its high ratio of volume to projected area. Whole-body studies provide an assessment of skeletal health; however, they may be less sensitive to changes in bone density due to the dominance of the head region. Reporting the subcranial skeleton, therefore, is more meaningful with regard to evaluating the bone status of children and adolescents and assessing the effects of dietary intervention. Calcium supplementation has been shown to exert a significant influence on bone mineral areal density of the skull and lower extremities during the bone modeling phase. Complete catch-up in bone mineral density of the skull has been observed during the bone consolidation phase of late adolescence, as compared to the long bones of the lower extremities; this suggests a site-specific difference in bone behavior as related to nutritional challenge.

INTRODUCTION

Dual-energy x-ray absorptiometry (DEXA) analyses of various skeletal regions of interest depend on the size, shape, and volumetric density of the measured bones. Because of its high ratio of volume to projected area, the skull is the densest part of the skeleton (Table I). It contributes significantly to the whole-body bone mineral areal density of growing individuals; therefore, whole-body DEXA scans of children may be less sensitive to small changes in bone mineral areal density. Moreover, the skull enlarges much less during adolescence than the long bones of the lower extremities [1]. This results in a decrease in its contribution to the whole-body bone mineral areal density as an individual grows during adolescence (Table I). In addition, biomechanical factors influence bone mass acquisition of the skull much less than they influence the lower extremities. Thus, a long-term calcium intervention during growth could have a different impact on these two skeletal regions of interest.

To evaluate the effectiveness of calcium supplementation on the bone mineral areal density of the skull and lower extremities, whole-body scans of young females who participated in a 7-year randomized controlled clinical trial were analyzed for regions of interest [2]. The study included the period of pubertal growth spurt, characterized by a high rate of bone modeling, as well as the post-puberty period when epiphyses are closed and bone consolidation dominates. Of particular interest was evaluating the bone behavior and trajectories of the skull and lower extremities as they relate to dietary intervention during growth.

TABLE I   Results of Regions of Interest Taken from Whole-Body DEXA Scans for Two Females

Age	YSM	Head	Arms	Legs	Trunk	Ribs	Pelvis	Spine	TBBMD	SCBMD	%Difference
6.0	—	1.307	0.495	0.680	0.562	0.481	0.632	0.600	0.733	0.602	21.7
10.5	−2.6	1.381	0.613	0.814	0.687	0.566	0.830	0.727	0.825	0.731	12.9
13.0	−0.1	1.459	0.712	1.002	0.804	0.612	0.991	0.874	0.946	0.874	8.2
15.5	+2.4	1.818	0.853	1.200	0.939	0.748	1.172	0.963	1.108	1.027	7.9
17.7	+4.6	2.029	0.889	1.343	1.005	0.789	1.226	1.078	1.196	1.106	8.1

Note: Data for age 6 are from one subject, while those for ages 10.5 through 17.7 are for longitudinal scans from a second subject. TBBMD = total-body bone mineral areal density; SCBMD = subcranial bone mineral areal density (total body without skull). The percent difference between the TBBMD and SCBMD analyses demonstrates the changing contribution of the skull to the whole-body bone mineral areal density.

METHODS

The study was conducted in a cohort $(n = 354)$ of young females who participated in a 7-year, randomized, double-blind, placebo-controlled clinical trial with calcium supplementation (calcium citrate–malate, 1000 mg/day; Procter & Gamble Company, Cincinnati, OH). A total of 177 subjects were randomly assigned to each arm of the trial. For this study, only subjects completing at least 7 of 15 semiannual visits were included $(n = 236)$. Inclusion criteria included: Caucasian, normal health (absence of previous history of chronic disease/treatment that might interfere with growth), pubertal stage 2 (either breast or pubic hair development), and calcium intake below the threshold level (1480 mg/day) [3]. The average cumulative dietary calcium intake among the study participants was between 800 and 900 mg/day and was considered a habitual dietary calcium intake of the study population [2]. All minors and their parents gave informed consent according to guidelines of the Human Subjects Committee at The Ohio State University.

Physical examination, anthropometry, nutritional status, and whole-body bone mineral density were obtained at baseline and every 6 months. The subject's weight and standing height were measured according to standard procedures described previously [4]. Pubertal stage based on breast development and pubic hair distribution was self-assessed by marking corresponding figures of sexual development (scale of 1–5). The timing of menarche was recorded. Nutritional status was assessed from 3-day dietary food records using Nutritionist III, v8.5 (Hearst Corp., San Bruno, CA) [4]. Total calcium intake in the supplemented group included dietary calcium plus pill calcium, adjusted for compliance. Bone mineral areal densities of the skull and lower extremities were obtained from the whole-body scan measured by DEXA (1.3q software, GE-Lunar DPX-L, Madison, WI).

The statistical analysis was conducted on an intent-to-treat basis to measure the effectiveness of calcium supplementation irrespective of compliance in average teenage females accustomed to dietary calcium intake between 800 and 900 mg/day for 7 years. Because this was a long-term study dealing with human growth and skeletal development from childhood to young adulthood, it was possible to evaluate the effectiveness of calcium supplementation on the bone accumulation profile and on the estimated peak bone mass at these two skeletal regions of interest. However, intent-to-treat analysis is not without controversy, as effectiveness is directly proportional to compliance, regardless of the efficacy of the treatment [5,6]. Therefore, in order to evaluate the biologic efficacy of calcium as related to bone accretion during growth, a subgroup analysis was conducted according to *post hoc* strata based on the average total (dietary and pill combined) cumulative calcium intake in the lower and upper tercile. As the onset of menarche is one of the most powerful markers for change in skeletal physiology in young women [7], all outcome variables were analyzed relative to menarche. With this approach, all individual growth profiles used the same biological clock. The intent-to-treat analysis involved fitting a linear mixed effect (LME) model to fixed group effects, but random subject effects, thus allowing a subject-specific bone accretion curve [8,9]. In order to allow adaptive shapes for individual profiles, natural splines were used to estimate bone mass accretion versus years since menarche (YSM). In this analysis, LME models were fitted to all subjects with a minimum of seven visits, as early dropouts cannot contribute to the long-term study outcome. In addition, 95% confidence bands for the difference in bone mass accretion profiles between the groups were obtained. These confidence bands provide the estimated range of YSM values during which the patterns under comparison differ significantly. Conservatively, when this confidence band contains zero, the difference at that time point is not significant. The S-plus 2000 package for Windows, Professional Release 3 (Insightful Corporation, Seattle, WA) was used for all the statistical analyses [10].

RESULTS

No significant differences were observed between the pill and the placebo arms at the baseline in any of the parameters [2]. The cohort with ≥7 visits had the same baseline characteristics for the two arms of the clinical trial. The average cumulative compliance with pills was the same between the two arms of the clinical trial (65.5%). The average total calcium intake in the supplemented arm was ~1500 mg/day and close to the calcium intake threshold for adolescents. Total calcium intake in the supplemented individuals declined by about 100 mg/day during the last 3 years of the study, primarily due to a drop in pill compliance. In addition, several placebo individuals had an average cumulative calcium intake comparable to the level of total calcium intake in the supplemented arm. The *post hoc* analysis of subgroups shows that 76 young females from the calcium arm and 4 from the placebo arm had an average total cumulative calcium intake in the upper tercile (>1305 mg/day), and 75 from the placebo and 3 from the calcium arm had a cumulative calcium intake in the lower tercile (<824 mg/day).

Bone mineral areal density of the skull is the highest of all the skeletal regions of interest, including the lower extremities (Table I). Bone mineral

TABLE II   Bone Mineral Areal Density of the Skull and Lower
Extremities Among 100 Young Females from 11 to 18 Years of Age

Age (years)	Skull BMD (g/cm^2)	Legs BMD (g/cm^2)
11	1.57 ± 0.15	0.88 ± 0.09
11.5	1.59 ± 0.16	0.91 ± 0.09
12	1.62 ± 0.17	0.96 ± 0.10
12.5	1.66 ± 0.17	0.99 ± 0.11
13	1.70 ± 0.17	1.04 ± 0.10
13.5	1.74 ± 0.18	1.07 ± 0.10
14	1.80 ± 0.19	1.10 ± 0.10
14.5	1.84 ± 0.19	1.12 ± 0.10
15	1.88 ± 0.18	1.14 ± 0.09
15.5	1.95 ± 0.18	1.16 ± 0.09
16	1.98 ± 0.18	1.18 ± 0.09
16.5	2.00 ± 0.18	1.19 ± 0.09
17	2.01 ± 0.18	1.20 ± 0.09
17.5	2.04 ± 0.18	1.20 ± 0.09
18	2.06 ± 0.17	1.21 ± 0.09

areal density increased steadily by 25% from the average age of 11 to about 16 years, after which the rate of increase declined to about 5% for the period from ages 16 to 18 years (Table II, Fig. 1). However, when the data were presented in time since menarche, there was a much higher rate of change from time 0 YSM to +2.5 YSM, with slower bone mineral accretion rates prior to and after this period (Fig. 2).

Contrary to the skull, bone mineral areal density of the lower extremities changed on average by ~40% from childhood to young adulthood. Bone mineral density of the lower extremities is 60% of the skull density, with the difference being maintained from age 11 to 18 years (Table II, Fig. 3). Analysis of the data according to the time since menarche revealed a slightly higher rate of bone accretion from about –2 YSM to +2 YSM, with a decreased rate thereafter (Fig. 4). This coincided with closure of the epiphyses and cessation of longitudinal bone growth.

Presentation of the data in time since menarche improved homogeneity and decreased variability of the bone variables and provided a continuous dataset based on bone biology. This supported use of the LME for longitudinal data analysis when evaluating the effect of intervention on bone accretion profiles. The LME showed that the bone mineral density of the skull in the calcium arm reached a higher level sooner than the placebo arm ($p < 0.0001$). However, only a minimal difference was observed during the bone consolidation phase (Fig. 5). This indicates almost complete catch-up in bone mineralization at the skull. Bone mineral density of the skull

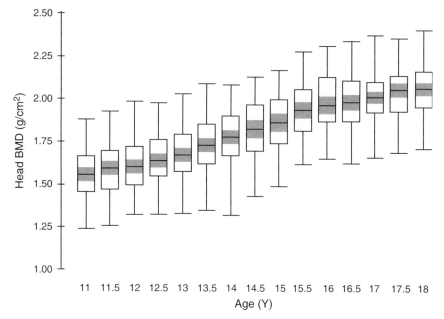

FIGURE 1 Boxplots of bone mineral areal density of the skull (g/cm^2) among 100 young females (placebo arm) from age ~11 to ~18 years. The outlined central box depicts the middle half of the data between the 25th and 75th percentiles. Median = horizontal line across the 95% confidence interval (shaded area); whiskers = highest and lowest connected data value.

analyzed according to subgroups (lower and upper terciles of the cumulative calcium intake over time) showed similar bone behavior, with complete catch-up in bone accretion of the placebo arm during the bone consolidation phase.

Calcium supplementation significantly influenced bone mineral density of the legs during the bone modeling phase of pubertal growth spurt (± 2 YSM). Profiles of the placebo and calcium-supplemented arms are significantly different from 0 during this time interval, with the calcium arm having denser bones (the 95% confidence bands do not include 0; $p < 0.0001$) (Fig. 6). Subgroup analysis based on the average cumulative calcium intake over time showed a significantly higher bone mineral density of the legs in young females with calcium intake in the upper tercile ($p < 0.0001$). The difference remains up to $+5$ YSM (Fig. 7). Further follow-up of this cohort is required to document the maintenance of the difference into young adulthood, as the current data points at $+6$ YSM are few.

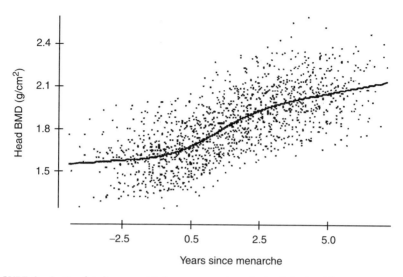

FIGURE 2 Scatterplot diagram with Lowess smooth analysis of the head bone mineral areal density with years since menarche.

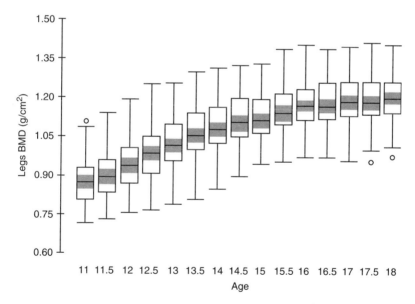

FIGURE 3 Boxplots of bone mineral areal density of the legs (g/cm^2) among 100 young females (placebo arm) from age ~11 to ~18 years. The outlined central box depicts the middle half of the data between the 25th and 75th percentiles. Median = horizontal line across the 95% confidence interval (shaded area); whiskers = highest and lowest connected data value; circles = outliers.

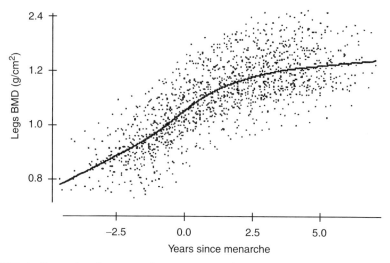

FIGURE 4   Scatterplot diagram with Lowess smooth analysis of lower extremity bone mineral areal density with years since menarche.

DISCUSSION

In children, the growth of the head is well advanced in development as compared to height. For example, by the age of 6 years, about 70% of adult height is reached, whereas the head has attained about 90% of its final size [11]. From about 10 to 15 years of age, height in an average teenage female changes by ~18%, subischial length by 19%, and head circumference by ~4% [1]. Thus, the skull occupies relatively more of the total skeletal mass during childhood than later in life. Contrary to this, subischial leg length changes more dramatically during the pubertal growth spurt due to longitudinal expansion of the long bones of the lower extremities [1]. This relationship is coupled with the fact that the bone mineral areal density of the skull is the highest of the regions of interest from the whole-body scan; therefore, the skull contributes a large portion of the whole body bone mineral areal density. Moreover, this contribution decreases rather significantly during growth from about 20% at age 6 to about 8% at age 13 and remains constant to age 18 (Table I).

Whole-body studies provide an assessment of skeletal health and body composition; however, as a result of the changing influence of the skull, they may be less sensitive to changes in bone density. Reporting bone mineral density results for the subcranial skeleton could, therefore, be a better

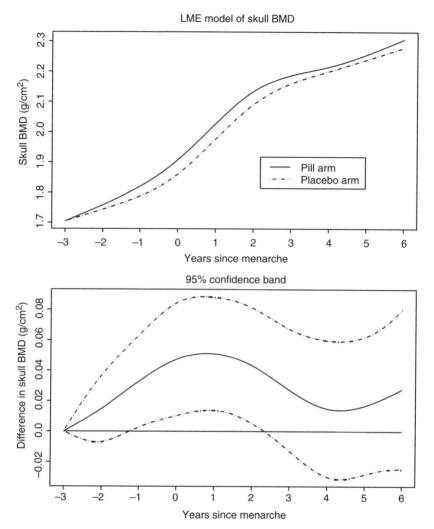

FIGURE 5   LME model of the skull bone mineral areal density change with time since menarche in the calcium supplemented (pill) and placebo arm (top). 95% confidence band for the difference between the groups (bottom).

option and more objective with regard to the assessment of skeletal health during growth.

This study also documented that calcium supplementation in addition to a habitual calcium intake of 800 to 900 mg/day increases bone mass acquisition during the pubertal growth spurt (bone modeling phase) but has much

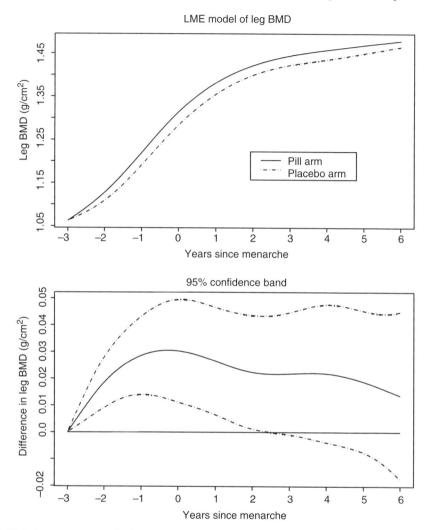

FIGURE 6 Linear mixed effect model of leg bone mineral areal density change with time since menarche in the calcium-supplemented (pill) and placebo arm (top); 95% confidence band for the difference between the groups (bottom).

less effect during late adolescence (skeletal consolidation). This was more prominent in the skull due to a catch-up phenomenon in bone mineral accretion. However, at the lower extremities, the difference produced during the bone modeling phase remained through young adulthood, implying the inability of bone accretion to fully catch up at this region. This was more

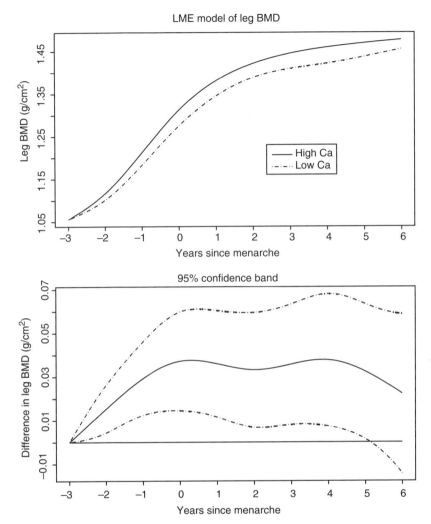

FIGURE 7 Linear mixed effect model of leg bone mineral areal density change with time since menarche in the high-calcium-intake subgroup (upper tercile) and low-calcium-intake subgroup (lower tercile) (top); 95% confidence band for the difference between the groups (bottom).

evident when data were analyzed according to calcium intake subgroups allowing for the analysis of biologic efficacy of calcium. Individuals in the upper tercile of total cumulative calcium intake (pill and dietary combined) were able to maintain the acquired difference in bone mass as compared to subjects in the lower tercile. The difference in bone behavior between the skull and legs could be due to a lower rate of bone modeling of the skull as compared to the long bones of the lower extremities. In addition, the mechanical stresses prone to influence the growth and mineralization of the femur and tibia may play a role as well. The bones of the skull have a more passive role and, presumably, could serve as a better reservoir for calcium in cases of skeletal needs.

The data from this study suggest unequal site-specific bone accretion profiles during growth. The assumption is that skeletal regions with a high rate of bone modeling and exposed to mechanical stress respond differently to calcium nutritional challenge than slow-growing, non-loaded sites. Changes in bone mineral areal density of the skeleton may be identified better from whole-body scans when only the subcranial skeleton is considered. This may help in assessing the efficacy of interventions involving bone mass. Additionally, calcium has a positive effect on bone mass acquisition, which is more pronounced in the early stages of adolescence, during the pubertal growth spurt.

ACKNOWLEDGMENTS

Supported by grants from the National Institutes of Health (NIH RO1 AR40736-01A1), National Institutes of Health Clinical Research Center (CRC-NIH M01-RR00034), National Research Initiative Competitive Grants Program/U.S. Department of Agriculture (NRICGP/USDA-37200-7586), Procter & Gamble Company, National Dairy Council, Ross Products Division Abbott Laboratories, and General Mills Company.

REFERENCES

1. Buckler, J.M.H. (1981). *A Reference Manual of Growth and Development*. Blackwell Scientific, Oxford.
2. Matkovic, V., Badenhop-Stevens, N.E., Landoll, J.D., Goel, P., and Li, B. (2002). Long-term effect of calcium supplementation and dairy products on bone mass of young females. *J. Bone Min. Res.* 17: S172.
3. Matkovic, V. and Heaney, R.P. (1992). Calcium balance during human growth: evidence for threshold behavior. *Am. J. Clin. Nutr.* 55: 992–996.
4. Ilich, J.Z., Skugor, M., Hangartner, T., Baoshe, A., and. Matkovic, V. (1998). Relation of nutrition, body composition, and physical activity to skeletal development: a cross-sectional study in preadolescent females. *J. Am. Coll. Nutr.* 17: 136–147.
5. Everitt, B.S. and Pickles, A. (1999). *Statistical Aspects of the Design and Analysis of Clinical Trials*. Imperial College Press, London.
6. Sommer, A. and Zeger, S.L. (1991). On estimating efficacy from clinical trials. *Statist. Med.* 10: 45–52.

7. Mobley, S.L., Landoll, J.D., Badenhop-Stevens, N.E., Ha, E.J., Andon, M., Rosen, C., Nagode, L., and Matkovic, V. (2001). Changes in bone biomarkers and IGF-I in time since menarche. *J. Bone. Min. Res.* 16: S466.
8. Laird, N.M. and Ware, J.H. (1982). Random-effects model for longitudinal data. *Biometrics* 38: 963–974.
9. Pinheiro, J.C. and Bates, D. (2000). *Mixed-Effects Models in S and S-PLUS.* Springer-Verlag, New York.
10. Everitt, B.S. and Rabe-Hasketh, S. (2001). *Analyzing Medical Data Using S-PLUS.* Springer-Verlag, New York.
11. Baughan, B., Demirjian, A., Levesque, G.Y., and Lapalme-Chaput, L. (1979). The pattern of facial growth before and during puberty as shown by French-Canadian girls. *Ann. Hum. Biol.* 6: 59.

CHAPTER 2

Calcium Retention in Adolescence as a Function of Calcium Intake: Influence of Race and Gender

Connie M. Weaver

Department of Foods and Nutrition, Purdue University, West Lafayette, Indiana, USA

ABSTRACT

The relationship between calcium intake and calcium retention can be used to determine calcium requirements. As calcium intake increases, calcium retention increases to a plateau, reflecting optimal conditions for increasing bone mass during the adolescent growth period. This relationship is understood for Caucasian adolescent girls consuming a Western diet, but it still must be determined for other populations and other lifestyles. Calcium kinetic studies are useful for studying the mechanisms at work that lead to differences in peak bone mass. Black girls retain more calcium than Caucasian girls on the same calcium intakes through increased absorption, net skeletal retention, and decreased excretion. Caucasian boys may be similarly efficient compared to girls.

INTRODUCTION

Adolescence is a period of dramatic skeletal growth when half of adult skeletal mass is accrued. Understanding the factors that modify calcium (*i.e.*, bone)

17

accretion during this period underlies the development of strategies aimed at increasing peak bone mass. The influence of endocrine, diet, and exercise on net calcium retention has been reviewed [1]. Previously, our group reported the use of metabolic balance studies and calcium stable isotope kinetics to determine the relationship between calcium intake and calcium retention in Caucasian girls in this age group [2,3]. This chapter reports racial differences in this relationship using the same approach and preliminary observations on gender differences.

METHODS FOR DETERMINING CALCIUM RETENTION AND METABOLISM

Controlled feeding studies are the preferred approach to studying quantitative effects of diet on measures of health or disease. We study the relationship between calcium intake and calcium retention in adolescents during summer research camps so that feeding quantitative diets can be supervised, isotopes can be administered, and excreta and blood can be collected. Each metabolic study is 3 weeks. The first week is an adjustment period and the second two weeks comprise the balance period. The relationship between calcium intake and calcium retention in Caucasian girls, as reported previously [3], exhibits a plateau. The calcium intake where no further significant increase in calcium retention occurs has been determined to be 1300 mg/day [4]. This intake has become the calcium requirement for all adolescents ages 9 to 18 in North America [5].

The use of stable calcium isotopes and kinetics analysis allows evaluation of the calcium physiological processes. An oral isotope and an intravenous isotope are given after subjects come into a steady state on the diet, which requires about 6 days. Isotopic tracer enrichment in urine, feces, and serum is subsequently measured by mass spectrometry. Data are fitted to curves and analyzed by a three-compartment model using the WinSAAM program (Windows version of Simulation, Analysis, and Modeling). Kinetic modeling showed that increasing calcium intake from 860 to 1900 mg/day resulted in a 145% increase in absorbed calcium and a 32% decrease in bone resorption which were approximately equal and offsetting in absolute amounts of calcium [6]. Thus, during this maximal period of bone turnover, calcium to the exchangeable pool is supplied from either diet or bone.

Using this framework, differences in the relationship between calcium intake and calcium retention in other populations can be determined as a basis to determine dietary calcium requirements of subpopulations. Similarly, the influence of other dietary variables and lifestyle factors can be evaluated by this approach.

RACIAL DIFFERENCES IN CALCIUM METABOLISM

African-Americans have higher femur bone mineral levels than do Caucasians [7]. Much of the evidence based on biochemical markers of bone turnover [8–11] and histomorphometry [12–14] suggests that blacks have more suppressed bone turnover than Caucasians across the lifespan, which was hypothesized to result in increased bone mass or at least reduction in bone loss. However, rates of age-related bone loss have been shown to be similar between black and Caucasian females ages 20 to 90, although bone mass was higher [15]. Thus, it appeared that racial differences in bone mass had already been achieved by the time the peak was attained, which points to adolescence, when almost half of this peak is acquired. Abrams used stable calcium isotope kinetics in girls ages 4.9 to 16.7 years on self-selected calcium intakes and reported higher, not lower, bone formation rates in black subjects compared to Caucasian subjects [16].

We undertook a study to compare calcium metabolism in adolescent black and Caucasian girls matched for sexual maturity and body size on controlled diets, where calcium and other nutrients were designed to be the same [17]. Subject characteristics are given in Table I. Figure 1 shows the striking racial differences in calcium metabolism under controlled conditions.

Black girls were much more efficient in utilization of calcium than Caucasian girls. Black girls had 70% higher calcium absorption efficiency and 46% urinary calcium excretion, resulting in 72% more calcium retention compared to Caucasians on calcium intakes of 1100 to 1300 mg/day. The projected racial difference in peak bone mass, using a nonlinear regression

TABLE I   Comparison of Baseline Anthropometric Characteristics

	Blacks	Caucasians
Age (years)	12.9 ± 1.0	13.6 ± 0.8
PMA (months)	12.2 ± 18.4	8 ± 15
Height (cm)	159 ± 7	157 ± 6
Weight (kg)	56 ± 11	53 ± 10
Total body fat (%)	25.0 ± 9.3	28.1 ± 8.9
Total body BMD (g/cm^2)	1.13 ± 0.09	1.03 ± 0.07[a]

[a] Means are significantly different ($p < 0.001$).

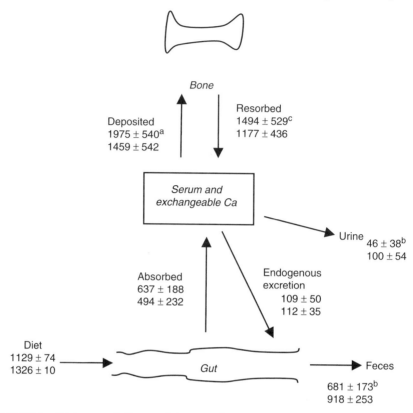

FIGURE 1 Calcium metabolism in adolescent girls. Upper values are for black girls and lower values are for Caucasian girls. Significance: a, $p < 0.05$; b, $p < 0.001$; c, $p < 0.07$.

model of the relationship between calcium retention and age [18], was 12% [17]. This value is similar to femur bone mass differences in adult black and Caucasian women participating in the National Health and Examination Survey (NHANES) III [7].

Determining the relationship between calcium intake and calcium retention is necessary in black girls to determine the threshold intake for maximal retention. It is clear from Fig. 1 that black girls will have higher bone mass than Caucasian girls on similar calcium intakes; however, the calcium intake required to maximize bone mass within their genetic potential might be similar for various races. Figure 2 shows our progress toward constructing the relationship in blacks.

Another mechanism by which blacks conserve calcium relative to Caucasians is through greater sodium retention on high-salt diets. Increased

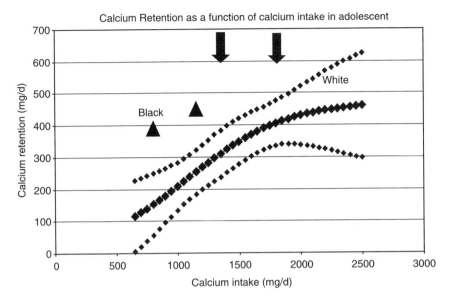

FIGURE 2   Calcium retention as a function of calcium intake in adolescent females. The three curves show the mean (bold) and 95% confidence interval for Caucasians, the triangles shows the mean for black girls at two calcium intakes, and the arrows show calcium intakes for which data analysis is in progress.

sodium retention in blacks may relate to the greater prevalence of salt sensitivity [19]. Conservation of sodium at the kidney also results in conservation of calcium. Sodium excretion in sweat during exercise, but not while sedentary, is also less in blacks compared to Caucasian adolescent girls under conditions of high-salt diets [20]. These differences result in higher total body sodium in black than Caucasian adults [21] in addition to higher total body calcium and bone mass.

GENDER DIFFERENCES IN CALCIUM METABOLISM

Boys accumulate more bone mass on average than do girls, resulting in larger adult skeletons [1]. Peak bone mineral velocity is higher in boys during puberty (406 versus 325 g/year) and occurs about 1.5 years later [22]. Endocrine regulation of sex difference in development of peak bone mass has been reviewed elsewhere [1]. Evaluation of the relationship between calcium intake and calcium retention for boys is underway. We have used the same approach described above for girls to study calcium retention for a range of intakes in boys. Each boy was studied twice on two levels of intakes using a cross-over design. To achieve their higher peak bone mass, boys may utilize calcium more efficiently than girls.

FUTURE DIRECTIONS

Quantitative nutrition approaches of metabolic balance studies coupled with calcium isotope kinetic studies enable us to determine racial and gender differences as well as the impact of lifestyle choices on calcium retention and metabolism. We have studied Caucasian and black girls and boys and the role of dietary salt during the adolescent growth period, but there is much more to do. Other races, other diets, the role of physical activity, and other conditions that perturb calcium metabolism all require further study. Quantitative nutrition techniques have been used sparingly to study similar questions in other age groups.

REFERENCES

1. Weaver, C.M. (2002). Adolescence: the period of dramatic bone growth. *Endocrine* 17: 48.
2. Weaver, C.M., Martin, B.R., and Peacock, M. (1995). Calcium metabolism in adolescent girls, in *Nutritional Aspects of Osteoporosis*, Vol. 7, Burckhardt, P. and Heaney, R.P., Eds., Serono Symposia International, New York, pp. 123–128.
3. Weaver, C.M., McCabe, G.P., and Peacock, M. (1998). Calcium intake and age influence calcium retention in adolescents, in *Nutritional Aspects of Osteoporosis*, Burckhardt, P., Dawson-Hughes, B., and Heaney, R.P., Eds., Springer-Verlag, New York, pp. 3–10.
4. Jackman, L.A., Millane, S.S., Martin, B.R., Wood, O.B., McCabe, G.P., Peacock, M., and Weaver, C.M. (1997). Calcium retention in relation to calcium intake and postmenarcheal age in adolescent females. *Am. J. Clin. Nutr.* 66: 327–333.
5. Institute of Medicine (1997). *Dietary Reference Intakes for Calcium, Phosphorus, Magnesium, Vitamin D, and Fluoride*, National Academy Press, Washington, D.C.
6. Wastney, M.E., Martin, B.R., Peacock, M., Smith, D., Jiang, X-Y., Jackman, L.A., and Weaver, C.M. (2000). Changes in calcium kinetics in adolescent girls induced by high calcium intake. *J. Clin. Endocrin. Metab.* 85: 4470–4475.
7. Looker, A.C., Wahner, H.W., Dunn, W.L., Calvo, M.S., Harris, T.B., Heupe, S.P., Johnston, Jr., C.C., and Lindsey, R. (1998). Updated data on proximal femur bone mineral levels of U.S. adults. *Osteoporosis Int.* 8: 468–489.
8. Bell, N.H., Yergey, A.L., Vieira, N., Oexmann, M.J., and Shary, J.R. (1993). Demonstration of difference in urinary calcium, not calcium absorption, in black and Caucasian adolescents. *J. Bone Miner. Res.* 8: 1111–1115.
9. Kleerekoper, M., Nelson, D.A., Peterson, E.L., Flynn, M.J., Pawluszka, A.S., Jacobsen, G., and Wilson, P. (1994). Reference data for bone mass, calciotropic hormones, and biochemical markers of bone remodeling in older (55–75) postmenopausal Caucasian and black women. *J. Bone Mineral Res.* 9: 1267–1276.

10. Bell, N.H., Greene, A., Epstein, S., Oexmann, M.J., Shaw, S., and Shary, J. (1985). Evidence for alteration of the vitamin D–endocrine system in blacks. *J. Clin. Invest.* 76: 470–473.
11. Meier, D.E., Lucky, M.M., Wallenstein, S., Lapinski, R.H., and Catherwood, B. (1992). Racial differences in pre- and postmenopausal bone homeostasis: association with bone density. *J. Bone Miner. Res.* 7: 1181–1189.
12. Parisien, M., Cosman, F., Morgan, D., Schnitzer, M., Liang, X., Nieves, J., Forese, L., Luckey, M., Meier, D., Shen, V., Lindsay, R., and Dempster, D.W. (1997). Histomorphometric assessment of bone mass, structure, and remodeling: a comparison between healthy black and Caucasian premenopausal women. *J. Bone Miner. Res.* 12: 948–957.
13. Weinstein, R.S. and Bell, N.H. (1988). Diminished rates of bone formation in normal black adults. *N. Engl. J. Med.* 319: 1698–1701.
14. Han, Z.H., Palnitkar, S., Rao, D.S., Nelson, D., and Parfitt, A.M. (1997). Effects of ethnicity and age or menopause on the remodeling and turnover of iliac bone: implications for mechanisms of bone loss. *J. Bone Mineral Res.* 12: 498–508.
15. Perry, III, H.M., Horowitz, M., Morley, J.E., Fleming, S., Jensen, J., Caccione, P., Miller, D.K., Kaiser, F.E., and Sundarum, M. (1996). Aging and bone metabolism in African-American and Caucasian women. *J. Clin. Endocrinol. Metab.* 81: 1108–1117.
16. Abrams, S.A., O'Brien, K.O., Liang, L.K., and Stuff, J.E. (1995). Differences in calcium absorption and kinetics between black and Caucasian girls aged 5–16 years. *J. Bone Mineral Res.* 10: 829–833.
17. Bryant, R.J., Wastney, M.E., Martin, B.R., Wood, O., McCabe, G.P., Morshidi, M., Smith, D.L., Peacock, M., and Weaver, C.M. (2003). Differences in bone turnover and calcium metabolism in adolescent females. *J. Clin. Endocrin. Metab.* 88(3): 1043–1047.
18. Weaver, C.M., Martin, B.R., Plawecki, K.L., Peacock, M., Wood, O.B., Smith, D.L., and Wastney, M.E. (1995). Differences in calcium metabolism between adolescent and adult females. *Am. J. Clin. Nutr.* 61: 577–581.
19. Wilson, D.K. Bayer, L., and Sica, D.A. (1996). Variability in salt sensitivity classifications in black male versus female adolescent. *Hypertension* 28: 250–255.
20. Palacios, C., Wigertz, K., Martin, B., and Weaver, C.M. (2003). Sweat mineral loss from whole body, patch and arm bag in Caucasian and black girls. *Nutr. Res.* 23(3): 401–411.
21. Aloia, J.F., Vaswani, A., Ma, R., and Flaster, E. (1997). Sodium distribution in black and Caucasian women. *Miner. Electrolyte Metab.* 23(2): 74–78.
22. Bailey, D.A., McKay, H.A., Mirwald, R.L., Crocker, P.R.E., and Faulkner, R.A. (1999). A six-year longitudinal study of the relationship of physical activity to bone mineral accrual in growing children: the University of Saskatchewan Bone Mineral Accrual Study. *J. Bone Miner. Res.* 14: 1672–1679.

CHAPTER 3

Longitudinal Study of Diet and Lifestyle Intervention on Bone Mineral Gain in School Children and Adolescents: Effects of Asian Traditional Diet and Sitting Style on Bone Mineral

Takako Hirota,[1] Tomoko Kusu,[1] Mizuho Hara,[1] and Kenji Hirota[2]

[1]*Research Laboratory, Tsuji Academy of Nutrition;* [2]*Department of Obstetrics and Gynecology, Nissei Hospital, Osaka, Japan*

ABSTRACT

Calcium supplements could increase bone mineral in children, but the effect of change in diet and other lifestyle factors is less clear. We investigated the effect of diet and lifestyle factors on accumulation of peak bone mass in adolescents. Male ($n = 286$) and female ($n = 858$) students ages 10 to 17 years were recruited. Bone status at the os calcis using quantitative ultrasound (QUS) and diet and lifestyle factors was assessed annually for five consecutive years, and the effect of educating students on behaviors to prevent osteoporosis was evaluated.

The greatest increase in QUS variables occurred between ages 11 to 13 years in girls and ages 12 and 15 years in boys. Peak bone status occurred by age 14 to 15 years in girls and after age 15 years in boys. Bone status was associated positively with body weight, height, and intake of dairy products, fruit, and small fish in both girls and boys, as well as with the Asian style of sitting on the floor; it was associated negatively with age at menarche in girls. Annual increases in bone status in girls were associated positively with increased intake of vegetables, fruit, and fish and Asian sitting style, and these same factors in boys were associated with increases in height and weight and increased intake of vegetables and small fish.

These results suggest that a dietary change incorporating an increased intake of small fish, fruit, and vegetables and an increased frequency of traditional Asian-style floor sitting could lead to an increased accrual of bone, resulting in a higher peak bone status among adolescents.

INTRODUCTION

Osteoporosis is a skeletal disease characterized by low bone mass, resulting in an increased incidence of fragility fractures. Bone mass is an important determinant of osteoporosis risk [1]. Maximizing the total bone mass acquired during childhood and adolescence is considered as important for osteoporosis prevention as slowing bone loss in older age [2,3]. About 50% of the variance in peak bone mass is attributable to genetics [4,5], but modifiable factors such as diet and physical activity also influence attainment of one's genetically programmed peak bone mass. Understanding factors that influence bone mass accumulation in childhood and maximizing peak bone mass in young adulthood, therefore, is important for designing preventive strategies to combat osteoporosis. Several experimental studies showed that calcium supplementation increases bone density in children and adolescents [6–9]. The baseline intake of calcium in Caucasian adolescents, however, has been much higher than in Japanese subjects [10]. Furthermore, only a few studies have made follow-up measurements after implementation of dietary improvements and changes in lifestyle factors. The purpose of this study was to examine longitudinally the effect of dietary and lifestyle changes on bone status in adolescent girls and boys who were educated about osteoporosis and to examine ways to improve bone mineral acquisition in adolescence.

SUBJECTS AND METHODS

All girls ($n = 262$) and boys ($n = 286$) ages 10 to 15 years attending public schools in a small seashore village and all girls ages 12 to 17 years ($n = 596$) attending a private high school in a metropolitan area were recruited in Japan for this study. Height and weight of subjects were similar to those reported by the National Nutritional Survey [10]. The mean menarcheal age of girls was 12.0 ± 1.0 years. In addition, 100 healthy 18- to 24-year-old students of average height and weight attending a nutrition academy were measured to provide information on quantitative ultrasound (QUS) peak bone status.

Informed consent was obtained, and the Educational Committee of Susami Town, Hatsusiba High School, and the Ethical Committee of Tsuji Academy approved the study.

Bone status was measured at the os calcis annually from 1995 to 1999. During each measurement session, students were informed of their bone status relative to population norms. Questionnaires and interviews were used to document current and past food intake and history of physical exercise and menstruation. Students were instructed on risk factors for osteoporosis and on the importance of a diet of calcium-rich foods and physical activity for early prevention of osteoporosis. Yearly changes in diet or physical activity were determined.

Bone status of the os calcis was measured with QUS using the Achilles A1000 ultrasonometer (GE Lunar; Madison, WI). The Achilles measures the speed of sound (SOS; meters per second) passing through the heel and the broadband ultrasound attenuation (BUA; decibels/megahertz), a measure of frequency-dependent attenuation of the ultrasound wave passing through the heel. The stiffness index (SI), a variable derived from a combination of SOS and BUA, is calculated according to the equation $0.67 \, BUA + 0.28 \, SOS - 420$. We used the SI for our measurement of bone status because this index has been shown to have the best correlation to bone mineral density (BMD) measured by dual energy x-ray absorptiometry (DEXA) and to fracture risk [11,12]. All analyses were performed using SPSS, v9.0 (SPSS, Inc.; Chicago, IL). Student's t-test was used to identify significant differences between boys and girls and variable means. The statistical significance of the differences among multiple groups was studied with one-way analysis of variance (ANOVA). Pearson's product–moment correlation coefficients were used to test for associations between lifestyle variables and QUS bone status. Lifestyle variables that showed a significant correlation with SI were chosen for multiple regression analyses. Results were expressed as means ± standard deviations, unless otherwise indicated; p values of < 0.05 were considered significant.

RESULTS

CROSS-SECTIONAL AND LONGITUDINAL OBSERVATIONS OF MEASUREMENT OF BONE STATUS WITH QUANTITATIVE ULTRASOUND

Results of bone measurements of girls and boys are shown in Fig. 1. Stiffness index values in girls ages 10 to 12 years were significantly higher than for

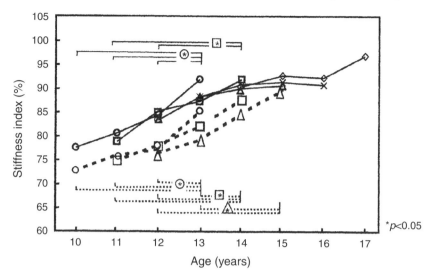

FIGURE 1   Longitudinal observation of os calcis bone status (stiffness index) from age 10 to 17 years in girls (solid lines) and 10 to 15 years in boys (broken lines).

boys of the same age. Longitudinal measurements showed that the os calcis SI at age 14 years in girls and age 15 years in boys was significantly higher than at younger ages. There was no significant change in SI between age 15 and 17 years in girls. Annual increases in SI were highest from age 11 to 14 years in girls and from age 12 to 15 years in boys (Fig. 1). The greatest increase in height occurred approximately one year prior to the greatest annual increment in the SI. This maximal increase occurred between ages 10 and 11 years in girls and between ages 11 and 14 years in boys.

FACTORS ASSOCIATED WITH INITIAL MEASUREMENTS OF OS CALCIS STIFFNESS INDEX

Factors associated with the initial bone mineral in girls ages 10 or 11 years (5th grade of school) were age at menarche, weight, height, intake of small fish and yogurt, and Japanese traditional sitting style on the floor (Table I). Weight, height, and intake of fruit were associated positively with the SI in boys. Lifestyle factors such as diet and traditional sitting style, as well as age at menarche, continued to show a significant association with the SI even after adjustment for body height and weight.

TABLE I   Factors Associated with Initial Os Calcis Bone Status (Stiffness Index) and Yearly
Changes from Ages 10 to 11 Years and from Ages 11 to 12 Years

	Girls		Boys	
	Factor	P	Factor	P
Initial bone minerals	Age at menarche (−)	***	Weight	**
	Weight	***	Intake of fruit	*
	Body mass index (BMI)	**	Body mass index (BMI)	*
	Intake of small fish	*	Height	*
	Intake of yogurt	*		
	Japanese sitting style on the floor	*		
Yearly change in bone minerals	Increased intake of fruit	***	Increase in height	**
	Increased intake of fish	**	Increase in weight	**
	Increased intake of vegetables	*	Increased intake of vegetables	*
	Japanese sitting style on the floor	*	Increased intake of small fish	*
			Intake of dairy products	**
			Intake of vegetables	*
			Knowledge of bone measurement	*

Note: *, $P < 0.05$; **, $P < 0.01$, ***, $P < 0.001$.

FACTORS ASSOCIATED WITH YEARLY INCREASE OF OS CALCIS STIFFNESS INDEX

Increased intake of fruit, fish, and vegetables and adherence to the traditional Japanese sitting style were associated with annual increases in the SI in girls. Increased intake of vegetables and small fish and height, weight, and knowledge of individual bone status were associated with an annual increase in the SI in boys (Table I).

CHANGES IN DIET, KNOWLEDGE OF BONE STATUS, AND STYLE OF SITTING ON THE FLOOR

Yearly increases in bone status were determined for subjects divided into subgroups depending on whether changes in diet or other lifestyle factor had occurred (Fig. 2). Annual increments in the os calcis SI were significantly higher in girls who had increased their intake of fish, fruit, and vegetables and in girls who showed an increased frequency of the Japanese sitting style on the floor. Girls who practiced sitting on the floor showed almost a doubling of the increase in heel SI compared with those who routinely sat in chairs. Moreover, annual increments of SI were significantly higher in boys who had

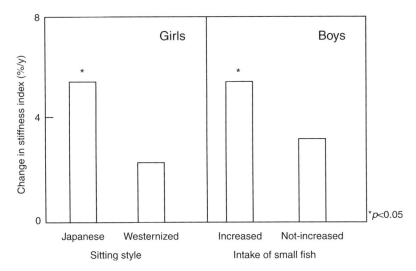

FIGURE 2   Bone status (stiffness index) changes from ages 10 to 11 years and from age 11 to 12 years in girls grouped by sitting style and in boys grouped by intake of small fish. Significant differences were observed between sitting style in girls and increased intake of small fish in boys.

increased their intake of small fish and vegetables and who had knowledge of their bone measurement results. Boys who expressed an awareness of their bone status results had significantly higher intakes of milk, cheese, and tofu (curdled soy protein), foods rich in calcium. Girls who were accustomed to sitting on the floor from early childhood had significantly lower bone fracture rates than girls who were not accustomed to the traditional style of sitting on the floor [13].

DISCUSSION

This is the first prospective study to investigate the relationship between dietary change and bone gain in adolescents. Bone measurement at the os calcis by QUS and education on measures to prevent osteoporosis through diet and physical activity were carried out annually for 5 consecutive years for girls ages 10 to 17 years and boys ages 10 to 15 years. Peak bone status measured by QUS was nearly attained by about 14 years of age in girls and later than 15 years of age in boys. The adolescent growth spurt in bone accumulation occurred around the ages of 11 to 14 years in girls and 12 to 15 years in boys (Fig. 1). These data were similar to reports for Caucasian adolescents [14,15].

Bone mineral status was associated with height, weight, age at menarche, and adherence to the Japanese sitting style in girls (Table 1). Annual positive increments in bone status were associated with increased intake of fish, small fish, vegetables, and fruit. Moreover, greater increases in bone were observed in girls who adhered to the style of sitting on the floor and in boys who were knowledgeable about their bone QUS values (Fig. 1).

Several prospective studies have shown a significant effect of calcium supplements on bone accumulation in early adolescence [6–9], as well as significant associations between milk intake in childhood and peak bone mass in adults by retrospective studies [16,17]. Few studies, however, have shown an effect on bone status of dietary change, knowledge of bone status, and osteoporosis education [18]. Our prospective study suggests a possible dietary effect of increased intake of vegetables, fruit, fish, and small fish on accumulation of bone in adolescence.

Most interesting is our finding that traditional Japanese customs, such as eating small fish and sitting directly on the floor instead of on a couch or sofa, as in Western countries, could result in an increase in bone accumulation that could strengthen bone and prevent fractures later in life. In fact, the hip fracture rates in Japanese women are much lower than in Western countries, in spite of a lower intake of calcium [19]. Adherence to the traditional Japanese style of sitting on the floor could stimulate increased bone formation in girls who otherwise lead a sedentary lifestyle compared with boys. The benefit of sitting on the floor probably results from the movement of standing up from the floor position, an activity that requires more muscular activity than standing up from a chair. The significantly lower fracture rate in these girls supports this theory [13].

Although the most important source of calcium in Western societies is dairy products, that is not true for the Japanese. The average daily intake of calcium from dairy products in Japanese subjects is only about 100 to 130 mg/day, but the total calcium intake is about 500 to 550 mg/day [10,16]. The Japanese custom of eating the whole bodies of small fish, including the head, skin, bone, and viscera, provides an important source of non-dairy calcium (490 mg/100 g fish) and vitamin D (61 μg/100 g fish). Dried small fish are also rich in $n-3$ polyunsaturated fatty acids and also provide icosapentaenoic acid and docosahexaenoic acid (0.47 and 0.99 g/100 g fish, respectively). These multiple sources of calcium-rich nutrients might be effective in improving the bone status of Japanese adolescents [20].

Recent data have shown that the intake of fruits and vegetables rich in potassium, magnesium, and vitamin C, but not calcium, was directly associated with bone mineral density in perimenopausal women and inversely related to bone loss in elderly men and women [21,22]. Our data support the beneficial effect of an increased intake of fruit and vegetables on bone accumulation in adolescents. The reason for this improved bone status among adolescents is not clear. Further study of the possible effect of potassium, magnesium, and vitamin C on bone metabolism is warranted.

Of considerable interest was our finding that awareness of one's bone status was a significant contributor among boys to an improved diet that included an increased intake of dairy food, tofu, and improved bone SI results. Results suggest that medical education at an early age might serve as preventive medicine for later in life.

Unfortunately, we had no validated method for defining sexual maturation for Asian populations similar to the Tanner stage method for Caucasian populations. Asian children follow a pattern of sexual maturation that is different from that of Caucasians. Another limitation of our study was that bone measurement was done by QUS, a method that is somewhat less accurate than dual energy x-ray absorptiometry (DEXA). Because of radiation injuries suffered in World War II, it is difficult to get informed consent from parents for measuring school children with procedures such as DEXA that utilize ionizing radiation. We were, however, able to show significant associations between bone status as measured by QUS and age, anthropometry, and food intake.

Our study of Japanese adolescent boys and girls found that measurements of bone status from an early age, followed up with medical and dietary information related to prevention of osteoporosis, should result in dietary changes, such as increased intake of vegetables, fruits, and small fish, that could accelerate bone accumulation and improve peak bone mass. These changes might prove to be beneficial in preventing osteoporosis later in life.

ACKNOWLEDGMENT

Part of this work has been supported by grants from the Japan Osteoporosis Foundation, the National Dairy Promotion and Research Association of Japan, and the Descente and Ishimoto Memorial Foundation for the Promotion of Sports Science. The authors thank C. Takeda and M. Asamoto in Susami Town and Teacher Y. Murotani and the principal in Hatsusiba Tondabayasi High School for continuous support of our research. We also thank Dr. Howard S. Barden of GE Lunar Co., for helpful editorial suggestions.

REFERENCES

1. Kanis, J.A., Melton, L.J., 3rd., Christiansen, C., Johnston, C.C., and Khaltaev, N. (1994). The diagnosis of osteoporosis. *J. Bone Miner. Res.* 9(8): 1137–1141.
2. Matkovic, V. (1992). Calcium and peak bone mass. *J. Intern. Med.* 231(2): 151–160.

3. Weaver, C.M., Peacock, M., and Johnston, C.C., Jr. (1999). Adolescent nutrition in the prevention of postmenopausal osteoporosis. *J. Clin. Endocrinol. Metab.* 84(6): 1839–1843.

4. Slemenda, C.W., Hui, S.L., Longcope, C., Wellman, H., and Johnston, C.C., Jr. (1990). Predictors of bone mass in perimenopausal women: a prospective study of clinical date using photon absorptiometry. *Ann. Intern. Med.* 112(2): 96–101.

5. Pocock, N.A., Eisman, J.A., Hopper, J.L., Yeates, M.G., Sambrook, P.N., and Eberl, S. (1987). Genetic determinants of bone mass in adults: A twin study. *J. Clin. Invest.* 80(3): 706–710.

6. Johnston, C.C., Jr., Miller, J.Z., Slemenda, C.W., Reister, T.K., Hui, S., Christian, J.C., and Peacock, M. (1992). Calcium supplementation and increases in bone mineral density in children. *N. Engl. J. Med.* 327(2): 82–87.

7. Lloyd, T., Andon, M.B., Rollings, N., Martel, J.K., Landis, J.R., Demers, L.M., Eggli, D.F., Kieselhorst, K., and Kulin, H.E. (1993). Calcium supplementation and bone mineral density in adolescent girls. *JAMA.* 270(7): 841–844.

8. Bonjour, J.-P., Carrié, A.L., Ferrari, S., Clavien, H., Slosman, D., Theintz, G., and Rizzoli, R. (1997). Calcium-enriched foods and bone mass growth in prepubertal girls: a randomized, double-blind, placebo-controlled trial. *J. Clin. Invest.* 99(6): 1287–1294.

9. Heaney, R.P. (2000). Calcium, dairy products and osteoporosis. *J. Am. Coll. Nutr.* 19(2): 83S–99S.

10. The Study Circle for Health and Nutrition Information (2002). *The National Nutrition Survey in Japan, 2001: Ministry of Health, Labour and Welfare, Japan.* Daiichishuppan, Japan.

11. Hans, D., Dargent-Molina, P., Schotto, A.M., Sebert, J.L., Cormier, C., Kotzki, P.O., Delmas, P.D., Pouilles, J.M., Breart, G., and Meunier, P.J. (1996). Ultrasonographic heel measurements to predict hip fracture in elderly women: the EPIDOS prospective study. *Lancet* 348(9026): 511–514.

12. Faulkner, K.G., McClung, M.R., Coleman, L.J., and Kingston-Sandahl, E. (1994). Quantitative ultrasound of the heel: correlation with densitometric measurements at different skeletal sites. *Osteoporosis. Int.* 4(1); 42–47.

13. Hirota, T., Kusu, T., Yamanishi, S., and Hirota, K. (2000). Traditional living style on tatami mat significantly increased bone mass in adolescent girls: 5-year follow-up study in a small village. *J. Bone Miner. Res.* 15: S540.

14. Bonjour, J.-P., Theintz, G., Buchs, B., Slosman, D., and Rizzoli, R. (1991). Critical years and stages of puberty for spinal and femoral bone mass accumulation during adolescence. *J. Clin. Endocrinol. Metab.* 73(3): 555–563.

15. Theintz, G., Buchs, B., Rizzoli, R., Slosman, D., Clavien, H., Sizonenko, P.C., and Bonjour, J.-P. (1992). Longitudinal monitoring of bone mass accumulation in healthy adolescents: evidence for a marked reduction after 16 years of age at the levels of lumbar spine and femoral neck in female subjects. *J. Clin. Endocrinol. Metab.* 75(4): 1060–1065.

16. Hirota, T., Nara, M., Ohguri, M., Manago, E., and Hirota, K. (1992). Effect of diet and lifestyle on bone mass in Asian young women. *Am. J. Clin. Nutr.* 55(6): 1168–1173.

17. Kalkwarf, H.J., Khoury, J.C., and Lanphear, B.P. (2003). Milk intake during childhood and adolescence, adult bone density, and osteoporotic fractures in U.S. women. *Am. J. Clin. Nutr.* 77(1): 257–265.

18. Hirota, T., Hara, M., Kito, Y., Shirokawa, N., Matsuda, M., Hosokawa, K., and Hirota, K. (1998). Change of lifestyle caused by health education improves ultrasound density of os calcis in osteopenic adolescents. *Bone* 23(5): S290.

19. Schwartz, A.V., Kelsey, J.L., Maggi, S., Tuttleman, M. Ho, S.H., Jonsson, P.V., Poor, G., Sisson de Castro, J.A., Xu, L., Matkin, C.C., Nelson, L.M., and Heyse, S.P. (1999). International variation in the incidence of hip fractures: cross-national project on osteoporosis for the World Health Organization program for Research on Aging. *Osteoporosis. Int.* 9(3): 242–253.

20. Kruger, M.C., Coetzer, H., de Winter, R., Gericke, G., and van Papendorp, D.H. (1998). Calcium, gamma-linolenic acid and eicosapentaenoic acid supplementation in senile osteoporosis. *Aging (Milano)* 10(5): 385–394.
21. Tucker, K.L., Hannan, M.T., Chen, H., Cupples, L.A., Wilson, P.W., and Kiel, D.P. (1999). Potassium, magnesium, and fruit and vegetable intakes are associated with greater bone mineral density in elderly men and women. *Am. J. Clin. Nutr.* 69(4): 727–736.
22. Hall, S.L. and Greendale, G.A. (1998). The relation of dietary vitamin C intake to bone mineral density: results from the PEPI study. *Calcif. Tissue Int.* 63(3): 183–189.

CHAPTER 4

A Co-Twin Calcium Intervention Trial in Premenarcheal Girls: Cortical Bone Effects by Hip Structural Analysis

Lynda Paton,[1] Thomas Beck,[2] Caryl Nowson,[3] Melissa Cameron,[4] Susan Kantor,[1] Heather McKay,[5] Mark Forwood,[6] and John D. Wark[7]

[1]Department of Medicine, Royal Melbourne Hospital, University of Melbourne, Victoria, Australia; [2]Department of Radiology, Johns Hopkins University School of Medicine, Baltimore, Maryland; [3]School of Health Sciences, Deakin University, Burwood, Victoria, Australia; [4]Cancer Council, Victoria, Australia; [5]School of Human Kinetics, University of British Columbia, Vancouver, British Columbia, Canada; [6]Anatomy and Developmental Biology, The University of Queensland, Brisbane, Australia; [7]Bone and Mineral Service, Department of Medicine, Royal Melbourne Hospital, University of Melbourne, Victoria, Australia

ABSTRACT

The reported responses of the growing skeleton to calcium are inconsistent. The mechanism(s) of the calcium effects are also uncertain, and influences on both remodeling and modeling have been proposed. We conducted a randomized, placebo-controlled trial of calcium supplementation (1200 mg daily as calcium carbonate) in female twins ages 10.4 ± 1.4 years (mean $\pm$ SD) at baseline, using a powerful co-twin control design. Bone properties were evaluated by hip structural analysis (HSA) of proximal femur densitometry scans in 33 twin pairs (18 monozygotic, 15 dizygotic) up to 18 months intervention. HSA parameters were measured at the narrowest segment of the

Nutritional Aspects of Osteoporosis, Second Edition

femoral neck (NN), intertrochanteric (IT), and upper femoral shaft (FS) sites. All data were adjusted for age, height, and weight. Height and weight did not differ between groups at any time point. By 18 months, the FS site showed significant within-pair percent differences when comparing calcium with placebo treated twins, respectively: areal bone mineral density (ABMD) ($+3.94\%$, $P = 0.019$), subperiosteal width (-2.55%, $P = 0.038$), endocortical diameter (-5.07%, $P = 0.015$), average cortical thickness ($+5.16\%$, $P = 0.015$), and average buckling ratio (-7.23%, $P = 0.014$). No consistent or major effects were seen at the NN and IT sites. Observed effects were limited to cortical bone at the femoral shaft with inhibition of modeling at both the endosteal and periosteal surfaces, resulting in narrowing of the femoral shaft and a thicker cortex. While changes in geometry were evident at the shaft, they resulted in increased ABMD without an apparent increase in either axial or bending strength.

INTRODUCTION

Osteoporosis is a disease characterised by low bone mass and microarchitectural deterioration of bone tissue, leading to enhanced fragility and a consequent increase in fracture risk [1]. Up to 80% of population variability in bone mass may be explained by additive genetic effects, with 20% variability in a given population explained by environmental factors such as nutrition and physical activity. Peak bone mass is the maximal lifetime amount of bone tissue accrued in the skeleton during growth. Low peak bone mass is now considered to be an important determinant of low bone mineral density (osteoporosis) in old age [2]. Maximizing peak bone mass during the first few decades of life is currently seen as a primary strategy in osteoporosis prevention.

The period of most rapid skeletal development occurs over several years in childhood and adolescence, accounting for 40 to 50% of the total accrual of skeletal mass. This period may provide not only the best opportunity to maximize peak bone mass but also to enhance the development of optimal bone geometry. A number of studies have assessed the effect of increased dietary calcium (as supplements) on bone density in children between the ages of 7 and 14 years [3–7]. These studies have all demonstrated increases in bone density with increased calcium intake. This positive effect on bone density, gain ranging from 1.6 to 5.1% compared to controls, has been seen when total calcium intake is increased to between 1200 and 1600 mg/day.

The effect of calcium supplementation on the biomechanical and material strength properties of bone has not been extensively investigated.

With the recent development of the HSA program [8–10], it is now possible to investigate the effect of calcium on measures of bone geometry and estimate strength of the proximal femur. Growing bone has the capacity to respond to physiological or mechanical stimuli by modeling and remodeling. Subperiosteal expansion due to apposition of new bone at the periosteal surface may confer increases in the cross-sectional moment of inertia (CSMI). The subsequent increase in the CSMI may increase the section modulus, a measure of bone stiffness, which is closely related to bending and torsional strength of bone [11]. Bone modeling may also occur by reduced bone resorption from the endocortical surface, resulting in reduced medullary expansion. The potential for these processes to increase cortical width, increase periosteal diameter, and minimize the increase in endosteal diameter may improve the overall strength of the proximal femur. These changes have not been detectable in the past with conventional dual-energy x-ray absorptiometry (DEXA), but with development of the HSA technique we can make use of the simple and safe DEXA technique to investigate the strength and geometry of bone and the changes in these properties with selected interventions.

We now report results from a randomized, co-twin, placebo-controlled, single-blind intervention study, measuring the effect of increased calcium intake on HSA-derived bone structural properties of the proximal femur in 33 pairs of premenarcheal female twins with a mean ± SD age at baseline of 10.4 ± 1.4 years and who completed 18 months of calcium supplementation at baseline. Our co-twin study design using female twins and determining within-pair differences in bone structural properties allows for greater control of environmental factors compared with most studies reported in the literature for which unrelated individuals were generally used. A major additional advantage of our co-twin study design is that it controls for all or, on average, half of the additive genetic effects on (changes in) bone structural properties at a stage of life when genetic variance in bone mineral density has been shown to increase [12]. For these reasons, our co-twin design confers a substantial advantage in statistical power compared with studies in unrelated individuals.

METHODS

PARTICIPANTS AND STUDY DESIGN

Twins (ages 8 to 13 years) enrolled with the Australian Twin Registry were approached from October 1995 through to March 2000 to participate in a calcium intervention trial. Fifty-one pairs of female twins (including 1 triplet

set) volunteered to participate and completed at least 6 months of intervention; 27 of the twin pairs were monozygotic, and 24 were dizyogtic. All
subjects were premenarcheal at baseline. The Clinical Research and Ethics
Committee of the Royal Melbourne Hospital and the Australian Twin Registry
approved the study. For each twin pair, informed consent was obtained
from at least one parent and the individual participants.

Twins completed visits to the study center at baseline and then at 6-month
intervals up to 18 months. At the baseline visit, members of each pair were
randomly assigned to receive either a calcium supplement (1200 mg of
calcium carbonate [caltrate]) or a matched placebo and were blinded to the
interventions. All tablets were generously supplied by Whitehall Pty. Ltd.
(Baukham Hills, Sydney, Australia). Twins were instructed to take two tablets
(600 mg each) nightly at approximately the same time. Tablet counts were
performed at the end of each 3-month period to assess compliance. At each
visit to the center, participants completed questionnaires to assess their
medical history, medication use, and physical activity. Calcium intake was
measured via a 4-day food record, assessed using the dietary analysis program
Diet 3 (Xyris Software). The food record was completed over 3 week days
and 1 weekend day and recorded in household measures with the option of
using scales if preferred. Physical activity was assessed as reported previously
[3]. Height (cm) and weight (kg) were measured at each visit.

BONE DENSITY AND HSA

At the baseline and at 6, 12, and 18 months, right proximal femur bone
density scans were acquired using a Hologic QDR 1000W densitometer (Waltham, MA). Proximal femur scans were assessed for structural
properties by the HSA program designed by Dr. Thomas Beck at The Johns
Hopkins University (Baltimore, MD). The method has been described elsewhere [8–10]. Three regions of the proximal femur were assessed: (1) the
narrow neck, narrowest segment of the femoral neck (NN); (2) the
intertrochanteric region (IT) along the bisector of the neck shaft angle; and
(3) the femoral shaft (FS), 2 cm distal to the midpoint of the lesser trochanter.
For each of these regions, the subperiosteal width (cm), bone cross-sectional
area (CSA, cm^2), and cross-sectional moment of inertia (CSMI, cm^4) were
determined from the bone mass profile. Estimates of the cortical thickness
were made. Section modulus (Z) was calculated as $Z = CSMI/y$, where $y = 1/2$
the subperiosteal width for the neck and shaft and the distance from
the centroid to the lateral cortical margin for the intertrochanteric region.
The buckling ratio was determined as the ratio of subperiosteal radius
(diameter/2) to estimated mean cortical thickness for each region.

STATISTICAL ANALYSES

For descriptive statistics, the mean, standard deviation (SD) or standard error of the mean (SEM) were reported. The within-pair difference in change over 18 months between calcium- and placebo-treated twins was expressed as the unit difference (see Table III) and 95% confidence interval and was assessed by a paired t-test. A P value less than 0.05 was considered to be statistically significant. All data were adjusted for age, height, and weight by linear regression (SPSS, version 11). The within-pair percentage difference in change over 18 months was expressed by dividing the change in the calcium-treated twin minus the change in the placebo-treated twin by the baseline value of the placebo-treated twin.

RESULTS

Thirty-three pairs of twins completed 18 months of calcium intervention and had HSA analysis performed on their right proximal femur scans. There was no difference in the mean values for the placebo or calcium groups for age, height, weight, or calcium intake (Table I) or physical activity (data not shown). There was no within-pair difference in height or weight at baseline or after 18 months of follow-up. HSA-derived measures of bone strength at the narrow neck, intertrochanteric, and femoral shaft regions at baseline are provided in Table II. There were no within-pair differences in any HSA-derived measures at baseline at the narrow neck, intertrochanteric, or femoral shaft regions. All measures changed over time in both the placebo and calcium groups.

   A significant difference was observed in several measures at the femoral shaft at 18 months (Table III). These significant differences in percent change from baseline were as follows (comparing placebo versus calcium-treated twins, respectively): areal bone mineral density (ABMD) ($+15.8\%$ versus

TABLE I   Baseline Descriptive Values for the Placebo and Calcium Groups

Variable	Placebo Mean (SD)	Calcium Mean (SD)
Age (years)	10.4 (1.4)	10.4 (1.4)
Height (cm)	142.04 (9.02)	141.81 (10.34)
Weight (kg)	36.72 (6.98)	37.48 (10.38)
Calcium intake/day (mg)[a]	721.78 (360.55)	714 .25 (353.41)

[a]Calcium as reported from 4-day food record.

TABLE II Structural Properties for Calcium and Placebo Groups at Baseline

	Placebo (n = 33) Mean ± SEM	Calcium (n = 33) Mean ± SEM
Narrow neck		
Neck length (cm)	4.24 ± 0.07	4.33 ± 0.05
Bone mineral density (g/cm²)	0.62 ± 0.01	0.62 ± 0.01
Cross-sectional area (cm²)	1.45 ± 0.3	1.47 ± 0.03
Subperiosteal width (cm)	2.50 ± 0.03	2.50 ± 0.03
Section modulus (cm³)	0.58 ± 0.01	0.59 ± 0.01
Estimated endosteal diameter (cm)	2.27 ± 0.03	2.26 ± 0.03
Estimated mean cortical thickness (cm)	0.12 ± 0.002	0.12 ± 0.002
Buckling ratio	16.37 ± 0.03	16.27 ± 0.27
Intertrochanter		
Bone mineral density (g/cm²)	0.62 ± 0.02	0.62 ± 0.02
Cross-sectional area (cm²)	2.40 ± 0.06	2.38 ± 0.06
Subperiosteal width (cm)	4.04 ± 0.04	4.05 ± 0.07
Section modulus (cm³)	1.60 ± 0.04	1.60 ± 0.05
Estimated endosteal diameter (cm)	3.55 ± 0.05	3.58 ± 0.07
Estimated mean cortical thickness (cm)	0.24 ± 0.006	0.24 ± 0.007
Buckling ratio	8.94 ± 0.28	9.24 ± 0.31
Femoral shaft		
Bone mineral density (g/cm²)	0.80 ± 0.01	0.79 ± 0.01
Cross-sectional area (cm²)	1.78 ± 0.03	1.80 ± 0.03
Subperiosteal width (cm)	2.34 ± 0.02	2.37 ± 0.03
Section modulus (cm³)	0.80 ± 0.02	0.81 ± 0.02
Estimated endosteal diameter (cm)	1.79 ± 0.03	1.82 ± 0.03
Estimated mean cortical thickness (cm)	0.27 ± 0.006	0.27 ± 0.006
Buckling ratio	4.39 ± 0.12	4.54 ± 0.15

TABLE III Hip Structural Properties (Mean [SD]) at the Femoral Shaft for Calcium and Placebo Groups After 18 Months of Intervention and Within-Pair Unit Difference in Change from Baseline to 18 months (95% CI)

	Placebo (n = 33)	Calcium (n = 33)	Within-Pair Difference
Bone mineral density (g/cm²)	0.92 (0.02)	0.95 (0.02)	0.03 (0.006 to 0.06)[a]
Cross-sectional area (cm²)	2.27 (0.04)	2.32 (0.04)	0.03 (−0.03 to 0.09)
Subperiosteal width (cm)	2.57 (0.03)	2.53 (0.02)	−0.6 (−0.12 to −0.004)[a]
Section modulus (cm³)	1.11 (0.03)	1.11 (0.03)	−0.02 (−0.6 to 0.02)
Estimated endosteal diameter (cm)	1.93 (0.04)	1.87 (0.03)	−0.09 (−0.16 to −0.02)[a]
Estimated mean cortical thickness (cm)	0.32 (0.007)	0.33 (0.007)	0.02 (0.003 to 0.03)[a]
Buckling ratio	4.16 (0.12)	4.01 (0.11)	−0.31 (−0.54 to −0.07)[a]

[a] $P < 0.05$.

+ 19.9%, $P = 0.019$), subperiosteal width ($+9.7\%$ versus $+7.1\%$, $P = 0.038$), endocortical diameter ($+7.7\%$ versus $+2.5\%$, $P = 0.015$), average cortical thickness ($+17.2\%$ versus $+22.8\%$, $P = 0.015$) and average buckling ratio (-5.1% versus -11.6%, $P = 0.014$). There were no differences in the change in HSA-derived measures for the NN or IT regions after 18 months of calcium intervention in this cohort (data not shown).

DISCUSSION

This is the first investigation of the effect of calcium supplementation on HSA-derived measures of bone geometry and strength in premenarcheal females. We have shown that the femoral shaft responded to calcium supplementation with a significantly greater gain in BMD and a thicker femoral shaft cortex, with reduced subperiosteal deposition and endosteal resorption. Endosteal resorption was inhibited more than subperiosteal apposition. The buckling ratio was significantly reduced in the calcium group but there was no difference in the change in section modulus and CSA. These changes were not associated with any change in indices of bone strength after 18 months of intervention. It is difficult to predict the later outcome on strength measures, so follow-up measures post-intervention will be particularly important in these subjects.

The difference in the change in buckling ratio is of interest. It is thought that fragility results in later life when the buckling ratio of a bone rises above a theoretical threshold. With increasing age, subperiosteal expansion occurs and tends to compensate for endocortical resorption, helping to maintain the bending strength of the bone. If calcium supplementation thickens the cortex in the long term, then it may take longer for a bone to reach the fragility threshold as it expands with age.

In this study we did not demonstrate a difference in the CSMI or section modulus of the femoral shaft with 18 months of intervention. The study may not have had sufficient power to detect a difference should it exist. This may also account for the lack of detectable differences at the NN and IT regions, where the cortex is thinner than the shaft, presumably making differences more difficult to detect.

Similarly, we did not detect differences in the rate of change of the HSA measures at the narrow neck and intertrochanteric regions. The changes seen in the femoral shaft in this study follow a pattern similar to those described at the femoral neck following an exercise intervention in young girls by Petit et al. [11], who reported a significant increase in the BMD, CSA, and cortical thickness but no change in the subperiosteal diameter with this exercise intervention.

The present study has not addressed the issue of pubertal status beyond restricting participation in the study to girls who were prepubertal at baseline. This maybe an important factor, as several studies have shown differences in BMD responses to calcium according to pubertal status [4,6,13,14].

We hope to address the issue of power by pooling the results of this study with our previously reported calcium intervention trial [3]. Expansion of the dataset will also aid in the assessment of the pubertal effect. We have undertaken post-intervention follow-up of these subjects. The analysis of these data will address important issues regarding the maintenance of the changes we have described at the femoral shaft and the effect of subsequent growth and maturation on the effects described here.

The HSA technique provides a valuable insight into the structural properties of bone but like all techniques it has limitations that must be considered. HSA is used to estimate three-dimensional structure from a two-dimensional DEXA image [15,16]. The estimation of the bone geometry is based on assumptions of the cross-sectional shape of each of the diverse regions being assessed. The assumptions underlying the HSA technique appear to be robust with respect to measurements at the femoral shaft; therefore, the finding of calcium-mediated changes in the geometry of the femoral shaft is likely to be valid. A second randomized, placebo-controlled, co-twin study of calcium supplementation in adolescent females has been undertaken and will provide independent validation of the present findings.

REFERENCES

1. WHO Study Group. (1994). Assessment of fracture risk and its application to screening for postmenopausal osteoporosis. *World Health Org. Tech. Rep. Ser.* 843: 5–6.
2. Consensus statement. Australian National Consensus Conference 1996. (1997). The prevention and management of osteoporosis. *Med. J. Australia* 7:167 Supple: 51–115.
3. Nowson, C.A., Green, R.M., Hopper, J.L., Sherwin, A.J., Young, D., Guest, C.S., Smid, M., Larkins, R.G., and Wark, J.D. (1997). A co-twin study of the effect of calcium supplementation on bone density during adolescence. *Osteoporosis Int.* 7: 219–225.
4. Johnston, C.C., Miller, J.Z., Slemensa, C.W., Reister, T.K., Christian, J.C., and Peacock, M. (1992). Calcium supplementation and increases in bone mineral density in children. *N. Engl. J. Med.* 327: 82–87.
5. Lloyd, T., Andon, M., Rollings, N., Martel, J.K., Landis J.R., Demers, L.M., Eggli, D.F., Kieselhorst, K., and Kulin, H.E. (1993). Calcium supplementation and bone mineral density in adolescent girls. *JAMA* 270: 841–844.
6. Lloyd, T., Martel, J., Rollings, N., Andon, M., Kulin, H., Demers, L., Eggli, D., Kieselhorst, K., and Chinchilli, V. (1996). The effect of calcium supplementation and tanner stage on bone mineral density, content and area in teenage women. *Osteoporosis Int.* 6: 276–283.
7. Bonjour, J.P., Carrie, A.L., Ferrari, S., Clavien, H., Slosman, D., Theinty, G., and Rizzoli, R. (1997). Calcium enriched foods and bone mass growth in prepubertal girls: a randomized, double-blind, placebo-controlled trial. *J. Clin. Invest.* 99(6): 1287–1294.

8. Beck, T.J., Ruff, C.B., Warden, K.E., Scott, W.W., Jr., and Rao, G.U. (1990). Predicting femoral neck strength from bone mineral data: a structural approach. *Invest. Radiol.* 25: 6–18.

9. Beck, T.J., Ruff, C.B., Scott, W.W.W., Plato, C.C., Tobin, J.D., and Quan, C.A. (1992). Sex differences in geometry of the femoral neck with aging: a structural analysis of bone mineral data. *Calcif. Tissue Int.* 50: 24–29.

10. Mourtada, F., Beck, T., Hauser, D., Ruff, C., and Bao, G. (1996). A curved beam model of the proximal femur for estimating stress using DXA derived structural geometry. *J. Orthop. Res.* 14: 483–462.

11. Petit, M.A., McKay, H.A., MacKelvie, K.J., Heinonen, A., Khan, K.M., and Beck, T.J. (2002). A randomized school-based intervention confers site and maturity-specific benefits on bone structural properties in girls: a hip structural analysis. *J. Bone Miner. Res.* 17: 363–372.

12. Hopper, J.L., Green, R., Nowson, C., Young, D., Larkins, R.G., and Wark, J.D. (1998). Genetic, common environment and individual specific components of variance for bone mineral density in 10–26 year old females: a twin study. *Am. J. Ep.* 147: 17–29.

13. Molgaard, C., Thomsen, B.L., and Michaelsen, K.F. (1999). Whole body bone mineral accretion in healthy children and adolescents. *Arch. Dis. Children* 81: 10–15.

14. Boot, A.M., De Ridder, M.A.J., Pols, H.A., Krenning, E.P., Muinck, D.E., and Keizer-Schrama, S.A.M. (1997). Bone mineral density in children and adolescents: relation to puberty, calcium intake and physical activity. *J. Clin. Endocrinol. Metab.* 28: 57–62.

15. Nelson, D.A. and Koo, W.W. (1999). Interpretation of absortiometric bone mass measurements in the growing skeleton: issues and limitations. *Calcif. Tissue Int.* 65: 1–3.

16. McKay, H.A., Petit, M.A., Bailey, D.A., Wallace, W.M., Schutz, R.W., and Khan, K.M. (2000). Analysis of proximal femur DXA scans in growing children: comparisons of different protocol for cross-sectional 8-month and 7-year longitudinal data. *J. Bone Miner. Res.* 15: 1181–1188.

CHAPTER 5

Calcium Carbonate Supplementation is Associated with Higher Plasma IGF-1 in 16- to 18-Year-Old Boys and Girls

Fiona Ginty,[1] A. Prentice,[1] A. Laidlaw,[1] L. McKenna,[1] S. Jones,[1] S. Stear,[1] and T.J. Cole[2]

[1]Elsie Widdowson Laboratory, MRC Human Nutrition Research, Cambridge, United Kingdom;
[2]Centre for Paediatric Epidemiology and Biostatistics, Institute of Child Health, London, United Kingdom

ABSTRACT

We have recently shown that calcium carbonate supplementation for 15 months resulted in significant increases in bone mineral content in 16- to 18-year-old girls and boys. A significant increase in height and bone size was also found in calcium-supplemented boys. In both studies, a reduction in bone turnover markers was observed, which may have accounted for the bone mineral gains but not the effects on bone size in boys. Because insulin-like growth factor I (IGF-1) is one of the principal anabolic hormones responsible for stimulating bone growth, the aim of this study was to determine whether IGF-1 was higher in calcium-supplemented subjects. In the girls' study, 131 girls age 17.3 (SD 0.3) years were randomized to receive either a calcium supplement (1000 mg calcium per day as $CaCO_3$) or matching placebo. In the boys' study, 143 subjects age 16.8 (SD 0.5) years were randomized to receive the same calcium supplement or matching placebo as the girls. Preliminary analysis has shown that at the end of the intervention period, plasma IGF-1 concentration was significantly higher in girls ($+9.3\%$, $P = 0.03$) and boys

Nutritional Aspects of Osteoporosis, Second Edition

($+6.8\%$, $P=0.02$) with tablet compliance greater than 50%. A similar result was obtained in girls and boys who had greater than 75% tablet compliance (girls: $+12\%$, $P=0.02$; boys: $+11\%$, $P=0.006$). The results of this study suggest that calcium carbonate supplementation is associated with higher production of IGF-1 in 16- to 18-year-old girls and boys. This differential may have resulted in greater bone mineral accretion in calcium-supplemented girls and boys and bone growth in boys.

INTRODUCTION

Optimization of peak bone mass during adolescence and early adulthood may be an effective means of offsetting age-related bone loss and thus reducing the risk of osteoporosis later in life [1]. The Cambridge Bone Studies were set up to address the lack of evidence on dietary and lifestyle determinants of bone health in older adolescent girls and boys. As a result of these studies, we have shown for the first time that calcium supplementation (1000 mg as calcium carbonate) of 16- to 18-year-old girls for 15 months results in a significant increase in whole-body and regional-size-adjusted bone mineral content (BMC) [2]. In a further similarly designed study in 16- to 18-year-old boys, significant BMC increases at the whole body, spine, and hip sites were also found [3]. Unexpectedly, bone size and height were also significantly increased in calcium-supplemented boys. Bone turnover markers were reduced in calcium-supplemented girls and boys [4,5], which may have accounted for the gains in bone mineral but not the effects on bone size. Therefore, it was hypothesized that calcium supplementation may result in higher production of insulin-like growth factor 1 (IGF-1), thus providing a mechanistic basis for the gains in bone size in boys.

Insulin-like growth factor 1 is a major determinant of bone growth and mineral content [6], and plasma concentrations are approximately 4 to 5 times higher in adolescents than in adults [7]. Animal and human studies have shown that hepatic IGF-1 production, plasma IGF-1 concentration, and the proportion of free IGF-1 (i.e., the portion not bound to its principal binding protein IGFBP-3) is regulated by dietary protein intake [8,9]. Increased milk consumption in adolescent girls [10] and elderly men and women [11] has been shown to result in significantly higher plasma IGF-1. In both studies, it was postulated that the higher protein content of milk mediated the rise in plasma IGF-1; however, it is currently unknown as to whether calcium intake has an independent stimulatory effect on hepatic or osteoblast production of IGF-1. Therefore, the aim of this study was to determine whether calcium carbonate supplementation of 16- to 18-year-old girls and boys resulted in a higher plasma concentration of IGF-1, thus providing a mechanistic basis for the greater gains in bone size in calcium-supplemented boys.

METHODS

SUBJECTS

For the girls' study, 144 healthy female students were recruited from sixth-form colleges in Cambridge, U.K. They were age 17.3 ± 0.3 years and were 4.7 ± 0.2 (mean $\pm$ SD) years postmenarche; 131 subjects completed the study. For the boys' study, 150 subjects with a mean age of 16.8 ± 0.5 years were also recruited from Cambridge sixth-form colleges and 143 subjects completed the study. Exclusion criteria for both studies included any medical problem, a history of eating disorders, and use of medication known to interfere with bone metabolism. Written informed consent was obtained from both the subjects and their parents or guardians. Approval for the study was given by the Ethical Committee of the MRC Dunn Nutrition Unit (of which the Nutrition and Bone Health Group of MRC Human Nutrition Research was formerly a part).

STUDY DESIGN

Details of the girls' study design have been previously published [2]. In summary, subjects were randomized, double-blind, to receive a calcium supplement (group S, $n = 65$) or matching placebo (group P, $n = 66$). Randomization was stratified by college and performed in permuted blocks of four. The calcium supplement was chewable, orange-flavored calcium carbonate containing 500 mg calcium per tablet (Calcichew® 500 mg); the placebo was indistinguishable in shape, taste, and texture (distributed by Shire Pharmaceuticals, U.K., and manufactured by Nycomed Pharma, Norway). Subjects were asked to consume one of their assigned tablets twice a day for 15 months (total supplement provided: 1000 mg calcium per day). Subjects were also randomly allocated to one of two exercise groups that were stratified by supplement group to ensure equal numbers consuming calcium and placebo. The exercise group (group E, $n = 75$) were invited and encouraged to attend three 45-minute exercise classes a week during term time. The remaining subjects (group N, $n = 56$) were not invited to these sessions. Details of subject numbers and study design are shown in Fig. 1. The total calcium intervention period was 15.5 months, with the exercise intervention lasting a total of 24 weeks.

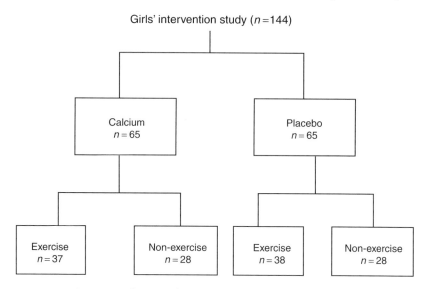

FIGURE 1   Subject numbers and design of girls' intervention study.

The design of the boys' study differed from the girls study in one respect in that it included an extra group with pre-existing high activity levels (group H, defined as >9 hours sport per week) who participated in the supplement intervention but were excluded from the exercise intervention [3]. The participants in the low activity group (group L, defined as <9 hours sport per week) were randomly allocated to one of two exercise groups, stratified by supplement group to ensure equal numbers consuming calcium and placebo. Details of the study design and subject numbers are provided in Fig. 2. The total duration of the calcium intervention was 12.7 ± 0.5 months, and the exercise intervention was of a similar duration as the girl's study.

BLOOD SAMPLE COLLECTION

To allow for the varying daily routines of the subjects, non-fasting blood samples (13 mL total, consisting of 10 mL lithium heparin and 2.5 mL potassium EDTA) were collected between 900 hr and 1900 hr. Time of blood sample collection and last meal were recorded, and the timing of the final blood sample was kept as consistent as possible with that of the baseline sample. Blood samples at baseline and final time points were successfully obtained from 102 subjects in the girls' study. In the boys' study, blood

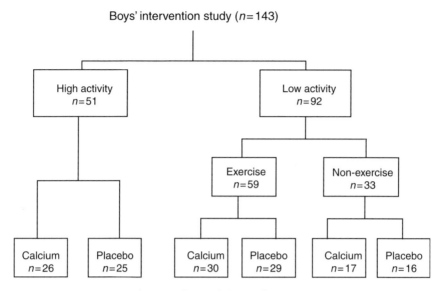

FIGURE 2   Subject numbers and design of boys' intervention study.

samples were obtained from 122 boys at baseline, interim (6 months), and final time points (12.7 months). Samples were kept cold after collection using cooler bags containing ice blocks or by refrigeration. They were centrifuged at 4°C (3000 rpm) within 2 hours of collection. Separated plasma was aliquoted and stored at –80°C

MEASUREMENTS

Height was measured to the nearest 0.1 cm using a wall-mounted stadiometer. Weight was measured to the nearest 0.1 kg using an electronic digital scale (Sauter weighing scales; Todd Scales Ltd., Norwich, U.K.). Dietary calcium intake, including supplement and antacid use, was assessed at baseline and final time points for the week prior to the measurement and over the previous year using the food frequency questionnaire "Calquest" (M. Nelson, King's College, London, U.K.). This is a validated dietary instrument in common use in the United Kingdom, based on the frequency of consumption of the main sources of calcium in the British diet: milk, dairy products, and calcium-fortified flour products [2].

Dietary protein intake was determined in boys and girls at baseline using 7-day food diaries. Portion sizes were matched against food photographs, and quantities were described in household measures. Subjects were also asked some supplementary questions about the type of milk they usually drank and whether they ate meat. The diet records were coded using the in-house program DIDO (Diet In Data Out) [12], and quantification of protein intake was determined using an in-house suite of programs based on the nutrient database of *McCance and Widdowson*, edition 5 [13].

Serum IGF-1 was measured by a two-site immunoenzymometric assay (OCTEIA® IGF-1; IDS Ltd., Boldon, U.K.). The method included a sample pretreatment step that denatured the IGF-1 binding proteins, allowing total IGF-1 to be measured. Samples from both time points were analyzed in duplicate within the same run. Kit controls with a low (50 to 100 µg/L) or high (200 to 400 µg/L) IGF-1 concentration, as well as an in-house plasma pool (which had an average IGF-1 concentration of 110 µg/L), were also measured in each run. Samples with a coefficient of variation greater than 10% were repeated. Inter-assay variation averaged 4.3% for the low control, 7.8% for the high control, and 6.7% for the in-house control.

STATISTICAL ANALYSIS

Statistical analysis was carried out using Data Desk 6.1.1 (Data Description, Inc.; Ithaca, NY). Summary statistics for all relevant variables at each time point are presented as mean (SD). Percent differences are presented as mean (SE). Differences across groups were assessed using analysis of variance (ANOVA). All continuous variables, excluding age, blood collection time, and difference between time of last meal and time of blood collection, were transformed to natural logarithms (ln) to allow the exploration of power relationships between continuous variables and to determine the proportional effects of discrete variables. Once transformed, all variables approximated normality. When the dependent variable is in natural logarithmic form, the multiplication of the regression coefficient by 100 corresponds closely to the percentage effect as defined by (difference/mean) ×100 [14]. All percentage differences shown in this paper were derived in this manner.

Multiple linear regression models were constructed to examine the effects of calcium supplementation on IGF-1. An interaction between the supplement and exercise interventions was also tested for. All subjects, irrespective of compliance, were initially included in the analysis (intention-to-treat model). The analyses were then restricted to those subjects with the higher tablet compliance (subjects who consumed more than 50 and 75% of the assigned tablets). These cutoffs were arbitrary but provided a reasonable compromise between high compliance and sample numbers.

All variables of interest were included in the initial model, including baseline values (to minimize the effects of regression toward the mean) and other likely confounders such as age, weight, height, and days since baseline measurement; age at menarche; days since last menstrual period; dietary calcium intake; and time of blood sample collection (for plasma markers). A consistent approach to variable selection was taken throughout by using the simultaneous procedure (Linear Model Type 3, DataDesk 6.1.1) with backward elimination of the least significant factors ($P > 0.05$) to produce a final parsimonious model.

RESULTS

SUBJECT CHARACTERISTICS AT BASELINE

Baseline summary statistics for girls and boys are shown in Tables I and II. No significant differences were found between the calcium- and placebo-supplemented subjects with respect to age, weight, height, daily protein and calcium intakes, and plasma IGF-1 concentration. In girls, age of menarche, time of blood sample collection, and time since last meal were not found to differ significantly between the calcium and placebo groups. In boys, time of blood sample collection was approximately 1 hour earlier in the calcium compared to placebo group (15.6 ± 2.2 hr versus 14.3 ± 2.8 hr, respectively; $P < 0.001$). However, there was no significant difference in time

TABLE I   Baseline Summary Statistics for Calcium- and Placebo-Supplemented Girls Who Provided a Blood Sample

	Calcium ($n = 50$) Mean (SD)	Placebo ($n = 52$) Mean (SD)
Age (yr)	17.4 (0.4)	17.3 (0.3)
Weight (kg)	57.6 (7.8)	56.2 (7.9)
Height (cm)	164.8 (6.5)	164.3 (7.3)
Age of menarche (yr)	12.7 (1.2)	12.6 (1.5)
Protein intake (g/day)	67.9 (19.4)	67.4 (13.8)
Calcium intake (g/day)	939 (295)	988 (307)
IGF-1 (µg/L)	243 (60)	223 (52)

Note: Variables include age, body weight and height, age of menarche, daily energy, protein and calcium intake, and plasma concentration of IGF-1 (µg/L). Food intake data are for 82 subjects who completed a food diary and provided a blood sample (i.e., 41 in both the calcium- and placebo-supplemented groups). No significant differences were found between groups (ANOVA).

TABLE II   Baseline Summary Statistics (mean (SD)) for Calcium- and Placebo-Supplemented Boys Who Provided a Blood Sample

	Calcium ($n=65$) Mean (SD)	Placebo ($n=57$) Mean (SD)
Age (yr)	16.8 (0.5)	16.8 (0.4)
Weight (kg)	69.4 (10.9)69.4	68.1 (9.4)
Height (cm)	177.8 (5.9)	177.3 (6.5)
Protein intake (g/day)	93.4 (25.0)	91.2 (23.7)
Calcium intake (g/day)	1245 (662)	1354 (737)
IGF-1 (µg/L)	214 (47)	214 (45)

Note: Variables include age, body weight and height, hours of sport per week, daily energy, protein and calcium intake, and plasma concentration of IGF-1 (µg/L). Food intake data are for 91 subjects who completed a food diary and provided a blood sample (i.e., 48 and 43 in the calcium- and placebo-supplemented groups, respectively). No significant differences were found between groups (ANOVA).

since last meal (3.4 ± 2.7 hr versus 3.4 ± 2.7 hr). Compared to girls, boys were younger, taller, and heavier and had a higher protein and calcium intake (all $P < 0.0001$). However, plasma IGF-1 was 7% higher in girls compared to boys (231 (SD 57) versus 213 (SD 47) µg/L, respectively; $P = 0.03$).

EFFECT OF CALCIUM SUPPLEMENTATION ON PLASMA IGF-1 IN GIRLS AND BOYS

Between baseline and final time points, there was a significant decrease in IGF-1 in girls (-14.7%, $P < 0.0001$) and boys (-19.7%, $P < 0.0001$), but the decrease was approximately 4% (NS) lower in calcium-supplemented subjects compared to placebo subjects (i.e., IGF-1 was higher in calcium-supplemented subjects). When the results of the girls and boys at final were combined and adjusted for baseline concentration, IGF-1 was significantly higher in calcium-supplemented subjects ($+6\%$, $P = 0.02$). The difference was greater in subjects with >75% tablet compliance ($+12.4\%$, $P = 0.003$). A significant difference in IGF-1 response to calcium supplementation between girls and boys was not found.

EFFECT OF CALCIUM SUPPLEMENTATION ON PLASMA IGF-1 IN GIRLS

Insulin-like growth factor I was marginally higher (NS) in all calcium-supplemented girls (ITT) ($+4.3 \pm 3.9\%$, $P = 0.30$). This difference was

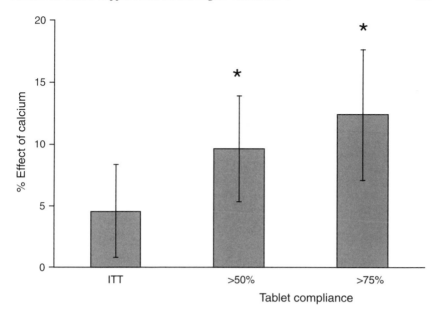

FIGURE 3   Percent effect of calcium supplementation on plasma IGF-1 after 15.5 months of calcium supplementation in girls. *$P \leq 0.05$.

significantly greater in subjects with tablet compliance >50% ($+9.4 \pm 4.1\%$, $P = 0.03$) and >75% ($+12.0 \pm +4.9\%$, $P = 0.02$) (Fig. 3). No significant effect of the exercise intervention on IGF-1 or a significant interaction with calcium supplementation was found. No significant differences between calcium- and placebo-supplemented subjects were observed (i.e., weight, height, calcium and protein intake, hours of sport/week, difference between time of blood sample collection and last meal, age at menarche) which might explain the difference in IGF-1 between the two groups.

EFFECT OF CALCIUM SUPPLEMENTATION ON PLASMA IGF-1 IN BOYS

After 6 months of calcium supplementation, IGF-1 was marginally higher (NS) in calcium-supplemented boys, compared to the placebo subjects (ITT: $+2.9 \pm 2.5\%$, $P = 0.25$; subjects with >50% tablet compliance: $+4.3 \pm 3.6\%$, $P = 0.23$; subjects with >75% tablet compliance: $+5.1 \pm 4.7\%$, $P = 0.29$) (Fig. 4). After 12 months supplementation, the difference between calcium and placebo supplemented subjects was significant in subjects with tablet

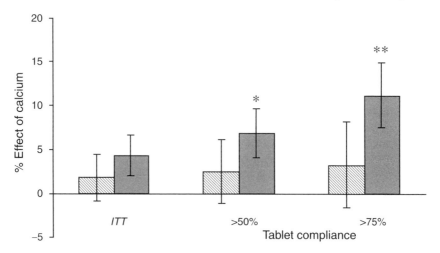

FIGURE 4   Percent effect of calcium supplementation on plasma IGF-1 after 6 months and 12 months of calcium supplementation in boys. $^*P \leq 0.05$; $^{**}P \leq 0.01$.

compliance >50% ($+6.8 \pm 3.0\%$, $p = 0.02$) and >75% ($+11.1 \pm 3.8\%$, $P = 0.006$) (Fig. 4). No significant effect of the exercise intervention was found on IGF-1 at either time point, and no significant interaction was found between the exercise intervention and the effects of the calcium supplementation on IGF-1. Similarly to the girls, no significant differences between calcium- and placebo-supplemented subjects were observed that might explain the differential in IGF-1 between the two groups.

DISCUSSION

Previous analysis of bone turnover markers in the girls and boys studies showed that calcium supplementation resulted in a significant reduction in plasma osteocalcin concentration and bone specific alkaline phosphatase activity in girls [4] and a transient reduction in parathyroid hormone (PTH) at the interim (6 months) time point in the boys, followed by a significant reduction in plasma osteocalcin at final (12 months) [5]. These changes show some similarity to those that have been found in studies of calcium-supplemented adults [15–17] but do not necessarily indicate that the increases in bone mineral that were found in both studies are a result of a reduction in bone turnover [18]. Comparison of the skeletal response to calcium between older adolescents and adults may not be appropriate, as the skeleton is still in an anabolic state, as indicated by ongoing bone growth and elevated markers of bone turnover that were observed in both studies.

The increases in bone size in the calcium-supplemented boys [3] indicate that a mechanism beyond a reduction in bone turnover occurred. This hypothesis would appear to be supported by the higher plasma IGF-1 concentration in calcium-supplemented subjects. IGF-1 is one of the principal anabolic factors mediating bone growth during puberty, reaching a peak concentration during puberty and then declining toward adult concentrations at the end of longitudinal growth [7,19]. Plasma IGF-1 concentration has been previously shown to be approximately 10% higher in 12-year-old girls who were supplemented with 1 pint of milk per day for 18 months compared to unsupplemented controls [20]. A similar effect on IGF-1 was observed in older men and women (55 to 85 years) who increased their milk intake by 720 mL/day [11]. In both studies, this increment in IGF-1 has been attributed to increased protein intake from milk.

In the present study, protein intake was not found to influence plasma IGF-1 concentration in either boys or girls. The higher plasma IGF-1 concentration in calcium-supplemented boys and girls suggests that either IGF-1 production was increased by calcium supplementation or that the age-related decline in IGF-1, observed in both groups, was attenuated in the calcium-supplemented group. This differential may have resulted in greater bone mineral accretion in girls and boys and greater gains in bone size in boys. Recently, it has been shown that selective knock-out of the IGF-1 receptor gene in mouse osteoblasts resulted in mice with normal bone size and weight but a decrease in the rate of mineralization of osteoid (Zhang et al., 2002). The authors suggested that osteoblast-derived IGF-1 might be essential for coupling collagen synthesis to sustained mineralization. The question remains whether the effects of calcium supplementation on bone mineral accumulation in this and other age groups is primarily mediated by a reduction in bone turnover rate or whether it is possible that an anabolic factor, such as IGF-1, maximizes mineral accretion.

CONCLUSIONS

In our preliminary analysis, calcium carbonate supplementation was found to be associated with higher plasma IGF-1 in girls and boys, and this differential may have mediated greater gains in bone mineral in girls and boys and bone size in boys. The mechanism by which IGF-1 was maintained at a higher concentration remains to be determined, and current analysis of IGF-1 binding proteins may assist in the interpretation of these findings.

ACKNOWLEDGMENTS

Funded by the Medical Research Council as an addition to work supported by awards from the Department of Health/Medical Research Council Nutrition Research Initiative (boys' study) and the Mead Johnson Research Fund (girls' study). The views expressed in this publication are those of the authors and not necessarily those of the sponsors.

REFERENCES

1. Heaney, R.P., Abrams, S., Dawson-Hughes, B., Looker, A., Marcus, R., Matkovic, V., and Weaver, C. (2000). Peak bone mass. *Osteoporosis Int.* 11: 985–1009.
2. Stear, S.J., Prentice, A., Jones, S.C., and Cole, T.J. (2003). Effect of a calcium and exercise intervention on bone mineral status of 16–18 year old adolescent girls. *Am. J. Clin. Nutr.* 77: 985–992.
3. Prentice, A., Stear, S.J., Ginty, F., Jones, S.C., Mills, L., and Cole, T.J. (2002). Calcium supplementation increases height and bone mass of 16–18 year old boys. *J. Bone Miner. Res.* 17: S397.
4. Ginty, F., Stear, S.J., Jones, S.C., Prentice, A., Stirling, D.M., Bennett, J., Laidlaw, A., and Cole, T.J. (2002). The effects of a 15 month calcium and exercise intervention on markers of bone and calcium metabolism in 16–18 year old girls. *J. Bone Miner. Res.* 17: 1341.
5. Ginty, F., Stear, S.J., Jones, S.C., Stirling, D.M., Bennett, J., Laidlaw, A., Cole, T.J., and Prentice, A. (2002). Impact of calcium supplementation on markers of bone and calcium metabolism in 16–18 year old boys. *J. Bone Miner. Res.* 17: S178.
6. Yakar, S., Rosen, C.J., Beamer, W.G., Ackert-Bicknell, C.L., Wu, Y., Liu, J.L., Ooi, G.T., Setser, J., Frystyk, J., Boisclair, Y.R., and LeRoith, D. (2002). Circulating levels of IGF-1 directly regulate bone growth and density. *J. Clin. Invest.* 110: 771–781.
7. Juul, A., Dalgaard, P., Blum, W.F., Bang, P., Hall, K., Michaelsen, K.F., Muller, J., and Skakkebaek, N.E. (1995). Serum levels of insulin-like growth factor (IGF)-binding protein-3 (IGFBP-3) in healthy infants, children, and adolescents: the relation to IGF-I, IGF-II, IGFBP-1, IGFBP-2, age, sex, body mass index, and pubertal maturation. *J. Clin. Endocrinol. Metab.* 80: 2534–2542.
8. Clemmons, D.R. and Underwood, L.E. (1991). Nutritional regulation of IGF-I and IGF binding proteins. *Ann. Rev. Nutr.* 11: 393–412.
9. Langlois, J.A., Rosen, C.J., Visser, M., Hannan, M.T., Harris, T., Wilson, P.W., and Kiel, D.P. (1998). Association between insulin-like growth factor I and bone mineral density in older women and men: the Framingham Heart Study. *J. Clin. Endocrinol. Metab.* 83: 4257–4262.
10. Cadogan, J., Blumsohn, A., Barker, M.E., and Eastell, R. (1998). A longitudinal study of bone gain in pubertal girls: anthropometric and biochemical correlates. *J. Bone Miner. Res.* 13: 1602–1612.
11. Heaney, R.P., McCarron, D.A., Dawson-Hughes, B., Oparil, S., Berga, S.L., Stern, J.S., Barr, S.I., and Rosen, C.J. (1999). Dietary changes favorably affect bone remodelling in older adults. *J. Am. Diet. Assoc.* 99: 1228–1233.
12. Price, G.M., Paul, A.A., Key, F.B., Harter, A.C., Cole, T.J., Day, K.C., and Wadsworth, M.E.J. (1995). Measurement of diet in a large national survey: comparison of computerised and manual coding in household measures. *J. Human Nutri. Diet* 8: 417–428.

13. Holland, B., Welch, A., Unwin, I., Buss, D., Paul, A., and Southgate, D. (1991). *McCance and Widdowson's The Composition of Foods.* Royal Society of Chemistry and Ministry of Agriculture, Fisheries and Food, London.
14. Cole, T.J. (2000). Sympercents: symmetric percentage differences on the 100 log(e) scale simplify the presentation of log transformed data. *Stat. Med.* 19: 3109–3125.
15. Blumsohn, A., Herrington, K., Hannon, R.A., Shao, P., Eyre, D.R., and Eastell, R. (1994). The effect of calcium supplementation on the circadian rhythm of bone resorption. *J. Clin. Endocrinol. Metab.* 79: 730–735.
16. Ginty, F., Flynn, A., and Cashman, K.D. (1998). The effect of short-term calcium supplementation on biochemical markers of bone metabolism in healthy young adults. *Br. J. Nutr.* 80: 437–443.
17. Kamel, S., Fardellone, P., Meddah, B., Lorget-Gondelmann, F., Sebert, J.L., and Brazier, M. (1998). Response of several markers of bone collagen degradation to calcium supplementation in postmenopausal women with low calcium intake. *Clin. Chem.* 44: 1437–1442.
18. Heaney, R.P. (2001). The bone remodeling transient: interpreting interventions involving bone-related nutrients. *Nutr. Rev.* 59: 327–334.
19. Wang, J., Zhou, J., and Bondy, C.A. (1999). IGF-1 promotes longitudinal bone growth by insulin-like actions augmenting chondrocyte hypertrophy. *FASEB J.* 13: 1985–1990.
20. Cadogan, J., Eastell, R., Jones, N., and Barker, M.E. (1997). Milk intake and bone mineral acquisition in adolescent girls: randomised, controlled intervention trial. *Br. Med. J.* 315: 1255–1260.
21. Zang, M., Xuan, S., Bouxsein, M.L., von Stechow, D., Akeno, N., Faugere, M.C., Malluche, H., Zhao, G., Rosen, C.J., Efstratiadis, A., and Clemens, T.L. (2002). Osteoblast-specific knockout of the insulin-like growth factor (IGF) receptor gene reveals an essential role of IGF signaling in bone matrix mineralization. *J. Biol. Chem.* 277: 44005–44012.

PART II

Dairy Products, Calcium Metabolism

Nutrients, Interactions, and Foods: The Importance of Source

ROBERT P. HEANEY

University Chair, Creighton University, Omaha, Nebraska

INTRODUCTION

When investigating the role of nutrition in the prevention, causation, or treatment of any disease, there is an inescapable tendency toward a reductionist approach, evaluating nutrients one by one, most often in isolation from what would be otherwise concurrent changes in other nutrients. While such an approach is necessary to a point, there is also a point beyond which nutrient interactions, both constructive and destructive, need to be evaluated. In an earlier symposium in this series, Dawson-Hughes remarked, quite correctly I believe, that one could not evaluate the calcium requirement in the absence of vitamin D repletion and could not evaluate the vitamin D requirement in the absence of calcium repletion. Yet, individuals ignorant of the underlying biology of the calcium and bone economies continue to attempt separate evaluations, as witnessed by the tendency in meta-analyses to exclude all calcium treatment trials that took pains to ensure vitamin D repletion [1].

Nutritional Aspects of Osteoporosis, Second Edition

It is now firmly established that several nutrients play roles in bone health, and it is appropriate, therefore, to look beyond individual nutrient effects and examine more closely both nutrient interactions and the effects of the food sources for those nutrients. This brief review touches on three distinct examples of this more integral approach to the relationship of nutrition and osteoporosis. Specifically, it describes the connection between the calcium content of a diet and its overall nutritional quality, it looks at the constructive interactions between calcium and protein, and finally it looks at a possibly destructive interaction between calcium supplementation and phosphorus nutrition.

CALCIUM AND DIET QUALITY

Several years ago Barger-Lux and Heaney published a study of 272 healthy Caucasian premenopausal women who had provided 7-day diet diaries as a part of the screening process for entry into various ongoing investigations at the Creighton Osteoporosis Research Center [2]. Using a scheme developed by Davis *et al.* [3], these diets were scored by giving one point for each of nine nutrients consumed at two-thirds or more of the recommended intake levels. The nutrients concerned were calcium; iron; magnesium; vitamins A, C, B_6, and B_{12}; thiamin; and riboflavin. These nutrients were selected because they had relatively low co-variance and were, therefore, reasonably good markers for *total* nutrient intake from a variety of sources. The nutrient intakes concerned were exclusively from food, not supplement sources, and, as is usual in the industrialized nations, calcium intakes at or above the recommended levels came mainly from dairy foods. The maximum possible score was 9, and scores of 4 or below were considered to represent "poor" diets [3].

The women were sorted on the basis of whether their calcium intake exceeded two-thirds of the recommended intake (*i.e.*, whether they had a calcium score of 0 or 1). Of these women, 151 (56% of the total) had calcium scores of 0, and 121 had calcium scores of 1. Figure 1 shows the distribution of diet scores for the two calcium intake groups and illustrates dramatically the difference in overall diet quality between them. The median diet score for those with low calcium intakes was 4; that is, they typically had "poor" diets, not simply because of the low calcium intake but because, on average, they had deficient intakes of at least four other nutrients as well. Five of the women had diets so poor that they had a total diet score of 0.

By contrast, women with calcium scores of 1 had a median diet score of 8, and roughly one-third had perfect diet scores. Approximately 90% of them, overall, had diets that could be characterized as "adequate"; that is, they had

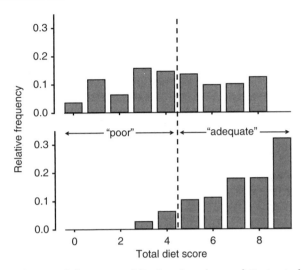

FIGURE 1 Distribution of diet scores, following the scheme of Davis *et al.* [3], for 151 premenopausal women with calcium intakes less than two-thirds of the RDA (top panel) and 121 premenopausal women with calcium intakes greater than two-thirds of the RDA (bottom panel). (Adapted from Barger-Lux and Heaney [2]. With permission.)

intakes that were nominally sufficient for five or more nutrients. To put it differently, 53% of the women with low calcium intakes had overall poor diets, while only 10% of the women with adequate calcium intakes had poor diets. The clear conclusion is that a low calcium intake is a marker for a poor diet. It follows inexorably that mononutrient supplemention with calcium constitutes an inadequate approach to the total nutritional need of such women.

What is especially noteworthy about this analysis is that the addition of a single serving of milk to the diets of those women with low calcium intakes would have pushed most of their diets from the "poor" into the "adequate" category, substantially increasing the intake of most of the index nutrients (with the exception of iron). Table I lists the nutrient content of a liter of low-fat milk, both in terms of the quantities of the nutrients concerned and the approximate percentages of the currently recommended intakes of those nutrients. Even cursory inspection of the table reveals both what a complete food milk is and how low is the calorie cost of getting an abundance of the other nutrients. It becomes clear, also, that repairing the "poor" diet status of women with low calcium intakes would not have been so easily possible with any other high-calcium source, particularly supplements. No other high-calcium source contains the unique mixture of phosphorus, protein, potassium, and magnesium that is found in milk.

TABLE I   Nutrient Content of One Liter of Reduced Fat (1%) Milk

Nutrient	Content	Percent (%) RDA[a]
Calcium (mg)	1276	~100
Phosphorus (mg)	1044	150
Protein (g)	35.5	68
Magnesium (mg)	118	37
Potassium (mg)	1715	44
Riboflavin (mg)	0.38	32
Vitamin B$_6$ (mg)	0.43	33
Vitamin B$_{12}$ (μg)	3.8	158
Vitamin D[b] (I.U.)	423	~100
Energy (kcal)	431	~20[c]

[a]For United States.
[b]For North America.
[c]Assuming a total energy need of 2200 kcalories/day.

It is not simply that these other nutrients are necessary for health, and milk is therefore an efficient way to get total nutrition; rather, there may well be other less clearly identified nutrients in milk that are important as well. Such a conclusion is strongly suggested by several studies evaluating the impact of milk as a calcium source on various nonskeletal disorders. For example, the 10-year CARDIA study in young adults [4] showed that dairy consumption was inversely associated with development of all of the components of the metabolic syndrome (obesity, hyperinsulinemia, and insulin resistance), with each daily dairy serving lowering the odds ratio of developing this syndrome by 21%. High dairy intakes reduced the transition from overweight to obesity by 30%, and the transition from normal blood pressure to hypertension by nearly two-thirds.

A similar effect is seen in the DASH studies [5], in which substantial reductions in blood pressure were achieved in mildly hypertensive individuals by a diet high in fruits and vegetables and low fat dairy products. The dairy products greatly augmented the effect of the fruit and vegetable component of the diet, and, what may be of even greater interest, the degree of blood pressure reduction/control achieved in DASH was substantially greater than had been reported for calcium supplements alone [6]. A comparable difference in effect between dairy and supplement calcium had been reported by Zemel [7] in his randomized controlled trial of calcium sources as an adjuvant to weight reduction. In this relatively small trial, dairy sources of calcium produced greater weight reduction, better sparing of lean body mass, and preferential loss of fat from the torso, all relative to the same calcium intake provided by a calcium carbonate supplement.

Whether these apparent augmentations of the effect of calcium alone are due to some other, unidentified ingredient in dairy foods or to constructive interactions of several of the nutrients contained in dairy foods is unknown; nevertheless, they underscore the importance of food sources. While it would be desirable to have more feeding studies such as DASH and, specifically, studies contrasting food sources with pure sources of those same nutrients, it is unlikely that many such will be done, inasmuch as they are expensive. But, any program emphasizing the role of nutrition in the health of various body systems would probably be well advised to seek out food sources of the nutrients of interest, rather than relying too heavily on supplement sources alone.

CALCIUM AND PROTEIN

Several facts with respect to calcium and protein seem well established: (1) calcium aids bone status by providing the mineral needed for bone mass accumulation during growth, by slowing age-related bone loss, and by reducing fracture risk in the elderly [8]; (2) protein increases urinary calcium loss [9–11]; and (3) protein aids recovery from hip fracture [12,13]. For the most part, the studies establishing these diverse and to some extent contradictory effects have been done by varying only the nutrient concerned.

For example, the calciuric effects of protein have been demonstrated most clearly in studies in which purified protein or protein hydrolysates were used, with each gram of protein resulting in an approximate 1 mg rise in urinary calcium excretion. Spencer et al., however, observed that, when the protein was fed as ground beef, urinary calcium did not rise, with the difference in response being due, presumably, to the fact that the meat contained substantial quantities of phosphorus [14]. On the other hand, Kerstetter et al. [15] have reported that high protein intakes enhance calcium absorption, an effect that would counter a calciuric effect (were there to be one). Not everyone has been able to reproduce this finding in chronic feeding studies [16], and it may be, to the extent that the phenomenon is operative, that it applies only acutely. Very recently Roughead et al. [17] in a controlled study found no effect of high and low protein intakes from meat (117 g/day versus 68 g/day) either on calcium balance or on urinary calcium excretion, a finding consistent with that of Spencer et al. [14] and Heaney [16], but at odds with that of Kerstetter [15]. The two diets in the Roughead study also differed in their content of phosphorus (1679 mg/day versus 1266 mg/day) and potassium (2887 mg/day versus 2249 mg/day), nutrients that would have accompanied protein ingested as meat and which may have countered a protein effect on urine calcium (as both tend to be hypocalciuric).

The very reproducible calciuric effect of pure protein or amino acids had led to the tentative conclusion that high protein intakes might be deleterious for the skeleton; however, not only do the studies involving food sources of protein, such as those just cited, not support that conclusion, but epidemiological studies, such as those from the Framingham osteoporosis cohort [18], indicate instead that age-related bone loss in postmenopausal women is *inversely* related to protein intake, not *directly*, as might have been predicted from a calciuric effect.

Against this background it is of interest to examine the interaction of protein and calcium intakes in the study of Dawson-Hughes and colleagues [19]. In their randomized controlled trial of calcium supplementation, the bone gain associated with the calcium was confined to individuals in the highest tertile of protein intake, while in the placebo group there was a nonsignificant trend toward worsening bone status as protein intake rose. This latter effect is what would be predicted if there were some degree of protein-induced calciuria without an offsetting increase in calcium intake. Protein intake in this study spanned only a relatively narrow range and was not randomly assigned to the subjects, so these results cannot be considered final. Nevertheless, they do exhibit two interesting features: (1) high protein intake clearly did not block the calcium effect, and (2) most of the protein was from animal sources (as was true for the Framingham osteoporosis cohort, as well). This latter point provides no support for the hypothesis that animal foods (as contrasted with vegetable protein sources), by increasing urinary calcium loss, artificially elevate the calcium requirement.

The importance of adequate protein intake is at least twofold. First, protein is a bulk constituent of bone. Because of extensive post-translational modification of the collagen molecule (*e.g.*, cross-linking, hydroxylation), many of the amino acids released in bone resorption cannot be recycled; hence, bone turnover requires a continuing supply of fresh protein. Second, protein elevates serum IGF-1 [20,21], which is trophic for bone [21].

The IGF-1 response has threshold characteristics; that is, above certain protein intakes no further increase in IGF-1 can be produced. This effect is analogous to calcium retention, which rises at suboptimal calcium intakes but which plateaus at or above the individual's calcium intake requirement. For both nutrients, a rise in retention (for calcium) or a rise in IGF-1 (for protein) can be taken as evidence that the pre-supplement intake of the corresponding nutrient was suboptimal. The fact that IGF-1 has not reached its plateau at intakes in the range of current RDAs has led some to conclude that the current RDA for protein is set too low, particularly for the elderly. In any case, it is important to understand this relationship of nutrient intakes to the respective response plateaus. Different studies would be expected to show more or less of a beneficial effect of increasing one or both nutrient intakes depending upon whether the pre-supplement intake were below or above the respective threshold level.

Because several published studies of increased protein intake have shown rises in serum IGF-1 [20,21], it may be tentatively concluded that protein intakes in the individuals concerned were suboptimal. To the extent that this is true and that both of the bulk constituents of bone (calcium and protein) are ingested at suboptimal intakes, then it follows that the true effect of either nutrient cannot be discerned in studies that do not ensure full repletion of the other.

In any event, it is generally agreed that the frail elderly frequently have low protein intakes and frequently manifest hypoproteinemia on admission to the hospital for hip fracture (or other medical or surgical conditions). Vigorous protein supplementation in such individuals has been demonstrated in randomized controlled trials to improve outcomes substantially [12,22]. Protein supplements after fracture in these patients not only improve recovery but also slow bone loss in the contralateral hip [13], a finding presumably due, at least in part, to their effect on serum IGF-1.

PHOSPHORUS AND CALCIUM

Phosphorus is, in some sense, a pariah among the nutrients. Phosphorus intake is a significant problem for patients with end-stage renal disease, and phosphorus retention is the single most important factor in extraosseous calcification in patients with renal failure. While this concern is irrelevant to individuals with adequate kidney function, it has nevertheless tended to color medicine's approach to the nutrient. Specifically, phosphorus has been indicted in the genesis of osteoporosis [23], even if not convincingly, and the phosphorus content of colas, despite the lack of convincing evidence that they exert any harmful effects, has been cited repeatedly as the means whereby carbonated beverages may contribute to the genesis of bony fragility [24]. It is interesting, in this regard, to note in passing that orange juice has essentially the same phosphorus content as do the colas, and in those countries with calcium fortification of orange juice the phosphorus content may rise to 5 times that of a typical cola. To my knowledge, however, no concern has been raised about the harmful effects of orange juice on the skeleton.

The facts are that: (1) bone mineral is predominantly calcium phosphate; (2) adequate quantities of ingested phosphorus (expressed as a serum phosphate concentration of 1–2 mmol/L) are essential for bone building; and (3) hypophosphatemia, from whatever cause, limits mineralization at new bone forming sites, impairs osteoblast function, and enhances osteoclastic resorption. Additionally, ingested phosphorus alters the operation of the calcium economy. As was noted in the preceding section, the phosphorus content of meats was judged to be the principal reason why protein taken as food did not produce the same degree of calciuria as did protein taken in pure form. Phosphorus is known to be hypocalciuric, and phosphorus supplements have been used therapeutically to reduce renal stone formation in patients with hypercalciuria.

At issue in the context of this symposium is whether a low phosphorus intake in any way contributes to the problem of osteoporosis. And a secondary consideration is: are phosphorus-containing supplements safe?

Phosphorus is a trace nutrient in the biosphere. Most phosphorus is tied up in protoplasm or in guano deposits. Phosphorus is vital for cellular life and activity, as it is involved in cell structure, information coding, energy transfer, functional activation, and, in short, virtually every aspect of cell function. Animals get the phosphorus they need by ingesting the protoplasm of other organisms (animal or plant), and plants obtain phosphorus by taking up into their roots phosphorus released during decay of other organisms into the superficial soil layers of the biosphere. As would be expected for a trace nutrient, phosphorus absorption by the human intestine is relatively efficient, with net absorption typically ranging between 55 and 80% (depending upon concurrent calcium intake and absorption; see below). Moreover, because phosphorus is widely distributed in many foods, adult human phosphorus intakes tend to be adequate.

Nevertheless, circumstances do exist in which phosphorus intake may be limiting in the management of patients with osteoporosis. Table II sets forth the values that define various percentiles of phosphorus intake for

TABLE II   Distribution of Phosphorus Intakes by Age and Percentiles (mg/day) in Non-Hispanic White Women in the United States

Ages (yr)	5th	10th	15th	25th	50th	75th	85th	90th	95th
30–39	434	581	677	761	1111	1457	1637	1804	2092
40–49	486	575	634	764	1027	1341	1564	1650	1797
50–59	451	525	596	739	976	1214	1375	1565	1892
60–69	399	482	586	727	998	1299	1497	1735	2183
70–79	415	478	550	679	902	1224	1397	1500	1748
80 +	353	431	486	581	833	1157	1286	1435	1686

Note: Italic type indicates less than 70% of adult RDA.

Source: From Alaimo, K. et al. (1994). Dietary Intake of Vitamins, Minerals, and Fiber of Persons 2 Months and Over in the United States: Third National Health and Nutrition Examination Survey (NHANES), Phase 1, 1988–91, Advance Data from Vital and Health Statistics, No. 258. National Center for Health Statistics, Hyattsville, MD.

non-Hispanic white women, ages 30 to over 80, in the United States from NHANES-III [25]. The RDA in the United States is 700 mg/day. As the table shows, the median intake for all ages is above that level, and for younger women substantially so; 10 to 15% of women at all ages ingest more than twice the RDA. (These relatively high intakes, overall, certainly place phosphorus in a category different from that of calcium, where the bulk of the population has an intake below the recommended intake.) However, as can be seen from inspection of Table II, 5% of adult women over age 30 have intakes on any given day that are less than 70% of the RDA, 10% of women over 60, and 15% of women over 80.

Even a rudimentary knowledge of food composition will suffice to demonstrate that phosphorus intakes below 70% of the RDA will necessarily be low in other key nutrients, as well, particularly calcium and protein. Hence the diets of women with low phosphorus intakes are multiply inadequate. The correct solution to their problem is for health professionals first to recognize it, and then to address it, either with a change in diet or with a polyvalent nutritional supplement. Unfortunately, this is not often done in medical practice, and frequently these women, particularly if they have osteoporosis, will be placed on bone active agents and encouraged to take a calcium and vitamin D supplement.

Figure 2 depicts this situation schematically and focuses attention on the intersection of the three sets where, manifestly, the likelihood is highest that phosphorus intake will be limiting. The matter of bone active therapy is important because, precisely to the extent that it may be effective, such therapy increases the phosphorus requirement and aggravates any potential deficiency. Calcium supplement use is important because the most commonly used calcium salts (carbonate and citrate) will bind food phosphorus in the gut and reduce its absorption. Each of these points will be discussed briefly in what follows.

Phosphorus released in bone resorption can be efficiently reutilized in bone mineralization; hence, simple maintenance of skeletal mass translates to zero phosphorus balance and places little or no demand on dietary phosphorus intake. Urinary phosphorus excretion can be reduced to extremely low levels, and even intakes well below the RDA should be able to sustain zero balance. Antiresorptive therapies change that picture somewhat. They typically produce a slow increase in bone mineral content on the order of 0.5 to 1.0% per year at the spine after an initial positive remodeling transient of $+4.5$ to $+5.5\%$ in the first year. The steady-state increase after year one creates a small phosphorus requirement, with daily phosphorus balance in the range of $+4.5$ to $+9$ mg/day. By contrast, new generation anabolic therapies, capable of increasing axial bone mineral content by up to 15% per year, call for a positive phosphorus balance of

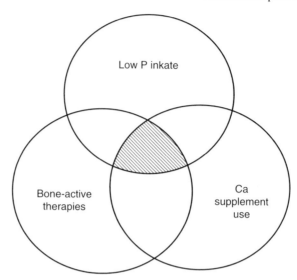

FIGURE 2   Venn diagram highlighting the portion of the elderly osteoporotic population most
likely to be susceptible to insufficient phosphorus intake; domain sizes are not drawn to scale.
(© Robert P. Heaney, 2003. Used with permission.)

up to $+45$ to $+90$ mg/day. (The foregoing estimates assume that values
measured in the axial skeleton in response to bone-active agents apply to the
whole skeleton and hence reflect a worst-case, or maximum possible,
phosphorus demand.)

Food phosphorus binding by co-ingested calcium is a well recognized
and utilized phenomenon, particularly in the management of phosphorus
absorption in patients with end-stage renal disease. Over a broad range of
intakes, roughly 90% of ingested calcium is unabsorbed and hence remains in
the intestinal lumen, capable of binding a variety of other substances. One of
these, of course, is phosphorus. Heaney and Nordin [26] have shown that
fecal phosphorus content (and therefore, inversely, absorbed phosphorus) is
determined primarily by fecal calcium content and to a lesser extent by
actual phosphorus intake. Dietary calcium and phosphorus together account
for nearly three-fourths of the variation in the quantity of phosphorus
absorbed. Briefly, each 500 mg of ingested calcium binds 166 mg of diet
phosphorus (95% CI: 144–188 mg).

Figure 3 shows the amount of food phosphorus that would be available
for absorption in a woman ingesting 70% of the phosphorus RDA
(i.e., the italicized cells in Table II) under varying conditions of calcium
supplementation. The calculations used in constructing Fig. 3 [26] assume
that the calcium supplements are co-ingested with the food phosphorus

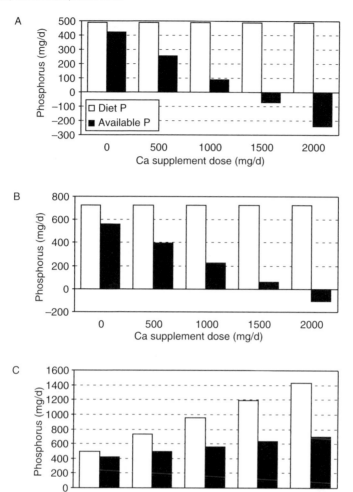

FIGURE 3 Total phosphorus intake and available phosphorus in individuals ingesting 70% of the RDA for phosphorus under varying conditions of calcium supplementation. (A) All supplemental calcium as the carbonate or citrate; (B) same as for A, except for the addition of a single serving of milk to the diet; and (C) same as for A, except that the calcium supplemental intake is in the form of tricalcium phosphate. (© Robert P. Heaney, 2003. Used with permission.)

(see below). Inspection of Fig. 3A demonstrates that, at a calcium supplement intake of between 1000 and 1500 mg/day, all of the food phosphorus is complexed by unabsorbed calcium and rendered non-available. Above that point, phosphorus absorption becomes negative; that is, phosphorus in digestive secretions and sloughed intestinal mucosa, estimated to be perhaps as much as 250 mg/day, will be complexed, as well, which converts the gut into a net excretory organ for phosphorus. Adding a single serving of milk to the diet of such women (Fig. 3B) effectively eliminates the problem. Alternatively, the use of a calcium phosphate supplement (Fig. 3C) provides the desired calcium, prevents the blocking of food phosphorus absorption, and ensures a generous supply of available phosphorus.

As noted, the foregoing calculations are for simultaneous ingestion of calcium and phosphorus, and the timing of the calcium supplement intake is therefore important for this relationship. The usual recommendation is to take supplements with meals, and this remains a sound stratagem. (By slowing gastric emptying the meal effect improves calcium absorption efficiency, and by spreading the dose out over the course of the day calcium absorption is improved further.) However, as just noted, this same stratagem maximizes phosphorus binding and minimizes phosphorus absorption. Schiller *et al.* [27] have shown, in a single meal design, that separation of the calcium supplement dose from the time of the meal substantially reduces the degree of phosphorus binding. This is, of course, to be expected for a process that involves nothing more complex than chemical binding. Figure 4

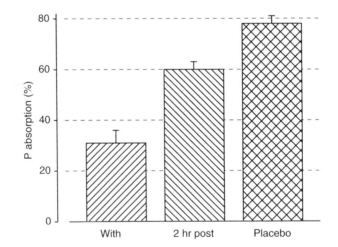

FIGURE 4 Percent phosphorus absorption from single meals with and without ingestion of supplemental calcium, showing the relationship to time of supplement ingestion. The phosphorus content of the test meal was 370 mg and the calcium supplement dose was 1000 mg, given as the acetate salt. With no calcium supplement, net phosphorus absorption averaged nearly 80%; with simultaneous ingestion, 31%; and when the calcium was delayed for 2 hours, 59%. (Drawn from the data of Schiller *et al.* [27]. (© Robert P. Heaney, 2003. Used with permission.)

plots some of the data from the paper of Schiller *et al.* showing both the degree of reduction in phosphorus absorption produced by simultaneous co-ingestion of calcium and phosphorus and the reduction in this effect by giving the calcium supplement 2 hours after the meal.

Very large calcium supplement doses, particularly if taken regularly with every meal, could create a negative phosphorus balance situation even for women who are not on anti-osteoporosis therapies; however, it is improbable that a regimen of invariable co-ingestion would be rigidly followed. Hence, without a bone-building demand for phosphorus, it is unlikely that phosphorus binding by calcium supplements would constitute a significant problem. However, once bone active agents, and particularly anabolic agents such as teriparatide, are employed, the situation changes. Figure 3 shows that at calcium supplement intakes in excess of 1200 mg/day there is effectively no diet phosphorus available to support bone building. This is less than the calcium supplement dose used in some teriparatide treatment studies.

Because of the likelihood of some irregularity of the co-ingestion of calcium supplements with foods, it may still be possible for women with low phosphorus intakes and receiving antiresorptive therapies to realize the small increase in bone mass that these therapies are able to produce. However, it is unlikely that this would be the case with the anabolic agents, with a phosphorus demand for bone mineralization that is roughly 10 times that of the antiresorptives. Under such circumstances, it would clearly be prudent to adjust the diet of the patient or to use a calcium phosphate product as the calcium supplement.

A final consideration relates to the safety of phosphate salts. This should not be an issue, as successful supplementation trials such as that of Chapuy *et al.* [28] used tricalcium phosphate as the supplement source without evident difficulty; Spencer *et al.* [29] showed that a 150% increase in phosphorus intake did not alter calcium balance at low, middle, or high calcium intakes, and supplement products based on bone-derived hydro-xyapatite have been in use worldwide for over 30 years. Nevertheless, one continues to encounter objections that increasing phosphorus intake will lead to an increase in parathyroid hormone (PTH) secretion with a consequent increase in bone resorption and presumably a corresponding increase in bony fragility [30].

To help resolve any lingering uncertainties, we addressed this problem in a small study involving 24 postmenopausal women with low usual intakes of calcium and phosphorus, employing three consecutive 1-week supple-mentation regimens. All meals were provided, and foods were selected to ensure total food phosphorus intakes of <600 mg/day. During the first week, no supplemental calcium was given; during the second week, 1800 mg calcium was given as carbonate; and during the third week, 1800 mg calcium was given as tricalcium phosphate (providing 930 mg of additional phosphorus and increasing phosphorus intake by more than 150%). At the end of each week, serum and urine were collected and analyzed for PTH and N-telopeptide (NTx), respectively. Relative to the baseline, when no calcium or phosphorus supplements were used, fasting PTH was reduced by 15% by both supplement sources ($P < 0.01$). The reduction was identical for the phosphate and the carbonate salts. Similarly, 24-hr urine NTx was reduced by 32% for both sources ($P < 0.01$), with no difference between them.

In brief, phosphate salts of calcium produce the same degree of PTH suppression and reduction in bone resorption as do carbonate sources. Thus, both relatively large-scale clinical use of phosphate-based supplements and metabolic experiments such as those just described indicate that there is essentially no cause for concern about the use of phosphate-containing calcium salts.

CONCLUSION

All three of the topics addressed in this brief review support a conclusion that food sources of key nutrients important for bone are not only nutritionally superior to use of isolated nutrients but also produce results that are at least quantitatively, and often directionally, different as well. Thus, calcium, phosphorus, vitamin D, and protein can be said to have additive effects on the skeleton. More attention needs to be paid to dietary status and to dietary quality in the evaluation of an elderly population prone to, or afflicted with, osteoporosis. Particular attention needs to be paid to improving the intake of good polynutrient sources such as dairy foods and the use of calcium supplement regimens that include sources containing phosphorus and vitamin D as well as calcium.

REFERENCES

1. Shea, B., Wells, G., Cranney, A., Zytaruk, N., Robinson, V., Griffith, L., Ortiz, Z., Peterson, J., Adachi, J., Tugwell, P., and Guyatt, G. (2002). Meta-analyses of therapies for postmenopausal osteoporosis. VII. Meta-analysis of calcium supplementation for the prevention of postmenopausal osteoporosis. *Endocr. Rev.* 23(4): 552–559.
2. Barger-Lux, M.J., Heaney, R.P., Packard, P.T., Lappe, J.M., and Recker, R.R. (1992). Nutritional correlates of low calcium intake. *Clin. Appl. Nutr.* 2(4): 39–44.
3. Davis, M.A., Murphy, S.P., Neuhaus, J.M. *et al.* (1990). Living arrangements and dietary quality of older U.S. adults. *J. Am. Diet. Assoc.* 90: 1667–1672.

4. Pereira, M.A., Jacobs, D.R., Jr., Van Horn, L., Slattery, M.L., Kartashov, A.I., and Ludwig, D.S. (2002). Dairy consumption, obesity, and the insulin resistance syndrome in young adults. *J. Am. Med. Assoc.* 287: 2081–2089.

5. Appel, L.J., Moore, T.J., Obarzanek, E., Vollmer, W.M., Svetkey, L.P., Sacks, F.M., Bray, G.A., Vogt, T.M., Cutler, J.A., Windhauser, M.M., Lin, P.-H., and Karanja, N. (1997). A clinical trial of the effects of dietary patterns on blood pressure. *N. Engl. J. Med.* 336: 1117–1124.

6. Birkett, N.J. (1998). Comments on a meta-analysis of the relation between dietary calcium intake and blood pressure. *Am. J. Epidemiol.* 148(3): 223–233.

7. Zemel, M.B., Thompson, W., Zemel, Morris, K., and Campbell P. (2004). Calcium and dairy acceleration of weight and fat loss during energy restriction in obese adults. *Obesity Res.* 12: 582–590.

8. Heaney, R.P. (2000). Calcium, dairy products and osteoporosis. *J. Am. Coll. Nutr.* 19(2): 83S–99S.

9. Heaney, R.P. and Recker, R.R. (1982). Effects of nitrogen, phosphorus, and caffeine on calcium balance in women. *J. Lab. Clin. Med.* 99: 46–55.

10. Johnson, N.E., Alcantara, E.N., and Linkswiler, H.M. (1970). Effect of protein intake on urinary and fecal calcium and calcium retention of young adult males. *J. Nutr.* 100: 1425–1430.

11. Chu, J.Y., Margen, S., and Costa, F.M. (1975). Studies in calcium metabolism. II. Effects of low calcium and variable protein intake on human calcium metabolism. *Am. J. Clin. Nutr.* 28: 1028–1035.

12. Delmi, M., Rapin, C.-H., Bengoa, J.-M., Delmas, P.D., Vasey, H., and Bonjour, J.-P. (1990). Dietary supplementation in elderly patients with fractured neck of the femur. *Lancet* 335: 1013–1016.

13. Schürch, M.-A., Rizzoli, R., Slosman, D., Vadas, L., Vergnaud, P., and Bonjour, J.-P. (1998). Protein supplements increase serum insulin-like growth factor-1 levels and attenuate proximal femur bone loss in patients with recent hip fracture. *Ann. Intern. Med.* 128: 801–809.

14. Spencer, H., Kramer, L., and Osis, D. (1978). Effect of a high protein (meat) intake on calcium metabolism in man. *Am. J. Clin. Nutr.* 31, 2167–2180.

15. Kerstetter, J.E., O'Brien, K.O., and Insogna, K.L. (1998). Dietary protein affects intestinal calcium absorption. *Am. J. Clin. Nutr.* 68: 859–865.

16. Heaney, R.P. 2000. Dietary protein and phosphorus do not affect calcium absorption. *Am. J. Clin. Nutr.* 72: 758–761.

17. Roughead, Z.K., Johnson, L.K., Lykken, G.I., and Hunt, J.R. (2003). Controlled high meat diets do not affect calcium retention of bone status in healthy postmenopausal women. *J. Nutr.* 133: 1020–1026.

18. Hannan, M.T., Tucker, K.L., Dawson-Hughes, B., Cupples, L.A., Felson, D.T., and Kiel, D.P. (2000). Effect of dietary protein on bone loss in elderly men and women: the Framingham Osteoporosis Study. *J. Bone Miner. Res.* 15: 2504–2512.

19. Dawson-Hughes, B. and Harris, S.S. (2002). Calcium intake influences the association of protein intake with rates of bone loss in elderly men and women. *Am. J. Clin. Nutr.* 75: 773–779.

20. Heaney, R.P., McCarron, D.A., Dawson-Hughes, B., Oparil, S., Berga, S.L., Stern, J.S., Barr, S.I., and Rosen, C.J. (1999). Dietary changes favorably affect bone remodeling in older adults. *J. Am. Diet. Assoc.* 99: 1228–1233.

21. Bonjour, J.P., Schüch, M.A., Chevalley, T., Ammann, P., and Rizzoli, R. (1997). Protein intake, IGF-1 and osteoporosis. *Osteoporos. Int.* 7(suppl. 3): S36–S42.

22. Bastow, M.D., Rawlings, J., and Allison, S.P. (1983). Benefits of supplementary tube feeding after fractured neck of femur. *Br. Med. J.* 287: 1589–1592.

23. Jowsey, J. (1976). Osteoporosis, its nature and the role of diet. *Postgrad. Med.* 60: 75–83.

24. Wyshak, G. and Frisch, R.E. (1994). Carbonated beverages, dietary calcium, the dietary calcium/phosphorus ratio, and bone fractures in girls and boys. *J. Adolescent Health* 15: 210–215.
25. Alaimo, K., McDowell, M.A., Briefel, R.R., Bischof, A.M., Caughman, C.R., Loria, C.M., and Johnson, C.L. (1994). Dietary Intake of Vitamins, Minerals, and Fiber of Persons 2 Months and Over in the United States: Third National Health and Nutrition Examination Survey, Phase 1, 1988–91, Advance Data from Vital and Health Statistics, No. 258. National Center for Health Statistics, Hyattsville, MD.
26. Heaney, R.P. and Nordin, B.E.C. (2002). Calcium effects on phosphorus absorption: implications for the prevention and co-therapy of osteoporosis. *J. Am. Coll. Nutr.* 21(3): 239–244.
27. Schiller, L.R., Santa Ana, C.A., Sheikh, M.S., Emmett, M., and Fordtran, J.S. (1989). Effect of the time of administration of calcium acetate on phosphorus binding. *N. Engl. J. Med.* 320: 1110–1113.
28. Chapuy, M.C., Arlot, M.E., Duboeuf, F., Brun, J., Crouzet, B., Arnaud, S., Delmas, P.D., and Meunier, P.J. (1992). Vitamin D$_3$ and calcium to prevent hip fractures in elderly women. *N. Engl. J. Med.* 327: 1637–1642.
29. Spencer, H., Menczel, J., Lewin, I., and Samachson, J. (1965). Effect of high phosphorus intake on calcium and phosphorus metabolism in man. *J. Nutr.* 86(2): 125–132.
30. Calvo, M.S. and Park, Y.K. (1996). Changing phosphorus content of the U.S. diet: potential for adverse effects on bone. *J. Nutr.* 126: 1168S–1180S.

PART III

Vitamins, Flavonoids

CHAPTER 7

Vitamin K and Bone Health

CEES VERMEER

Department of Biochemistry, University of Maastricht, The Netherlands

ABSTRACT

Vitamin K is required for the synthesis of two proteins involved in calcium and bone metabolism: osteocalcin (OC), which is synthesized exclusively by osteoblasts, and matrix Gla protein (MGP), which is a product of chondrocytes in cartilage and of smooth muscle cells in the vasculature. In experimental animals, vitamin K-antagonists induce bone malformations and excessive calcification of cartilage and arteries. Population-based evidence suggests that in humans low vitamin K status is associated with low bone mass, increased hip fracture risk, and increased cardiovascular mortality. Recently, the results of the first vitamin K intervention trials have been completed, and they demonstrate a synergy of vitamins K, D, and minerals in decreasing the rate of postmenopausal bone loss. Moreover, vitamin K completely abolished the age-related loss of vascular elasticity during the 3-year intervention period. The desirability and safety of large-scale vitamin K supplementation is discussed.

Nutritional Aspects of Osteoporosis, Second Edition

INTRODUCTION

Compounds with vitamin K activity share a common methylated naphtho-quinone group but may vary with respect to the structure of an aliphatic side chain attached to the 3-position of the aromatic ring system. Natural K vitamins can be classified into vitamin K_1 (phylloquinone) and vitamin K_2 (menaquinones). Whereas the side chain is invariably phytyl in K_1, vitamin K_2 can be further subclassified, depending on the length of its side-chain; the various forms are denominated as MK-n, where n stands for the number of isoprenyl residues in its side chain. The most relevant K_2 compounds in the diet are MK-4, MK-7, MK-8, and MK-9. In the human diet, vitamin K_1 is found in green leafy vegetables and some margarines and vegetable oils [1,2], while K_2 is found in meat and animal livers, in milk products such as curd and cheese, in eggs, and in the Japanese food natto [3]. Evidence suggests that K_1 can be endogenously converted to MK-4 [4].

Vitamin K functions as a cofactor in the post-translational carboxylation of a limited number of well-defined glutamate (Glu) residues into gamma-carboxy glutamate (Gla). Gla is an unusual amino acid that serves as a calcium-binding group in a number of proteins; such proteins are generally designated as Gla proteins [5,6]. Whereas at one time Gla proteins were thought to participate exclusively in blood coagulation, new members of the Gla protein family — with completely different functions — have been discovered during recent years.

The development of sensitive analytical techniques to identify Gla and Gla proteins has facilitated the identification of vitamin-K-dependent proteins. Such proteins may be detected among many others by the presence of their Gla residues. In that way, proteins such as osteocalcin and matrix Gla protein (MGP) were discovered in ethylene diamine tetraacetic acid (EDTA) extracts of bone [7,8]. On the other hand, the number of Gla-residues per mature protein molecule is fixed for each protein with, for instance 10 residues for the blood coagulation factor prothrombin, 3 residues for osteocalcin, and 5 residues for MGP. Therefore, vitamin K insufficiency may be readily detected by establishing the degree of under-carboxylation in Gla proteins. The most practical technique is to determine the ratio between the fractions of non-carboxylated and carboxylated Gla protein using conformation-specific antibodies. Tissue-specific vitamin K insufficiency may be established by measuring tissue-specific Gla proteins (e.g., prothrom-bin for liver and osteocalcin for bone vitamin K status). Osteocalcin has turned out to be the most sensitive marker for low vitamin K intake known at this time, and the ratio between non-carboxylated and carboxylated osteocalcin is therefore the most reliable marker for vitamin K adequacy [9].

Whereas the functions of various Gla proteins may vary widely, a common aspect is that in the non-carboxylated form their function is lost. Intermediately carboxylated Gla proteins may exhibit partial biological activity, but in general their activity is low. Severe vitamin K insufficiency leading to a defective coagulation system and risk of spontaneous bleeding is found among newborn babies and breast-fed infants and may also occur in adults with impaired bile secretion and fat malabsorption [6]. In healthy adults, however, vitamin K insufficiency to a degree affecting the hemostatic system is unknown.

Oral anticoagulants are antagonists of vitamin K that are widely used for the treatment and prophylaxis of thromboembolic disease. The clinical effectiveness of these drugs derives from their ability to block post-translational gamma-carboxylation of the four vitamin-K-dependent procoagulants (factors II, VII, IX, and X). The treatment thus results in the production of dysfunctional, under-carboxylated species of coagulation factors [10]. Oral anticoagulant treatment also affects the synthesis and functional activity of a number of other Gla proteins, including the anticoagulant protein C [11] and non-coagulation proteins such as osteocalcin in bone [10] and MGP in cartilage and the arterial vessel walls [12,13].

SITES OF VITAMIN K ACTION

The enzyme involved in Gla formation is the vitamin-K-dependent gamma-glutamyl carboxylase, an enzyme that has been found in a wide variety of tissues and cell types [5]. Despite at least two decades of research, the number of identified Gla proteins produced by these cells has remained surprisingly low. Hepatocytes produce a number of blood coagulation factors, most of which are unique for this cell type. The Gla content of prothrombin, the most abundant of these clotting proteins, is generally used as a marker for vitamin K status of the liver.

Osteocalcin is a Gla protein uniquely synthesized in osteoblasts (and to a very small part by odontoblasts). Part of the newly synthesized osteocalcin is not bound to bone but is set free in the circulation, where it may be quantified as osteocalcin total antigen (a bone formation marker). Fractions of carboxylated and under-carboxylated osteocalcin (cOC and ucOC, respectively) may be determined by sandwich enzyme-linked immunosorbent assay (ELISA) techniques using conformation-specific antibodies as the second antibodies [14]. Osteocalcin-deficient mice have shown that the protein is a negative regulator of bone growth and plays a role in the orderly deposition of the hydroxyapatite matrix in bone [15].

Matrix Gla protein is a 10-kDa protein containing 5 Gla residues, and it is synthesized in low amounts in many different cells [16]. In high quantities, it is produced by chondrocytes and vascular smooth muscle cells, where it acts of a strong inhibitor of cartilage and arterial calcification. Transgenic MGP-deficient mice exhibited a massive calcification of all large arteries, which started soon after birth and resulted in death by spontaneous rupture of the thoracic or abdominal aorta before the eighth week of life [17]. Gla residues are absolutely required for the calcification-inhibitory activity of MGP, which was demonstrated by treating rats with the vitamin K antagonist warfarin in such a way that only the extra-hepatic Gla formation was blocked. This resulted in arterial calcification within 4 weeks of treatment and in complete calcification of the epiphyses and other cartilages within several months [13].

Protein S is a coagulation inhibitor serving as a cofactor for protein C. It is synthesized in both the liver and in endothelium, the latter being responsible for about 40% of the circulating protein S. Obviously, the high surface-to-volume ratio will lead to relatively high local protein S concentrations in the capillary bed. The reason for this is currently unclear, but it may be a mechanism to prevent the formation of micro-thrombi during the low blood flow conditions in the capillary system. Several other mammalian Gla proteins have been described, including the growth arrest sequence protein 6 (Gas6) and two proline-rich Gla proteins. The function of these proteins *in vivo* is not known, however.

SIMILARITIES BETWEEN CALCIUM METABOLISM IN BONE AND ARTERIES

MOLECULAR MECHANISMS

Recent studies have shown that on a molecular basis the calcified vascular matrix shares many similarities with bone and cartilage [18–20]. The smooth muscle cells in the normal, healthy artery have a contractile phenotype and constitutively express proteins inhibiting mineralization; these proteins are also produced in cartilage (MGP) and bone (osteopontin, osteonectin). Vascular calcification is associated with differentiation of vascular smooth muscle cells into osteoblast-like cells, thus producing other bone-associated proteins including bone morphogenetic proteins, bone sialoprotein, osteo-calcin, and the bone-specific alkaline phosphatase. Moreover, calcium is deposited in the vessel wall as hydroxyapatite, the major calcium constituent of bone. Finally, typical lamellar bone-like tissue is common in calcified coronary arteries. Most of the various proteins mentioned above are expressed constitutively, and their activity cannot easily be regulated by simple interventions. The two exceptions are osteocalcin and MGP, the biological activity of which depends on a subject's vitamin K status.

INFLAMMATORY DISEASES

Rheumatoid arthritis (RA) is a systemic immune and inflammatory disease associated with increased morbidity and mortality. The median life expectancy of patients with RA is 17 years less than that of the general population, and most of the excess mortality is attributable to cardiovascular disease [21]. Atherosclerosis is a disease characterized by inflammation of the arterial intima, macrophage invasion, foam cell formation, smooth muscle cell differentiation, and deposition of calcium salts in the vasculature. The presence of RA is generally recognized as a major risk factor for atherosclerosis, which shares many similarities with synovial inflammation in RA, including activation of inflammatory cells and increased expression of cytokines, tumour necrosis factor-α, interleukin-1, adhesion molecules, growth factors, and matrix metalloproteases [22]. Whereas population-based studies have demonstrated a close association between atherosclerosis and RA, a causal relation has not been demonstrated. Alternatively, the presence of common risk factors may induce both diseases according to similar principles and mechanisms. Recent data have demonstrated that vitamin K insufficiency characterized by high circulating ucOC concentrations is a common factor in both diseases.

NON-INFLAMMATORY CALCIFICATIONS

Besides in relation to atherosclerosis, vascular calcification may also result from a disease generally known as Mönckeberg's media sclerosis. Whereas atherosclerosis results from an inflammatory injury of the intima, Mönckeberg's sclerosis is not associated with inflammation and originates around the elastin fibers and smooth muscle cells of the arterial media. It is especially common in diabetes mellitus and end-stage renal disease. Goodman et al. reported that more than 80% of young dialysis patients (ages 20 to 30 years) already developed severe and progressive coronary calcifications [23]. Remarkably, a vast number of population-based studies have demonstrated (1) a strong correlation between osteoporotic bone loss and arterial calcification [24], and (2) a similar correlation between arterial calcification and articular cartilage calcification such as in osteoarthritis [25].

POTENTIAL ROLE FOR GLA PROTEINS?

The tissues involved in the most common diseases associated with pathological calcium metabolism are bone, cartilage, and arterial vessel wall, and accumulating evidence suggests that the same principles and mechanisms seem to control the release or accumulation of calcium in all three tissues. It should be emphasized, however, that many details are currently incompletely understood — for instance, why apparently similar mechanisms result in opposite effects (*e.g.*, bone loss in osteoporosis goes together with increased calcification in vascular disease). Calcification-regulatory Gla proteins are synthesized in all three tissues mentioned (OC in osteoblasts, MGP in chondrocytes and vascular smooth muscle cells), and there is evidence for under-carboxylation of these proteins in the healthy population. As is detailed below, a growing body of evidence suggests that vitamin K insufficiency may be even more pronounced in osteoporosis, osteoarthritis, and arterial calcification.

VITAMIN K STATUS AND BONE HEALTH

Several papers have reported the relationship between vitamin K intake, bone mass, and hip fracture. In the Nurses' Health Study, over 72,000 women between 38 and 63 years of age were recruited and their dietary vitamin K intake was monitored by food frequency questionnaires [26]. On average, vitamin K intake over the 10-year study period was 192 µg/day, and 270 hip fractures were reported (fracture incidence = 38.4/100,000 person-years). The incidence of hip fracture in women in the higher quintiles for vitamin K intake was lower than that in the lowest quintile, with a relative risk of 0.70. After adjustment for hormone replacement therapy, the relative risk in the higher quintiles decreased further to 0.67. Much older women (average age of 75 years) were analyzed in the Framingham cohort [27]. Their average vitamin K intake was assessed to be 155 µg/day, and there was a significant reduction of hip fracture risk in the highest quartile for vitamin K intake relative to the lowest quartile (relative risk: 0.35). Further, a study in the Framingham Offspring cohort among younger women (average age of 59 years) demonstrated a positive correlation in women between K_1 intake and bone mineral density [28]. In other studies, hip fracture incidence was investigated in elderly institutionalized persons. The vitamin intake in this population is relatively low, and it was shown that in these subjects the hip fracture risk is much higher than in homedwellers, with low vitamin K intake as an independent risk factor [29,30]. Natto is a fermented soybean food notably appreciated in some parts of Japan, and it is extremely rich in vitamin K. In a Japanese study, postmenopausal women in areas with a traditionally high natto intake (northern Japan) were compared with women from areas where natto is not a common food (southern Japan), and it was found that natto consumption was associated with a markedly decreased hip fracture risk [31].

Whereas food frequency questionnaires provide evidence about food intake, no information is obtained about vitamin K sufficiency or insufficiency of bone tissue. Such information must be acquired from the carboxylation degree of the bone Gla protein osteocalcin. In a 3-year follow-up study, Szulc et al. demonstrated that the risk of hip fracture in elderly women is higher among those with elevated ucOC concentrations, with a relative risk ranging from 3.1 [32] to 5.9 [33] for women whose ucOC was above the premenopausal upper normal limit of 1.65 ng/mL. These data were confirmed by other studies among elderly women showing that women in whom the fraction of cOC relative to total osteocalcin was low were at risk of osteoporotic fractures [34,35], and that women with a high ucOC fraction were characterized by a low bone mineral density [36,37]. Whereas all these population-based studies provide accumulating evidence for high vitamin K intake as an independent factor decreasing the risk of post-menopausal osteoporosis and hip fracture, final proof for the importance of vitamin K in bone health must come from well-designed clinical intervention trials.

VITAMIN K STATUS AND CARDIOVASCULAR HEALTH

In a population-based study among 356 women ages 55 to 75 years of age (the EPOZ cohort), Jie et al. observed an inverse correlation between vitamin K_1 intake and aortic calcification as determined by x-ray analysis of the abdominal aorta [38]. In a subsequent analysis of the much larger Rotterdam study cohort (4500 men and women ages 55 years and over), a similar but much stronger correlation was found between vitamin K_2 intake and both myocardial infarction and cardiovascular mortality, with a 50% decreased infarction risk for the highest tertile of K_2 intake [39]. Consistently, the same study demonstrated a 25% decrease in all-cause mortality in the group with the highest vitamin K_2 intake. The data from the Rotterdam study suggest the major importance of vitamin K_2 for vascular health, which is remarkable as only 20% of the human dietary vitamin K intake is K_2. Plausible explanations for these observations are the better absorption of K_2 vitamins and the different plasma transport mechanisms for vitamins K_1 and K_2 resulting in targeted delivery to either the liver or extrahepatic tissues [40].

VITAMIN K INTERVENTION STUDIES

Extremely high doses (45 to 90 mg/day) of vitamin K_2 (invariably MK-4) have been used for the treatment of postmenopausal osteoporosis in Japan for several years [41–43]. After the positive outcomes of the first clinical trials, the treatment is now used on a large scale; thus far, no adverse side effects have been reported. The treatment has also been reported to be successful in other groups at risk for bone loss such as hemodialysis patients and those treated with corticosteroids. It remains to be seen whether similar beneficial effects of high MK-4 intake will be observed outside Japan for populations whose predisposition to osteoporosis differ with respect to hereditary as well as lifestyle factors such as calcium intakes. Because of the high doses applied, the use of vitamin K in these studies must be regarded as pharmacological rather than nutritional and falls outside the scope of this paper.

Nutritional doses of vitamin K will be defined in this paper as doses that may be obtained by eating a selected number of foods within the range of foods common in the western diet. Vitamin-K-rich vegetables such as kale or spinach contain 4 to 7 µg of vitamin K per gram. A 250-g portion of these foods may be large for the majority of the population, but it is not exceptional; therefore, we will use a value of 1 mg per day as an upper limit for what may be regarded as a nutritional supplement. This dose is about 8 times the current dietary reference intake for vitamin K. Thus far, two intervention trials with doses up to 1 mg of vitamin K have been completed, and in both cases K_1 was used.

The Dundee Bones and Vitamins Intervention Study (D-BAVIS) was a 2-year intervention study among 244 women ages 60 to 87 years [44]. Participants were stratified by age and randomly assigned to one of four supplement groups: (1) placebo, (2) vitamin K_1 (200 µg/day), (3) vitamin D_3 (10 µg/day + calcium 1 g/day), and (4) vitamin D_3 (10 µg/day + calcium 1 g/day + vitamin K_1 200 µg/day). The primary endpoint was bone densitometry by dual-energy x-ray absorptiometry (DEXA). Unfortunately, potential effects of treatment on hip BMD were obscured by the fact that at this site the loss of bone mass in the placebo group was much lower than expected. Therefore, the authors focused on changes in the ultra-distal radius. It was concluded that at this site combined supplementation with vitamins K_1 and D_3 at dietary relevant intakes significantly improved bone mineral density at the highest trabecular bone site measured and that equivalent supplementation in high osteoporotic risk groups may be beneficial.

In the Maastricht Osteostudy, 188 postmenopausal women ages 50 to 60 years were recruited and treated for 3 years with daily supplements [45]. The first group received placebo (maltodextrine), the second one received minerals (500 mg/day calcium, 150 mg/day magnesium, and 10 mg/day zinc) and 8 μg/day vitamin D_3, and the third group received minerals plus vitamin D_3 and an additional 1 mg/day of vitamin K_1. The primary endpoint was bone densitometry of the femoral neck by DEXA. During the 3-year treatment, a regular decrease of bone mineral density (BMD) was observed in the placebo group, and only a transient decrease of bone loss in the minerals + vitamin D group. Optimal osteoprotective effects were obtained if vitamin K was used in combination with minerals and vitamin D. Although no complete prevention was achieved, the rate of bone loss had decreased by 35 to 40% as compared to the placebo and minerals plus vitamin D groups. It may be calculated that if the observed effects continue over decades, lifelong supplementation could postpone fractures by up to 10 years. Vascular elasticity was taken as a secondary endpoint in the Maastricht Osteostudy, and it was found that in the placebo and minerals plus vitamin D group vascular stiffening had significantly progressed with a loss of elasticity by 10% during the 3-year study period [46]. No loss of elasticity was observed in the group also receiving vitamin K_1, where even a tendency to increased elasticity was reported. This study is the first clinical trial showing that vitamin K taken as a dietary supplement may help improve vascular health.

DIETARY VITAMIN K REQUIREMENTS FOR BONE AND VASCULAR HEALTH

There is no conclusive evidence that at nutritionally relevant doses the physiological functions of vitamins K_1 and K_2 are different: both are capable of functioning as a cofactor for the gamma-glutamyl carboxylase, and differences may only be expected with respect to pharmacokinetics and tissue distribution. This may be the reason why some menaquinones seem to have a greater effect in preventing arterial calcification than K_1. In the Western diet, K_1 from green vegetables forms around 80% of the total vitamin K intake, but because of low bioavailability the contribution of K_1 to total vitamin K status is commonly overestimated [3,47]. At this time dietary reference intake (DRI) values for vitamin K have only been set in the United States and the United Kingdom, and were recently increased from 1 to 1.5 μg/kg body weight per day. These recommendations are based on the function of vitamin K in blood coagulation rather than that in bone and vascular metabolism and may be too low to support full carboxylation of all extrahepatic Gla proteins. From the available dietary data, it would appear that daily intakes of between 200 and 500 μg/day of dietary vitamin K may be required for optimal gamma-carboxylation of OC, which may in turn benefit bone health. These amounts are not met by the majority of the healthy population without taking supplements. Bioavailability studies have demonstrated that vitamin K from supplements may be absorbed up to 5 times better than that from vegetables such as spinach or broccoli. Hence, comparable benefits might be obtained from supplements containing dosages of around 100 μg/day. The mean vitamin K intake $(K_1 + K_2)$ in the upper quartile for intake in the Rotterdam Study population was around 400 μg/day which is comparable with the vitamin K content of 100 g of spinach, but which is 3 to 4 times higher than current guidelines. In 2002, a number of experts in the fields of vitamin K and calcium and bone metabolism formulated a consensus standpoint concerning the optimal vitamin K intake, and it was concluded that higher dietary intakes than those generally consumed would probably be beneficial, and that *supplemental* levels of around 100 μg/day may improve vitamin K status in the majority of the population. European legislation defines the maximum supplementary dose of vitamin K_1 that can be administered via over-the-counter (OTC) supplements, and in most countries the addition of 100 μg/day is already allowed. We would propose that such legislation should be extended to the common menaquinones found in the human diet (*i.e.*, MK-4, MK-7, MK-8, and MK-9).

SAFETY AND POTENTIAL ADVERSE SIDE EFFECTS OF VITAMIN K SUPPLEMENTS

Vitamin K has a very wide safety range, which was acknowledged by the U.S. Institute of Medicine, which stated: "A search of the literature revealed no evidence of toxicity associated with the intake of either the phylloquinone (vitamin K_1) or menaquinone (vitamin K_2) form of vitamin K" [49]. Even in the large Japanese trial where doses of 45 mg/day and 90 mg/day have been administered for several years, no adverse side effects have been reported. A common misunderstanding is that high doses of vitamin K would increase the risk of thrombosis. Except for subjects under oral anticoagulant treatment, this is not true; the only potential risk of vitamin-K-containing foods or food supplements is their interference with oral anticoagulant therapy. This therapy is based on the use of coumarin derivatives (such as warfarin and acenocoumarol), which act as vitamin K antagonists. Coumarins are frequently used during episodes of increased thrombosis risk — for instance, after surgery, myocardial infarction, and pulmonary embolism. High intakes of vitamin K (notably as supplements) may interfere with this form of treatment. In a recent study among 12 anticoagulated volunteers, it was demonstrated that supplements up to 150 μg/day did not significantly affect the level of anticoagulation [50]. It was concluded from this study that vitamin K supplements in doses of 100 μg/day or lower are safe and may be distributed for use in adults independent of other medications.

REFERENCES

1. Bolton-Smith, C., Price, R.J.G., Fenton, S.T., Harrington, D.J., and Shearer, M.J. (2000). Compilation of a provisional UK database for the phylloquinone (vitamin K_1) content of foods. *Br. J. Nutr.* 83: 389–399.
2. Booth, S.L., Sadowski, J.A., Weihrauch, J.L., and Ferland, G. (1993). Vitamin K_1 (phylloquinone) content of foods: a provisional table. *J. Food Comp. Anal.* 6: 109–120.
3. Schurgers, L.J. and Vermeer, C. (2000). Determination of phylloquinone and menaquinones in food: effect of food matrix on circulating vitamin K concentrations. *Haemostasis* 30: 298–307.
4. Ronden, J.E., Drittij-Reijnders, M.J., Vermeer, C., and Thijssen, H.H.W. (1998). Intestinal flora is not an intermediate in the phylloquinone-menaquinone-4 conversion in the rat. *Biochim. Biophys. Acta* 1379: 69–75.
5. Vermeer, C. (1990). Gamma-carboxyglutamate-containing proteins and the vitamin K-dependent carboxylase. *Biochem. J.* 266: 625–636.
6. Shearer, M.J. (1995). Vitamin K. *Lancet* 345: 229–234.
7. Hauschka, P.V. and Reid, M.L. (1978). Vitamin K dependence of a calcium-binding protein containing gammacarboxyglutamic acid in chicken bone. *J. Biol. Chem.* 253: 9063–9068.
8. Price, P.A. and Williamson, M.K. (1985) Primary structure of bovine matrix Gla protein, a new vitamin K-dependent bone protein. *J. Biol. Chem.* 260: 14971–14975.
9. Vermeer, C., Jie, K.-S.G., and Knapen, M.H.J. (1995). Role of vitamin K in bone metabolism. *Annu. Rev. Nutr.* 15: 1–22.
10. Vermeer, C. and Hamulyák, K. (1991). Pathophysiology of vitamin K deficiency and oral anticoagulants. *Thromb. Haemostas.* 66: 153–159.
11. Simmelink, M.J., de Groot, P.G., Derksen, R.H., Fernandez, J.A., and Griffin, J.H. (2002). Oral anticoagulation reduces activated protein C less than protein C and other vitamin K-dependent clotting factors. *Blood* 100: 4232–4233.
12. Price, P.A., Williamson, M.K., Haba, T., Dell, R.B., and Jee, W.S. (1982) Excessive mineralization with growth plate closure in rats on chronic warfarin treatment. *Proc. Natl. Acad. Sci. USA* 79: 7734–7738.
13. Price, P.A., Faus, S.A., and Williamson, M.K. (1998). Warfarin causes rapid calcification of the elastic lamellae in rat arteries and heart valves. *Arterioscler. Thromb. Vasc. Biol.* 18: 1400–1407.
14. Koyama, N., Ohara, K., Yokata, H., Kurome, T., Katayama, M., Hino, F., Kato, I., and Akai, T. (1991). A one step sandwich enzyme immunoassay for gamma-carboxylated osteocalcin using monoclonal antibodies. *J. Immunol. Meth.* 139: 17–23.

15. Ducy, P., Desbois, C., Boyce, B., Pinero, G., Story, B., Dunstan, C., Smith, E., Bonadio, J., Goldstein, S., Gundberg, C., Bradley, A., and Karsenty, G. (1996). Increased bone formation in osteocalcin-deficient mice. *Nature* 382: 448–452.

16. Fraser, J.D. and Price, P.A. (1988). Lung, heart, and kidney express high levels of mRNA for the vitamin K-dependent matrix Gla-protein. Implications for the possible functions of matrix Gla-protein and for the possible distribution of the gamma carboxylase. *J. Biol. Chem.* 263: 11033–11036.

17. Luo, G., Ducy, P., McKee, M.D., Pinero, G.J., Loyer, E., Behringer, R.R., and Karsenty, G. (1997). Spontaneous calcification of arteries and cartilage in mice lacking matrix GLA protein. *Nature* 386: 78–81.

18. Shanahan, C.M., Cary, N.R.B., Salisbury, J.R., Proudfoot, D., Weissberg, P.L., and Edmonds, M.E. (1999). Medial localization of mineralization-regulating proteins in association with Mönckeberg's sclerosis. *Circulation* 100: 2168–2176.

19. Dhore, C.R., Cleutjens, J.P.M., Lutgens, E., Cleutjens, K.B.J.M., Geussens, P., Kitslaar, P.J.E.H.M., Tordoir, J.H.M., Spronk, H.M.H., Vermeer, C., and Daemen, M.J.A.P. (2001). Differential expression of bone matrix regulatory proteins in human atherosclerotic plaques. *Arterioscl. Thromb. Vasc. Biol.* 21: 1998–2003.

20. Fitzpatrick, L.A., Turner, R.T., and Ritman, E.R. (2003). Endochondral bone formation in the heart: a possible mechanism of coronary calcification. *Endocrinology* 144: 2214–2219.

21. Wong, M., Toh, L., Wilson, A., Rowley, K., Karschimkus, C., Prior, D., Romas, E., Clemens, L., Dragicevic, G., Harianto, H., Wicks, I., McColl, G., Best, J., and Jenkins, A. (2003). Reduced arterial elasticity in rheumatoid arthritis and the relationship to vascular disease risk factors and inflammation. *Arthrit. Rheum.* 48: 81–89.

22. Kaplan, M.J. and McCune, W.J. (2003). New evidence for vascular disease in patients with early rheumatoid arthritis. *Lancet* 361: 1068–1069.

23. Goodman, W.G., Goldin, J., Kuizon, B.D., Yoon, C., Gales, B., Sider, D., Wang, J., Chung, J., Emerick, A., Greaser, L., Elashoff, R.M., and Salusky, I.B. (2000). Coronary-artery calcification in young adults with end-stage renal disease who are undergoing dialysis. *N. Engl. J. Med.* 342: 1478–1483.

24. Kiel, D.P., Kauppila, L.I., Cupples, L.A., Hannan, M.T., O'Donnell, C.J., and Wilson, P.W. (2001). Bone loss and the progression of abdominal aortic calcification over a 25 year period: the Framingham Heart Study. *Calcif. Tissue Int.* 68: 271–276.

25. Rutsch, F. and Terkeltaub, R. (2003). Parallels between arterial and cartilage calcification: what understanding artery calcification can teach us about chondrocalcinosis. *Curr. Opin. Rheumatol.* 15: 302–310.

26. Feskanich, D., Weber, P., Willett, W.C., Rockett, H., Booth, S., and Colditz, G.A. (1999). Vitamin K intake and hip fractures in women: a prospective study. *Am. J. Clin. Nutr.* 69: 74–79.

27. Booth, S.L., Tucker, K.L., Chen, H., Hannan, M.T., Gagnon, D.R., Cupples, L.A., Wilson, P.W.F., Ordovas, J., Schaefer, E.J., Dawson-Hughes, B., and Kiel, D.P. (2000). Dietary vitamin K intakes are associated with hip fracture but not with bone mineral density in elderly men and women. *Am. J. Clin. Nutr.* 71: 1201–1208.

28. Booth, S.L., Broe, K.E., Gagnon, D.R., Tucker, K.L., Hannan, M.T., McLean, R.R., Dawson-Hughes, B., Wilson, P.W.F., Cupples, A., and Kiel, D.P. (2003). Vitamin K intakes and bone mineral density in women and men. *Am. J. Clin. Nutr.* 77: 512–516.

29. Tse, S.L.S., Chan, T.Y.K., Wu, D.M.Y., Cheung, A.Y.K., and Kwok, T.C.Y. (2002). Deficient dietary vitamin K intake among elderly nursing home residents in Hong Kong. *Asia Pac. J. Clin. Nutr.* 11: 62–65.

30. Simonen, O. and Mikkola, T. (1991). Senile osteoporosis and femoral neck fractures in long-stay institutions. *Calcif. Tissue Int.* 49: S78–S79.

31. Kaneki, M., Hedges, S.J., Hosoi, T., Fujiwara, S., Lyons, A., Crean, S.J., Ishida, N., Nakagawa, M., Takechi, M., Sano, Y., Mizuno, Y., Hoshino, S., Miyao, M., Inoue, S., Horiki, K., Shiraki, M., Ouchi, Y., and Orimo, H. (2001). Japanese fermented soybean food as the major determinant of the large geographic difference in circulating levels of vitamin K2: possible implications for hip-fracture risk. *Nutrition* 17: 315–321.
32. Szulc, P., Chapuy, M.-C., Meunier, P.J., and Delmas, P.D. (1996). Serum undercarboxylated osteocalcin is a marker of the risk of hip fracture: a three year follow-up study. *Bone* 18: 487–488.
33. Szulc, P., Chapuy, M.-C., Meunier, P.J., and Delmas, P.D. (1993). Serum undercarboxylated osteocalcin is a marker of the risk of hip fracture in elderly women. *J. Clin. Invest.* 91: 1769–1774.
34. Vergnaud, P., Garnero, P., Meunier, P.J., Breart, G., Kamihagi, K., and Delmas, P.D. (1997). Undercarboxylated osteocalcin measured with a specific immunoassay predicts hip fracture in elderly women: the EPIDOS Study. *J. Clin. Endocrinol. Metab.* 82: 719–724.
35. Luukinen, H., Käkönen, S.-M., Petterson, K., Koski, K., Laippala, P., Lövgren, T., Kivelä, S.-L., and Väänänen, H.K. (2000). Strong prediction of fractures among older adults by the ratio of carboxylated to total serum osteocalcin. *J. Bone Miner. Res.* 15: 2473–2478.
36. Szulc, P., Arlot, M., Chapuy, M.-C., Duboeuf, F., Meunier, P.J., and Delmas, P.D. (1994). Serum undercarboxylated osteocalcin correlates with hip bone mineral density in elderly women. *J. Bone Miner. Res.* 9: 1591–1595.
37. Knapen, M.H.J., Nieuwenhuijzen Kruseman, A.C., Wouters, R.S.M.E., and Vermeer, C. (1998). Correlation of serum osteocalcin fractions with bone mineral density in women during the first 10 years after menopause. *Calcif. Tissue Int.* 63: 375–379.
38. Jie, K.-S.G., Bots, M.L., Vermeer, C., Witteman, J.C.M., and Grobbee, D.E. (1995). Vitamin K intake and osteocalcin levels in women with and without aortic atherosclerosis: a population-based study. *Atherosclerosis* 116: 117–123.
39. Geleijnse, J.M., Vermeer, C., Schurgers, L.J., Grobbee, D.E., Pols, H.A.P., and Witteman, J.C.M. (2001). Inverse association of dietary vitamin K-2 intake with cardiac events and aortic atherosclerosis: the Rotterdam Study. *Thromb. Haemostas* (suppl., July): P473.
40. Schurgers, L.J. and Vermeer, C. (2002). Differential lipoprotein transport pathways of K-vitamins in healthy subjects. *Biochim. Biophys. Acta* 1570: 27–32.
41. Orimo, H., Shiraki, M., Tomita, A., Morii, H., Fujita, T., and Ohata, M. (1998). Effects of menatetrenone on the bone and calcium metabolism in osteoporosis: a double-blind placebo-controlled study. *J. Bone Mineral Metab.* 16: 106–112.
42. Shiraki, M., Shiraki, Y., Aoki, C., and Miura, M. (2000). Vitamin K_2 (menatetrenone) effectively prevents fractures and sustains lumbar bone mineral density in osteoporosis. *J. Bone Mineral Res.* 15: 515–521.
43. Iwamoto, J., Takeda, T., and Ichimura, S. (2001). Effect of menatetrenone on bone mineral density and incidents of vertebral fractures in postmenopausal women with osteoporosis: a comparison with the effect of etidronate. *J. Orthop. Sci.* 6: 487–492.
44. Bolton-Smith, C., Mole, P.A., McMurdo, M.E.T., Paterson, C.R., and Shearer, M.J. (2001). Two-year intervention study with phylloquinone (vitamin K_1), vitamin D and calcium: effect on bone mineral content. *Ann. Nutr. Metab.* 45(suppl. 1): 246.
45. Braam, L.A.J.L.M., Knapen, M.H.J., Geusens, P., Brouns, F., Hamulyák, K., Gerichhausen, M.J.W., and Vermeer, C. (2003). Vitamin K1 supplementation retards bone loss in postmenopausal women between 50 and 60 years of age. *Calcif. Tissue Int.* 73: 21–26.
46. Braam, L.A.J.L.M. (2002). Effects of High Vitamin K Intake on Bone and Vascular Health. Ph.D. thesis, Maastricht University, The Netherlands (ISBN 90-5681-145-2).
47. Gijsbers, B.L.M.G., Jie, K.-S.G., and Vermeer, C. (1996). Effect of food composition on vitamin K absorption in human volunteers. *Br. J. Nutr.* 76: 223–229.

48. Schurgers, L.J., Geleijnse, J.M., Grobbee, D.E., Pols, H.A.P., Hofman, A., Witteman, J.C.M., and Vermeer, C. (1999). Nutritional intake of vitamins K-1 (phylloquinone) and K-2 (menaquinone) in The Netherlands. *J. Nutr. Environm. Med.* 9: 115–122.
49. Food and Nutrition Board, Institute of Medicine. (2001). Vitamin K, in *Dietary Reference Intakes for Vitamin A, Vitamin K, Arsenic, Boron, Chromium, Copper, Iodine, Iron, Manganese, Molybdenum, Nickel, Silicon, Vanadium, and Zinc,* National Academy Press, Washington, D.C., pp. 5/1–5/27.
50. Schurgers, L.J. (2002). Studies on the role of Vitamin K1 and K2 in Bone Metabolism and Cardiovascular Disease: Structural Differences Determine Different Metabolic Pathways, Ph.D. thesis, Maastricht University, The Netherlands (ISBN 90-5681-138-X).

CHAPTER 8

Dietary Vitamin A is Negatively Related to Bone Mineral Density in Postmenopausal Women

Jasminka Z. Ilich,[1] Rhonda A. Brownbill,[1] Harold C. Furr,[2] and Neal E. Craft[2]

[1]School of Allied Health, University of Connecticut, Storrs, Connecticut; [2]Craft Technologies, Inc., Wilson, North Carolina

ABSTRACT

Limited evidence suggests that higher vitamin A intake is associated with lower bone mineral density (BMD) and higher risk of hip fractures. The purpose of this study was to evaluate the relationship between serum and dietary vitamin A and BMD of various skeletal sites in over 100 generally healthy postmenopausal women not taking medications known to affect bone. The subjects were part of a larger study investigating effects of sodium on BMD and were followed for 18 months. Bone mass and dietary vitamin A, including supplements, were assessed at 6-month intervals, while serum retinoic acid (RA) and retinol concentrations were analyzed only at baseline. Over 50% of subjects were taking vitamin A supplements, bringing the total average intake to >11,000 IU, or ~2200 µg/day, throughout the study. Serum RA and retinol concentrations were 4.9 ± 1.1 ng/mL and 0.75 ± 0.15 µg/mL, respectively. There was a positive significant correlation between vitamin A intake and serum retinol, but not with total RA, and the latter had no association with BMD. Multiple regression models (controlled

Nutritional Aspects of Osteoporosis, Second Edition

for age, body mass index, calcium, sodium, and energy intake) were utilized at each time point and showed negative relationships between dietary vitamin A and BMD of various skeletal sites. Repeated-measures analysis of covariance (ANCOVA; adjusted for the same confounders) compared groups divided below and above the median of total cumulative vitamin A intake over time and revealed significant negative association between vitamin A intake and BMD of total femur, shaft, proximal forearm, and total body. We conclude that higher intakes of vitamin A (>11,000 IU/day) might be detrimental for bone; therefore, vitamin A supplements should be carefully chosen by older women. Serum RA and retinol are homeostatically regulated and therefore may not be sensitive enough indicators of subclinical hypervitaminosis. More research is needed to elucidate their relationship with dietary vitamin A.

INTRODUCTION

Although calcium (Ca) and protein have been studied most extensively in relation to bone health and osteoporosis, other minerals and vitamins are crucial in carrying out reactions and metabolic processes in bone [1]. The interest in vitamin A in relation to bone health commenced relatively recently along with other antioxidant vitamins that may protect the skeleton from the toxicity of smoking. However, the retinoic acid nuclear receptors were found in both osteoblasts (bone forming cells) and osteoclasts (bone resorbing cells) [2,3], implying a role in bone remodeling, rather than just that of antioxidative nature. Accordingly, hypervitaminosis A may cause excessive binding of retinoic acid receptors to their response elements in osteoblasts, resulting in increased production of cytokines, which act as messengers to recruit osteoclast precursors from bone marrow. This eventually leads to an imbalance in bone turnover and higher resorption rates [4]. Other evidence in animals and humans suggests that vitamin A, through a separate mechanism, antagonizes the action of vitamin D and consequently may interfere with intestinal Ca absorption and its normal serum level [5,6].

Recent epidemiological findings point toward adverse association of even subclinical hypervitaminosis A and bone fractures/density. The results from the prospective 18-year follow-up analysis from the Nurse's Health Study revealed that women in the highest quintile of vitamin A intake (>3000 µg/day) had a significantly higher relative risk (1.48; 95% CI, 1.05–2.07; P for trend 0.003) for hip fracture compared to the women in the lowest quintile (RR, 1.00) [7]. In a sample of Swedish women, Melhus et al. found that for every milligram increase in daily intake of retinol, the risk of hip fracture increased by 68% over a 64-month period [8]. In a prospective study including about 1000 elderly women and men, a negative association was found between dietary and supplemental retinol intake (total average 4156 IU) and BMD in several skeletal sites [9]. Subsequently, another epidemiological study in over 2000 middle-age men reported a positive relationship between serum retinol and fracture incidents documented during a 30-year follow-up [10]. It needs to be emphasized that vitamin A intake in those studies was not at the toxic level and was below the upper limits of safety.

Little information has been published on the relationship between dietary intake of vitamin A and tissue/serum levels of retinoids and even less so in the context of bone health. Ballew et al. examined data from the National Health and Examination Survey III (NHANES III) and found no significant associations between fasting retinyl ester concentrations and any measure of bone mineral status [11]. Although serum retinol is frequently used as a measure of vitamin A status, its levels are homeostatically controlled, except in instances of frank vitamin A deficiency, and it is judged by some to be of limited usefulness in assessing vitamin A status. Retinoic acid is involved in control of gene expression and as such it may be a more useful *functional* indicator of vitamin A status than is retinol [12]. Very limited evidence in humans [13,14] and animals (rats [15], calves, [16]) indicates that retinoic acid concentration in serum is responsive to vitamin A intake; therefore, determination of both retinol and retinoic acid might provide a more comprehensive measure for functional status of vitamin A.

The purpose of this study was to evaluate the relationship between vitamin A intake and bone mineral status in postmenopausal women within 18 months of follow-up. At the baseline assessment, serum retinol and retinoic acid concentrations were measured as potential biological markers of vitamin A status and evaluated with regard to dietary vitamin A, as well as to bone mineral density of several skeletal sites.

METHODS

DESIGN AND SUBJECTS

The study was conducted in over 100 Caucasian, generally healthy postmenopausal women, free of chronic diseases or medications known to affect bone, including hormone replacement therapy. The subjects' recruitment and characteristics have been described in detail previously [17]. They were participants of a larger longitudinal study evaluating the effects of dietary sodium (Na) on bone mass. As per the protocol of the larger study, after the baseline assessment, half of the participants were instructed to reduce sodium intake to about 1500 to 2000 mg/day, while the other half were not limited in Na intake, averaging at about 3000 to 4000 mg/day. After initial screening, both groups were supplemented with calcium and vitamin D (Citracal®; Mission Pharmacal, San Antonio, TX) at about 630 mg/day and 200 IU/day, respectively. At baseline assessment, the 136 women were ages 57.4 to 88.6 years. In the subsequent evaluations at 6, 12, and 18 months, both the whole population and the subjects from the control group ($n = \sim 68$) were considered separately for the purpose of this study. Because the results had similar trends, we report only data from the whole population (controlled for Na intake). The study protocol was approved by the Human Subjects Review Board at the University of Connecticut, and an informed consent was signed by each participant.

ANTHROPOMETRY AND BONE DENSITOMETRY

Weight (kg) and standing height (cm) were recorded in light, indoor clothing without shoes, and the body mass index (BMI, kg/m^2) was calculated. Bone mineral density (BMD) was measured by dual-energy x-ray absorptiometry (DEXA) with a Lunar DPX–MD instrument (GE Medical Systems, Madison, WI) using specialized software for different skeletal regions, as described earlier [18]. The measured skeletal sites were total body, lumbar spine, both femurs (neck, trochanter, Ward's triangle, shaft, and total femur), and forearm (ulna and radius at ultradistal and one-third distal region measured from the styloid process). Quality assurance of the densitometer was performed daily; the *in vitro* and *in vivo* stability, as well as the coefficients of variation, in our laboratory have been reported previously [18].

SERUM ANALYSIS

The serum samples from the baseline assessment were analyzed for retinol and retinoic acid concentrations. Retinol was determined following protein precipitation with ethanol/acetonitrile (50/50) containing butylated hydroxytoluene (BHT) as an antioxidant and retinyl acetate as an internal standard. The supernatant was analyzed directly by reversed-phase high-performance liquid chromatography (HPLC) with ultraviolet (UV) detection at 325 nm. The limit of detection was 25 ng/mL using a 50-μL serum sample. Retinoic acid was determined using a modification of the extraction procedure of De Leenheer and Nelis [19]. Serum samples (500 µL) were first extracted under alkaline conditions to remove potential interfering components, then RA was extracted under acidic conditions. The isomers were separated by reversed-phase HPLC and detected by UV at 350 nm. The limits of detection were 0.2 ng/mL (5:1 signal-to-noise ratio) and below typical human serum concentrations of 1.2 to 4.5 ng/mL [12]. Both analyses were performed by Craft Technologies, Inc. (Wilson, NC).

DIETARY ASSESSMENT

Dietary intake was assessed by a 3-day dietary record (2 week days and 1 weekend day) at baseline and 6, 12, and 18 months into the study. A registered dietitian instructed participants individually on how to complete the records and advised them to choose typical days for reporting, as described previously [17]. The diets were analyzed using Food Processor® (ESHA Research, Salem, OR). Mean daily intake, including total energy (kcal/day) and all other macro- and micronutrients, was calculated. The intake of supplements was carefully recorded, as well, and included in the nutrient analysis, as described previously [18]. Therefore, each nutrient was expressed as dietary, supplemental, and/or total (food plus supplement).

DATA ANALYSIS

All data are presented as mean ± standard deviation (SD), unless otherwise noted, and analysis was performed using SPSS, version 10.0, and Data Desk® (Data Description, Inc., Ithaca, NY). Vitamin A was evaluated both as continuous and categorical variable by stratifying subjects below and above the median of intake. Repeated-measures ANCOVA (adjusted for age, BMI, and energy and calcium intake, as well as for sodium intake for analyses at 6, 12, and 18 months) was used to compare the groups over time. Multiple regression models were utilized at each time point to assess relationships between vitamin A metabolites (either dietary or serum for baseline) and bone mineral density or content of various skeletal sites. Diagnostics and residual plots for these models were analyzed to examine for heteroskedascisity and/or non-normality. Each model was controlled for age, body size (as BMI), and energy and calcium intake. Sodium intake was added as a confounder in the 6-, 12-, and 18-month analyses, as half of the subjects, as per intervention protocol in the original study, were consuming reduced Na. Various vitamin A metabolites (one at a time) were entered into the basic model as the independent variable. The overall accepted level of significance was set at $P \leq 0.05$. However, because we measured several skeletal sites, our interpretation of the results from multiple regression models took into account those sites and how much each explanatory variable contributed to the variance of the model.

RESULTS

BASELINE EVALUATION

Table I presents anthropometric and BMD data of subjects at baseline. Baseline assessment included 136 subjects of whom 58.8% ($n = 80$) and 69.8% ($n = 95$) were taking vitamin A (from 1000 to 15,000 IU/day) and Ca (from 25 to 2500 mg/day) supplements, respectively (see Table II). Vitamin A intake from food (8930 ± 5799 IU/day) and total from food and supplements (11969 ± 6568 IU/day) was above the recommended level of ~ 3500 IU but still under the tolerable upper limits of ~ 15000 IU. In a simple linear correlation, dietary vitamin A, carotenoids, and β-carotene showed a negative relationship with BMD of various hip and forearm sites.

TABLE I Descriptive Characteristics for Anthropometrics and Bone Variables in Population at Baseline

Variable	Mean ± SD	Min. − Max.
Age (years)	68.6 ± 7.1	57.4–88.6
Years since menopause	18.5 ± 8.4	5–41
Weight (kg)	68.0 ± 11.3	44.8–104.9
Height (cm)	161.7 ± 6.8	143.9–179.0
Body mass index (kg/m^2)	26.0 ± 3.8	17.2–38.0
TBBMD (g/cm^2)	1.077 ± 0.095	0.770–1.302
TBBMC (g)	2291 ± 397.3	1281–3338
Lumbar spine BMD (g/cm^2)	1.075 ± 0.196	0.786–1.900
Hip BMD (g/cm^2)	0.857 ± 0.132	0.581–1.269
Forearm UD BMD (g/cm^2)	0.275 ± 0.048	0.159–0.389
Forearm 1/3 BMD (g/cm^2)	0.591 ± 0.079	0.372–0.789

Note: TBBMD is total body bone mineral density, TBBMC is total body bone mineral content, hip BMD is BMD of total hip, forearm UD BMD is the BMD of the ultra-distal region of the forearm, and forearm 1/3 BMD is the BMD of the one-third distal region of the forearm (radius and ulna) measured from the styloid process.

TABLE II   Average Daily Intake of Vitamin A, Calcium, Energy, and Protein from Food Only, Supplements, and Total plus Serum Values for Retinol and Retinoic Acid (RA) in Population at Baseline

Variables	Mean ± SD	Min. – Max.
Vitamin A (IU):		
Food	8930 ± 5799	1021–27,483
Supplements	5165 ± 2246	1000–15,000
Total	11969 ± 6568	1021–32,483
Vitamin A (RE)	1228 ± 606	226–3298
Retinol (RE)	292 ± 168	13–761
Carotenoids (RE)	693 ± 587	29–2575
β-Carotene (µg)	3639 ± 3218	90–13,763
Calcium (mg):		
Food	873 ± 365	284–2204
Supplements	723 ± 491	25–2500
Total	1378 ± 632	307–3351
Energy (Kcal)	1691 ± 382	798–2699
Protein (g)	71 ± 19	24–125
Retinol (µg/mL)	0.75 ± 0.15	0.37–1.33
3-*cis* retinoic acid (ng/mL)	2.28 ± 0.56	1.32–5.07
9-*cis* retinoic acid (ng/mL)	1.36 ± 0.35	0.61–2.77
trans retinoic acid (ng/mL)	1.27 ± 0.39	0.56–2.72
Total retinoic acid (ng/mL)	4.91 ± 1.05	3.02–9.44

Serum RA was 4.9 ± 1.1 ng/mL, slightly above normal, while serum retinol of 0.75 ± 0.15 µg/mL was in the upper normal range. There was a positive significant relationship between serum retinol and all metabolites of retinoic acid, the highest one with the 9-*cis* RA ($r = 0.260$, $P = 0.0042$). A weak positive correlation was found between total vitamin A intake (food and supplement) and serum13-*cis* RA and retinol. Dietary retinol, however, was negatively related to 13-*cis* RA, while dietary carotenoids and β-carotene were negatively related to 9-*cis* RA. Total serum RA was significantly negatively related to BMI, body weight, and total body fat, but no relationship was found with BMD or bone mineral content (BMC) of any of the skeletal sites; however, serum retinol showed significant positive relationship with BMD of the spine ($r = 0.208$, $P = 0.0233$), total body, and all sites of forearm, with r ranging from 0.176 to 0.270 ($P \le 0.05$).

Multiple regression models (controlled for age, BMI, and energy and calcium intake) with BMD of femoral shaft as dependent and total vitamin A intake as independent variables are presented in Table III. Other skeletal sites (total femur, forearm) showed borderline significance and are not presented.

TABLE III Multiple Regression Models for BMD and BMC of Different Skeletal Sites as Dependent and Dietary Metabolites of Vitamin A as Independent Variables

Assessment Time	Dependent Variable	$r^2_{(adj)}$ for the Model	Vitamin A	Coefficient	t Ratio	P Level	$r^2_{(adj)}$ with Added Variable
Baseline	Femoral shaft	21.7	Total	$-3.8\ e^{-6}$	-2.03	0.0441	23.6
6 months	Femoral shaft	22.3	Total	$-4.3\ e^{-6}$	-2.86	0.0051	26.9
			From food	$-4.5\ e^{-6}$	-2.61	0.0106	26.0
			β-Carotene	$-6.5\ e^{-6}$	-2.17	0.0323	24.7
	Total femur	22.9	Total	$-2.9\ e^{-6}$	-2.30	0.0230	25.7
			From food	$-3.0\ e^{-6}$	-2.03	0.0444	24.9
	Total body	17.9	Total	$-2.1\ e^{-6}$	-2.33	0.0218	20.9
			From food	$-2.2\ e^{-6}$	-2.09	0.0393	20.2
			β-Carotene	$-3.0\ e^{-6}$	-2.03	0.0445	20.0
	Forearm (radius)	17.4	Total	$-1.3\ e^{-6}$	-2.06	0.0413	19.7
			From food	$-1.7\ e^{-6}$	-2.38	0.0192	20.6
12 months	Trochanter (BMC)	13.7	Total	$-6.2\ e^{-6}$	-1.90	0.0604	15.7
			From food	$-8.8\ e^{-5}$	-2.07	0.0412	16.2
18 months	Femoral shaft	17.2	Total	$-4.6\ e^{-6}$	-2.64	0.0098	22.1
	Total femur	16.7	Total	$-3.05\ e^{-6}$	-2.39	0.0190	20.7
	Total body	15.4	Total	$-4.0\ e^{-6}$	-4.09	≤ 0.0001	27.6
	Forearm (ulna and radius)	15.1	Total	$-1.6\ e^{-6}$	-2.69	0.0084	20.4

Note: The models were controlled for age and body mass index, as well as for calcium, sodium (except at baseline), and energy intake. BMC = bone mineral content.

Six, Twelve, and Eighteen-Month Evaluations

Almost all subjects taking vitamin A supplements at baseline continued to do so at the 6-month ($n = 69$ of 124, or 55.6%), 12-month ($n = 65$ of 117, or 55.6%) and 18-month ($n = 60$ of 101, or 59.4%) evaluations, in about the same amount and frequency. Figure 1 presents vitamin A intake from food and total throughout the follow-up. When the 6, 12, and 18-month intakes were regressed on baseline intake, 23.3, 15.9, and 19.7% of variance in vitamin A intake at those time points, respectively, could be explained by the intake at baseline. In the further evaluation of the relationship between vitamin A intake and BMD, we analyzed separately the control group only and the whole population. The trend in vitamin A metabolites intake remained proportionally the same over time and there was no statistical difference (ANOVA) in intake in any of the metabolites between visits. Figure 2 presents calcium intake from food and total throughout the follow-up. While almost 70% of subjects were taking Ca supplements from various sources at baseline, once they were enrolled into the study all started taking calcium citrate with vitamin D (as per the larger study protocol). The amount provided was 630 mg Ca + 200 IU vitamin D per day, with average compliance of about 90%, bringing total Ca above the recommendations of 1200 mg/day [20].

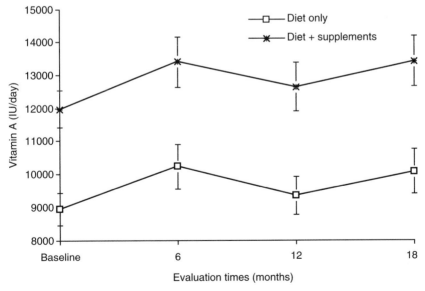

FIGURE 1   Intake of vitamin A from food and total over time (Mean ± SEM).

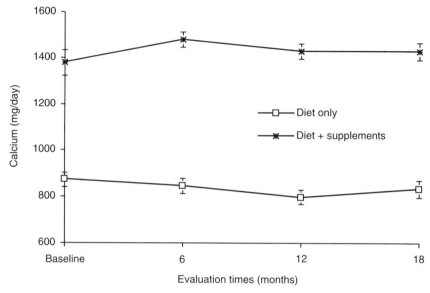

FIGURE 2   Intake of calcium from food and total over time (Mean ± SEM).

Separate multiple regression models were created for the 6-, 12-, and 18-month evaluations with BMD of various skeletal sites as dependent and vitamin A intake metabolites as independent variables. Each metabolite was entered into the model separately, due to high colinearity. Again, the models were controlled for age, BMI, and energy, calcium, and, in these cases, Na intake. Table III presents coefficients and P values for the most significant models.

Repeated-measures ANCOVA, with subjects divided by median of cumulative total vitamin A intake (11,199 IU), was used to examine the longitudinal relationship between vitamin A and BMD of various skeletal sites. Confounders were age, BMI, and energy, Ca, and Na intake. These data are presented in Figs. 3 and 4.

DISCUSSION

Based on our cross-sectional and longitudinal data, higher intakes of vitamin A — above the current dietary reference intake (DRI) of 700 to 900 μg retinyl equivalents (RE) or ~3500 IU but still below the tolerable upper limit of 3000 μg RE or ~15000 IU per day [21] — are associated with lower BMD of total body, hip, and forearm sites in this group of postmenopausal

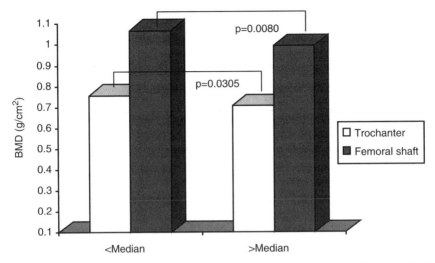

FIGURE 3   Bone mineral density (BMD) of femoral trochanter and shaft in subjects stratified below and above the median (11,199 IU) of total cumulative vitamin A intake (mean ± SEM adjusted for age, BMI, calcium, energy, and sodium intake).

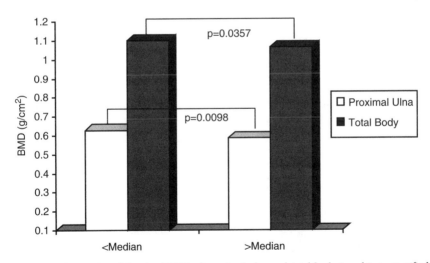

FIGURE 4   Bone mineral density (BMD) of proximal ulna and total body in subjects stratified below and above the median (11,199 IU) of total cumulative vitamin A intake (mean ± SEM adjusted for age, BMI, calcium, energy and sodium intake).

women. There was no relationship with lumbar spine BMD. Our findings are in agreement with two studies examining the association between vitamin A intake and BMD in older men and women [9] and women of wide age range [8]. In both studies, the intake was lower than in our population but higher than the recommended daily allowance (RDA). Because BMD is considered as a proxy for fracture, higher vitamin intake might increase incidents of hip fractures in these women, as has already been shown in other populations [7,8].

Humans obtain vitamin A in various forms, depending on the source. Green, red, orange, and yellow vegetables and fruits contain carotenoids. Of about 600 forms found in nature, 50 are known to have vitamin A function and the most potent one is β-carotene. Animal products such as egg yolks, butter, whole milk, liver, and fish oils contain retinoids (mostly different retinol esters). In the United States, skim and low fat milk, some juices, and breakfast cereals are all supplemented with vitamin A, rendering ~500 IU/serving [21]. Supplements may contain from 100 to 500% of the daily value either in the form of vitamin A esters or β-carotene. Even the generic one-a-day, multivitamin/mineral supplements contain 100% of the daily value for vitamin A. Therefore, due to food fortification, as well as massive supplement consumption, many people end up with excessive amounts of vitamin A which over time may have adverse effects on their bones. Particularly vulnerable might be the elderly, who have diminished vitamin A metabolism and clearance by liver [4].

Food Processor® software, used in our study to analyze dietary records, expresses vitamin A metabolites as vitamin A in IU, vitamin A in RE, carotenoids in RE, retinol in RE, and β-carotene in µg, and this is how we have presented our data (Table II). According to the software manufacturer, vitamin A expressed in IU seems to be the most complete assessment, as most of the food labels (from which the database is derived) express vitamin A content in IU. Additionally, vitamin A in supplements is also expressed in IU, and because more than half of the participants in our study were taking supplements throughout expressing vitamin A in IU was the best way to account for this amount. The conversion factors for metabolites vary depending on the source, and recently, a new retinol activity equivalent (RAE) was established [21]. Accordingly, 1 RE = 1 µg retinol, 6 µg β-carotene, and 12 µg other provitamin A carotenoids, while 1 RAE = 1 µg retinol, 12 µg β-carotene, and 24 µg other provitamin A carotenoids. Also, 1 RAE = 1 RE for retinol, or RE*0.5 for carotenoids. Approximately, 1 RE = 3.3 IU from animal products, 3.5 IU from cheese, 4.1 IU from yogurt, 5 IU from mixed foods, and 10 IU from plants. In our estimates and discussion, we used a conversion factor of 5 (as an average from mixed foods and supplements) to compare levels expressed in RE and IU.

We performed calculations using all metabolites of vitamin A (from carotenoids, retinol, β-carotene) separately; however, total vitamin A intake (food and supplements), expressed in IU, always had the strongest significance. The weaker relationship or lack of the relationship with other metabolites and BMD was probably due to the incomplete databases for those components of vitamin A, rendering less accurate assessment of its intake. In our multiple regression models, performed at each time point, vitamin A was repeatedly negatively associated with BMD of total femur and shaft, along with total body and forearm sites (Table III). This association with several skeletal sites strengthened our conclusions about the overall relationship. Additionally, adding vitamin A to the basic models containing age, BMI, and Ca, Na, and energy intake contributed from 1.9 to 12.2% of variance for a given BMD. Therefore, even if only borderline significance was reached for one of the skeletal sites, it could still be interpreted as influential. Dividing subjects by the median of their cumulative vitamin A intake showed us the longitudinal relationship and negative association between BMD and vitamin A of subjects above the median (Figs. 3 and 4).

The weak, positive relationship between serum retinol and BMD of some skeletal sites in our study is surprising, as it was also positively related to vitamin A intake. It is also in contrast to the Michaelsson et al. study [10] (although their outcomes were fractures), in which each SD increase in serum retinol was associated with a 26% increase in overall fracture risk in 50-year-old men. The serum retinol in that study, however, was measured only once during the 30-year follow-up, and it correlated only weakly with the dietary assessment of vitamin A obtained 20 years later [10]. Because the above-mentioned relationship in our study was weak, it just might be due to statistical chance or the fact that levels of serum retinol slightly elevated by vitamin A intake were not high enough to produce adverse effects on bone.

A positive weak correlation was found between serum 13-cis RA (but not total RA) and total vitamin A intake and no significant relationship between serum RA and BMD or BMC of any of the skeletal sites. Recently, Ballew et al. examined data from the NHANES III study and found no significant associations between fasting retinyl ester concentrations and any measure of bone mineral status [11]. Generally, studies involving RA and its relationship to dietary vitamin A intake are scarce. In a rare study that measured retinoic acid, Copper et al. [13] showed significant increases in plasma concentrations of retinol, all-trans retinoic acid, and 13-cis retinoic acid in cancer patients given treatments of daily doses of 300,000 IU retinyl palmitate. Such intake is many-fold higher than the DRI and therefore is not representative of typical dietary intakes. van Vliet et al. [14] found an increase in plasma concentrations of retinoic acid metabolites after consumption of dietary vitamin A, although this study provided a single meal instead of considering long-term dietary consumption. The latter two studies did not investigate relationship with bone mass but are mentioned here as the rare examples that include measurements of retinoic acid as a potential marker of vitamin A status (by relating it with vitamin A intake). It could be that both serum RA and retinol are homeostatically regulated and in cases of subclinical hypervitaminosis A, as in our case, are not sensitive enough as indicators of higher intake.

SUMMARY AND CONCLUSIONS

In summary, intake of vitamin A (>11,000 IU or ~2200 µg/day) in our population might be detrimental for bone, and vitamin A supplements should be carefully chosen by older women. Several foods, such as milk, cereals, and some juices, are currently fortified with vitamin A and their re-evaluation may be warranted. Future studies are needed to clarify the impact of chronic subclinical hypervitaminosis A on bone density/fractures. Based on the current understanding, it appears that either too high or too low levels of vitamin A are detrimental to bone and it is not clear what intake would be optimal for bone health. The range of optimal intake might be very narrow, and more studies are needed to define it. Because vitamin A comes in many forms and its dietary assessment is difficult, establishing a reliable serum metabolite as a potential biomarker of vitamin A status would be important. Therefore, future studies are also needed to determine the relationship between dietary vitamin A and serum retinol and retinoic acid as biological markers of vitamin A status.

ACKNOWLEDGMENTS

This study was funded in part by NRI/USDA 2001-00836, Donaghue Medical Research Foundation DF98-056, Mission Pharmacal, San Antonio, TX, and the University of Connecticut Office for Sponsored Programs.

REFERENCES

1. Ilich, J.Z. and Kerstetter, E.J. (2000). Nutrition in bone health revisited: a story beyond calcium. *J. Am. College Nutr.* 19: 715–737.

2. Kindmark, A., Torma, H., Johansson, A., Ljunghall, S., and Melhus, H. (1993). Reverse transcription-polymerase chain reaction assay demonstrates that the 9-cis retinoic acid receptor alpha is expressed in human osteoblasts. *Biochem. Biophys. Res. Commun.* 192: 1367–1372.
3. Saneshige, S., Mano, H., Tezuka, K., Kakudo, S., Mori, Y., Honda, Y., Itabashi, A., Yamada, T., Miyata, K., Hakeda, Y. *et al.* (1995). Retinoic acid directly stimulates osteoclastic bone resorption and gene expression of cathepsin K/OC-2. *Biochem. J.* 309: 721–724.
4. Anderson, J.J.B. (2002). Oversupplementation of vitamin A and osteoporotic fractures in the elderly: to supplement or not to supplement with vitamin A. *J. Bone Mineral Res.* 17: 1359–1362.
5. Rohde, C.M., Manatt, M., Clagett-Dame, M., and Deluca, H.F. (1999). Vitamin A antagonizes the action of vitamin D in rats. *J. Nutr.* 129: 2246–2250.
6. Johansson, S. and Melhus, H. (2001). Vitamin A antagonizes calcium response to vitamin D in man. *J. Bone Mineral Res.* 16: 1899–1905.
7. Feskanich, D., Singh, V., Willett, W.C., and Colditz, G.A. (2002). Vitamin A intake and hip fractures among postmenopausal women. *JAMA* 2: 47–54.
8. Melhus, H., Michaelsson, K., Kindmark, A., Bergstrom, R., Holmberg, L., Mallmin, H., Wolk, A., and Ljunghall, S. (1998). Excessive dietary intake of vitamin A is associated with reduced bone mineral density and increased risk for hip fracture. *Ann. Intern. Med.* 129: 770–778.
9. Promislow, J.H.E., Goodman-Gruen, D., Slymen, D.J., and Barret-Connor, E.L. (2002). Retinol intake and bone mineral density in the elderly: the Rancho Bernardo study. *J. Bone Mineral Res.* 17: 1349–1358.
10. Michaelsson, K., Lithell, H., Vessby, B., and Melhus, H. (2003). Serum retinol levels and the risk of fractures. *N. Engl. J. Med.* 348: 287–294.
11. Ballew, C., Galuska, D., and Gillespie, C. (2001). High serum retinyl esters are not associated with reduced bone mineral density in the Third National Health and Nutrition Examination Survey, 1988–1994. *J. Bone Mineral Res.* 16: 2306–2312.
12. Blaner, W.S. and Olson, J.A. (1994). Retinol and retinoic acid metabolism, in *The Retinoids*, Sporn, M.B., Roberts, A.B., and Goodman, D.S., Eds., Raven Press, New York, pp. 229–255.
13. Copper, M.P., Klaassen, I., Teerlink, T., Snow, G.B., and Braakhuis, B.J. (1999). Plasma retinoid levels in head and neck cancer patients: a comparison with healthy controls and the effect of retinyl palmitate treatment. *Oral Oncol.* 35: 40–44.
14. van Vliet, T., Boelsma, E., de Vries, A.J., and van den Berg, H. (2001). Retinoic acid metabolites in plasma are higher after intake of liver paste compared with a vitamin A supplement in women. *J. Nutr.* 131: 3197–3203.
15. Johansson, S. (2002). Subclinical hypervitaminosis A causes fragile bones in rats. *Bone* 31: 685–689.
16. Nonnecke, B.J., Horst, R.L., Hammell, D.C., and Franklin, S.T. (2000). Effects of supplemental vitamin A on retinoic acid concentrations in the plasma of preruminant calves. *Int. J. Vitamin Nutr. Res.* 70: 278–286.
17. Ilich, J.Z., Brownbill, R.A., and Tamborini, L. (2003). Bone and nutrition in elderly women: protein, energy, and calcium as main determinants of bone mineral density. *Eur. J. Clin. Nutr.* 57: 554–565.
18. Ilich, J.Z., Zito, M., Brownbill, R.A., and Joyce, M.E. (2000). Change in bone mass after Colles' fracture: a case report of unique data collection and long-term implications. *J. Clin. Densitometry* 3: 383–389.

19. De Leenheer, A.P. and Nelis, H.J. (1990). High performance liquid chromatography in blood. *Meth. Enzymol.* 189: 50–59.
20. Institute of Medicine. (1997). Dietary reference intakes for calcium, phosphorus, magnesium, vitamin D, and fluoride, in National Academy Press, Washington, D.C.
21. Institute of Medicine. (2001). Dietary reference intakes for vitamin A, vitamin K, arsenic, boron, chromium, copper, iodine, iron, manganese, molybdenum, nickel, silicon, vanadium, and zinc, in National Academy Press, Washington, D.C.

CHAPTER 9

Hesperidin, a Citrus Flavanone, Improves Bone Acquisition and Prevents Skeletal Impairment in Rats

MARIE-NOËLLE HORCAJADA and VÉRONIQUE COXAM

Unité des Maladies Métaboliques et Micronutriments, Groupe Ostéoporose, INRA de Theix, France

ABSTRACT

Flavonoids are a large family of compounds associated with many biological activities (*e.g.*, antioxidant, estrogenic, antiinflammatory properties). Until now, the most examined (iso)flavonoids with respect to bone health are the soy isoflavones, which have been shown to prevent bone loss in the ovariectomized rat and attenuate spinal bone loss in postmenopausal women.

Citrus fruits are rich in flavanones. Hesperidin (Hp), is one of the main flavanones in oranges. We investigated its effect on bone metabolism in intact and ovariectomized rats. The study was carried out on 40 3-month-old Wistar female rats; 20 were sham operated (SH), while the others were ovariectomized (OVX). Among each group, 10 sham-operated (TSH) and 10 ovariectomized (TOVX) rats were fed a standard diet for 90 days following surgery, and the 20 remaining animals received the same regimen but with 0.5% hesperidin added (10 HpSH, 10 HpOVX). At necropsy, the ovariectomy-induced uterine weight decrease did not differ between TOVX and HpOVX rats. Hesperidin consumption totally prevented the ovariectomy-induced demineralization (bone mineral density TOVX: −6.2% versus TSH; HpOVX versus TSH: NS; HpOVX: +10.7% versus TOVX), and significantly improved femoral metaphyseal density (HpSH: +11.5% versus TSH) in intact rats as well. The femoral diaphyseal density was also significantly enhanced by hesperidin in both SH and OVX rats, while an improvement of bone strength was only observed in ovariectomized animals. Plasma osteocalcin concentrations were higher in HpOVX ($P < 0.05$ versus HpSH). Urinary deoxypyridinolin excretion was reduced ($P < 0.01$) in both HpSH and HpOVX rats compared to their controls. Finally, the plasma concentration of hesperetin (the aglycone form) was 12.53 ± 2.48 µM in hesperidin fed rats, while the molecule stayed undetectable in control rats. These results indicate that, under our experimental conditions, hesperidin consumption was able to improve bone mass acquisition in intact rats and exhibited a significant protection against ovariectomy-induced bone impairment.

INTRODUCTION

Osteoporosis is a major public health problem and, with predicted demographic changes, its prevalence is expected to rise dramatically in the coming decades [1]. This disease is mainly due to estrogen deficiency which leads to bone loss through increased osteoclastic function (see Reference 2 for a review). However, the mechanisms by which estrogen deficiency induces bone resorption are still unclear. Several inflammatory cytokines, such as interleukin-1 (IL-1), IL-6, tumor necrosis factor alpha (TNF-α), have been implicated [3], those molecules being linked to the presence of reactive oxygen species [4]. It has been shown in vitro and in rodents that free radicals are involved in bone resorption [5,6]. In MC3T3-E1 cells (a preosteoblastic cell line), treatment with inducers of oxidative stress (hydrogen peroxide and xanthine/xanthine oxidase) results in inhibition of the differentiation [7]. More recently, Lean et al. [8] suggested that estrogen-deficiency-induced bone loss would be connected to a lowering of thiol antioxidants in osteoclasts, leading to enhanced expression of cytokines, which promote osteoclastic resorption. Moreover, a link between increased oxidative stress (stimulation of lipid peroxidation) and reduced bone mineral density in humans has been established [9].

Food provides not only essential nutrients needed for life but also other bioactive compounds for health benefits and prevention of degenerative disease [10]. Several studies revealed that diets rich in fruits and vegetables are protective against chronic, degenerative diseases [11,12] and the beneficial effects are hypothesized to be related, in part, to the antioxidants properties of their constituents [13–16]. More precisely, over the past several years, a high consumption of fruits and vegetables has been shown to have a strong positive link to bone health (related to a decrease in osteoporosis risk fracture) [17,18]. Nevertheless, the role of micronutrients, especially those with antioxidant and/or antiinflammatory properties, in bone metabolism remains unknown.

Among the extensive family of polyphenols, flavonoids comprise a large group of naturally occurring compounds that are found in a wide variety of edible plants. These molecules represent one of the most interesting classes of biologically active compounds with health-related properties [19]. Until now, the most examined (iso)flavonoids with respect to bone health have been the soy isoflavones, which have been shown to prevent or lower bone loss in the ovariectomized rat and attenuate spinal bone loss in postmenopausal women (see Ref. 20 for review). Attention has also focused on the possible role of other polyphenols. The potential effect of tea beverages in osteoporosis prevention in relation to their antioxidants phenolic compounds has been reported in adults [21,22]. Mühlbauer's team [23,24] has shown that vegetable consumption can affect bone resorption in the rat, the strongest effect being observed with onions, which are particularly rich in flavonols, a subfamily of flavonoids that includes quercetin and kaempferol. In a previous study, we reported that rutin, a quercetin glycoside, inhibits ovariectomy-induced osteopenia in rats [25]. Moreover, recent *in vitro* data also showed that quercetin and kaempferol exert a potent inhibitory effect on the bone resorbing activity of osteoclasts [26]. Also, a promoting effect of kaempferol on the differentiation and mineralization of MC3T3-E1 cells was demonstrated [27].

Among all of the flavonoids, another interesting subgroup, flavanones, is present in our diet almost exclusively from citrus fruits and some aromatic herbs. The most eaten flavonoid (28.3 mg/day), according to a study carried out on polyphenol intake in Finland, was hesperetin, corresponding to 30% of the total dietary flavonoid intake [28]. The content of hesperidin (hesperetin-7-O-rutinoside) in orange juices ranges from 200 to 590 mg/L [29], and because citrus fruits or juices are widely consumed, the daily intake of hesperidin should be quite high in the rest of the world. Hesperidin has been reported to exhibit antioxidant and radical scavenging properties (but with moderate action when compared to other flavonoids). Significant anti-inflammatory and analgesic effects were also attributed to this molecule [30]. This flavanone also regulates plasma and hepatic cholesterol through HMG-CoA reductase inhibition [31]. Because a higher bone mineral density (BMD) has been reported in patients treated with statins (cholesterol-lowering agents) [32], hesperidin could be involved in cardiovascular disease prevention and/or bone sparing effects. Indeed, very recently, an inhibition of bone resorption associated with decreased serum and hepatic lipids in ovariectomized mice has been reported [33].

Adult bone health is predominantly determined by two factors: maximum attainment of peak bone mass and rate of bone loss occurring with aging; consequently, in this study, we investigated the ability of hesperetin, in its glycoside form, on both bone acquisition in intact growing rats and osteopenia in ovariectomized rats (*i.e.*, an animal model for human osteoporosis) [34].

METHODS

Design

The study was conducted in accordance with current legislation on animal experiments in France. Forty 3-month-old virgin female Wistar rats, weighing 266 ± 2 g were purchased from a laboratory colony (National Institute of Agricultural Research [INRA], Clermont-Ferrand/Theix, France). Among them, 20 were surgically ovariectomized (OVX) and the other 20 were sham operated (SH) under anesthesia using chloral hydrate (Fluka Chemie AG, Buchs, Switzerland; 80 g/L in saline solution; 0.4 mL/100 g body weight, intraperitoneally). Each rat was housed individually in a plastic cage that allowed separation and collection of urine and feces; the temperature was maintained at 21°C; and a 12-hour light/12-hour dark cycle was used.

After an adaptation period of 1 week with a semipurified standard diet (INRA, Jouy en Josas, France), the animals were fed the same diet, which contains 0.4% calcium (Ca) and 0.3% phosphorus (P), but it was either supplemented with the flavanone or not supplemented. Hesperidin (from Sigma, L'Isle d'Abeau, Chesnes, France) was added to the diet (5 g/kg diet) of 10 sham-operated rats (HpSH) and 10 ovariectomized rats (HpOVX) (Table I). Diets were prepared every week and stored at 4°C. In order to prevent hyperphagia induced by castration, the diet consumed by each rat was weighed daily and every animal received the mean level consumed by SH rats the previous day. Thus, the daily mean consumption during the entire experimental period (90 days) was 19.25 ± 0.15 g. Urine of each animal was collected over a 24-hour period on days 0, 45, and 85 to measure urinary excretion of deoxypyridinoline, a marker for bone resorption.

At necropsy, on day 90, blood samples were harvested at 9 a.m. After centrifugation, plasma was collected to determine both osteocalcin concentration, a marker for osteoblastic activity, and the levels of hesperetin (the aglycone form of hesperidin). The success of ovariectomy was

TABLE I   Composition of Diets

	Control Diet (g/100 g dry feed)	0.5% Hesperidin Diet (g/100 g dry feed)
Casein	15	15
Rapeseed oil	5	5
Wheat starch	74.03	73.5
Calcium phosphate (2H$_2$O)	1.68	1.68
Sodium chloride	0.65	0.65
Potassium citrate	1.14	1.14
Magnesium sulfate	0.5	0.5
Trace elements mix	1	1
Vitamin mix	1	1
Hesperidin	—	0.5

confirmed by a marked atrophy of uterine horns in OVX and HpOVX rats. Femurs were separated from adjacent tissue, cleaned, and used for physical measurements.

PHYSICAL MEASUREMENTS

Body Composition and Femoral Mineral Density

One week before necropsy, lean and fat mass were measured on each animal under light anesthesia by dual-energy x-ray absorptiometry (DEXA) [35] using a Hologic QDR 4500A x-ray densitometer (Hologic, Massy, France). Femoral mineral density (g/cm^2) was also determined by DEXA. The total femoral bone marrow density (T-BMD) and two subregions were assessed: one corresponding to the distal metaphyseal zone (M-BMD), which is rich in cancellous bone, and the other to the diaphyseal zone (D-BMD), mainly cortical bone [36].

Femoral Mechanical Testing

Immediately after collection in NaCl (9 g/L), the length of the right femur and the mean diameter of the diaphysis were measured using a precision caliper (Mitutoyo, Shroppshire, U.K.). Because of the irregular shape of the femoral diaphysis, the diameter used in the calculation was the mean of the greatest and the smallest diaphysis diameters. Femoral failure load was determined using a three-point bending test. Each bone was secured on the two lower supports (diameter, 4 mm; separation, 20 mm) of the anvil of a

114 Nutritional Aspects of Osteoporosis

Universal Testing Machine (Instron 4501; Instron, Canton, MA). An upper cross-head roller (diameter, 6 mm) was applied in front of the middle of the shaft of the bone and advanced at 0.5 mm/min. The load at rupture (Newtons) was automatically determined and recorded by Instron 4501 software. This test method was previously validated by using Plexiglas® standard probes [37].

BIOCHEMICAL ANALYSIS

Marker of Bone Resorption

Deoxypyridinoline (DPD) was measured in urine by competitive radio-immunoassay (Pyrilinks D kit; Metra Biosystems, Mountain View, CA). The assay requires a rat monoclonal antibody against DPD, which is coated to the inner surface of a polystyrene tube and ^{125}I-labeled DPD. In our experimental conditions, the sensitivity was 2 nmol/L, and the intra- and inter-assay variations were 4 and 6%, respectively. Results are expressed as DPD (nM) per creatinine (mM) to avoid the possible influence of glomerular filtration rate [38]. The creatine assay (Bio Merieux SA, Marcy L'étoile, France) is based on a modified Jaffé's method in which picric acid forms a yellow compound with creatinine presence.

Marker of Osteoblastic Activity

Plasma osteocalcin (OC) concentration was measured by homologous radioimmunoassay using rat osteocalcin (OC) standard, goat anti-rat OC antibody, ^{125}I-labeled rat OC, and donkey anti-goat second antibody (Biochemical Technologies kit, Stoughton, MA).The lowest limit of detection for this assay was 0.01 nmol/L, and the intra- and inter-assay variations were 6.8% and 8.9%, respectively.

Plasma Hesperetin Levels

Plasma samples (180 µL) were acidified with acetic acid to pH 4.9 and incubated 5 hr at 37°C in the presence of 1000 units of β-glucuronidase and 45 units of sulfatase (from Helix pomatia; Sigma G0876, L'Isle d'Abeau, Chesnes, France). Samples were then mixed with 4 volumes of methanol:HCl (200 mmol/L) and centrifuged 5 min at 12500 g. The supernatant was analyzed by high-performance liquid chromatography (HPLC). The HPLC analysis was performed using a system consisting of two pumps (Model 580; ESA, Chelmsford, MA) for high-pressure gradient, a temperature-controlled autosampler (Gilson, Villiers-le-Bel, France), a 150 × 4.6-mm Hypersil BDS C_{18}-5μ column (Touzard et Matignon, Les Ulis, France), a thermostatic chamber, and eight-channel CoullArray detector (Model 5600; Eurosep, Cergy, France). Mobile phases consisted of a 30-mmol/L NaH_3PO_4 buffer (pH 3) containing 20% acetonitrile (A) or 40% acetonitrile (B). Separation was achieved using a gradient elution (35°C, 0.8 mL/min): 0 to 3 min, 100% A; 3 to 30 min, linear gradient from 100% A to 100% B; 30 to 35 min, 100% B; 35.01 to 45 min, 100% A. Potentials were set at 50, 350, 480, 550, 700, 760, 820, and 850 mV (Pd as reference). Hesperetin was quantified using the sums of height obtained on electrodes 2 and 3.

STATISTICS

Results are expressed as means ± SEM. A parametric one-way analysis of variance (ANOVA) was used to test for any difference among the groups. If the result was found to be significant ($P < 0.05$), the Student–Newman–Keuls multiple comparison test was then used to determine specific differences between group means. If a parametric ANOVA was not feasible (e.g., significant differences between the SD groups, as tested by the Kolmogourov–Smirnov test), a Kruskall–Wallis test followed by the Mann–Whitney–Wilcoxon U-test was performed to compare differences between groups.

RESULTS

BODY COMPOSITION AND UTERINE WEIGHT

During the entire experimental period, the animals kept growing, and the same pattern of body weight evolution was observed in each group from day 0 to day 90 (data not shown). Nevertheless, on day 85, no significant difference in body composition (% fat mass) between ovariectomized rats (27.7 ± 1.6) and intact rats (23.2 ± 1.2) was detected, and hesperidin consumption (25.7 ± 4.3 in HpSH; 27.7 ± 1.2 in HpOVX) had no effect on this parameter (Fig. 1A). The mean uterine weight decrease was 78% ($P < 0.01$ versus SH animals) in both ovariectomized groups when compared to intact rats. This measurement allowed validation of successful ovariectomies. Moreover, in our experimental conditions, the hesperidin diet elicited any uterotrophic activity (Fig. 1B).

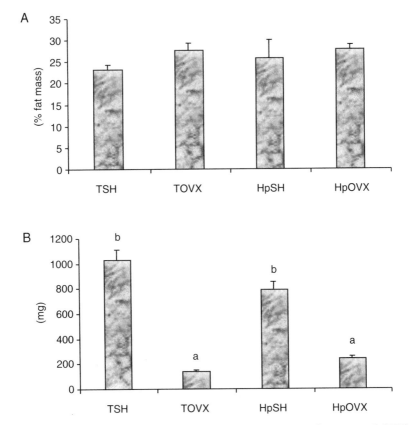

FIGURE 1   (A) Body fat mass and (B) uterine weight measured in sham-operated (TSH) or ovariectomized rats (TOVX) given a standard diet and in sham-operated (HpSH) or ovariectomized (HpOVX) hesperidin-supplemented animals (means ± SEM; a: $P < 0.01$ versus TSH and HpSH; b: $P < 0.01$ versus TOVX and HpOVX).

BONE MINERAL DENSITY

As expected, ovariectomy induced a significant decrease in T-BMD (TOVX: -5.2% versus TSH; $P < 0.05$). The M-BMD was also lower in TOVX animals (-6.2%; $P < 0.01$). Bone loss was totally reversed with the hesperidin diet in OVX rats, in both total and metaphyseal areas (HpOVX: $+14.9$ and $+10.7\%$ versus TOVX, respectively). Moreover, this parameter was significantly improved by hesperidin consumption in intact rats (HpSH: $+10.6$ and $+11.5\%$ versus TSH in T-BMD and M-BMD, respectively; $P < 0.01$ (Fig. 2A,B). Finally, despite no reduced density in the diaphyseal

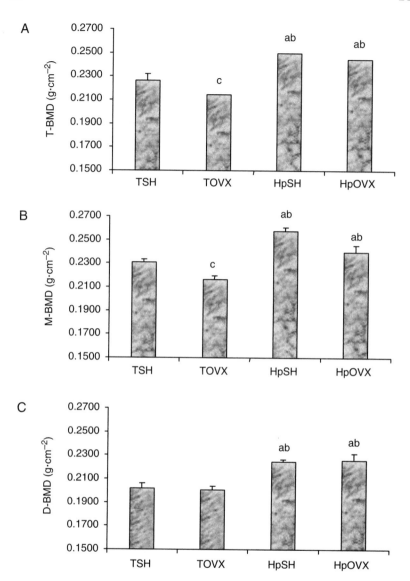

FIGURE 2 (A) Total (T-BMD), (B) metaphyseal (M-BMD), and (C) diaphyseal (D-BMD) femoral density measured in sham-operated (TSH) or ovariectomized rats (TOVX) given a standard diet and in sham-operated (HpSH) or ovariectomized (HpOVX) hesperidin-supplemented animals (means ±SEM; a: $P < 0.01$ versus TSH; b: $P < 0.01$ versus TOVX; c: $P < 0.05$ versus TSH).

TABLE II   Femoral Length, Mean Femoral Diameter, and Femoral Failure Load Measured
in Sham-Operated Control Rats (TSH), Ovariectomized Control Rats (TOVX), Sham-
Operated and Hesperidin-Treated (HpSH) Rats, or Ovariectomized and Hesperidin-Treated
(HpOVX) Rats

	TSH (Mean ± SEM)	TOVX (Mean ± SEM)	HpSH (Mean ± SEM)	HpOVX (Mean ± SEM)
Length (mm)	36.2 ± 0.3	36.3 ± 0.3	35.9 ± 0.3	36.4 ± 0.3
Diameter (mm)	3.48 ± 0.06	3.58 ± 0.05	3.61 ± 0.04	3.71 ± 0.05
Failure load (N)	109.5 ± 3.3	102.2 ± 2.9	106.3 ± 5.3	112.4 ± 3.4[a]

[a]$P < 0.05$ versus TOVX.

compartment in control OVX, D-BMD was enhanced in hesperidin groups (HpSH: +11.8% versus TSH; HpOVX : +12.7% versus TOVX; $P <$ 0.01) (Fig. 2C).

BONE SIZE AND STRENGTH

The length (mm) and the diameter (mm) of the femur were not different between groups. Concerning femoral failure load (N), the only significant difference in femoral strength was in HpOVX rats ($P < 0.05$ versus TOVX) despite a trend toward an increase in HpSH animals (Table II).

BONE TURNOVER AND PLASMA HESPERETIN CONCENTRATION

On day 90, osteocalcinemia (ng/mL) appeared not to be different between groups (TSH: 25.3 ± 1.9; TOVX: 33.1 ± 2.8; HpSH: 32.6 ± 3.7; NS), except in HpOVX rats for which a higher concentration was measured (HpOVX: 38.5 ± 2.6; $P < 0.05$ versus TSH), indicating an anabolic effect of hesperidin only in ovariectomized (Fig. 3A). Also, urinary DPD excretion was increased in OVX control rats (TOVX: +35% versus TSH; $P < 0.01$), a finding that was completely inhibited by the Hp diet (HpOVX: –38 % versus TOVX; $P < 0.01$). Moreover, bone resorption was also reduced by hesperidin in sham-operated rats (HpSH: –16% versus TSH; $P < 0.01$) (Fig. 3B). Finally, quantification of hesperetin in plasma has been performed after total hydrolysis of samples by β-glucuronidase/sulfatase using multi-electrode coulometric detection (Fig. 4). Mean plasma concentration of hesperetin was 12.53 ± 2.48 μM in hesperidin rats, while it was not detectable in plasma of control rats.

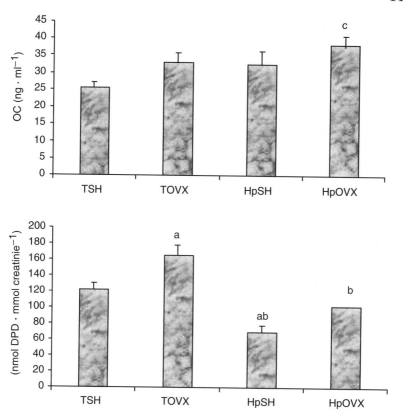

FIGURE 3   (A) Plasma osteocalcin and (B) urinary deoxypyridinoline (DPD) concentrations measured on day 90 in sham-operated (TSH) or ovariectomized rats (TOVX) given a standard diet and in sham-operated (HpSH) or ovariectomized (HpOVX) hesperidin-supplemented animals (means ±SEM; a: $P < 0.01$ versus TSH; b: $P < 0.01$ versus TOVX; c: $P < 0.05$ versus TSH).

DISCUSSION

Involutional osteoporosis is considered as one of the most serious diseases occurring among the aging population with a relative high penetrance [2], and preventive strategies need to be designed. Consumption of fruits and vegetables carries a large public health potential [12], and it has been strongly associated with reduced risk of cardiovascular disease, cancer, diabetes, and age-related functional decline [40]. Thus, a positive link with bone health has also been suggested [18]; besides calcium, micronutrients such as phenolic compounds have been cited for their putative role in dietary health

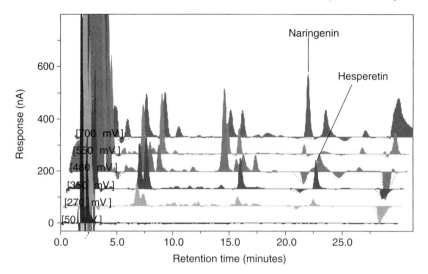

FIGURE 4   Representative HPLC–Coularray chromatograms of a hesperidin-supplemented rat plasma collected after 90 days of exposure (0.5% hesperidin in the diet). Naringenin was used as the internal control. The chromatographic conditions and the potentials applied are given in the Methods section of the text.

intervention in the nutritional prevention of osteoporosis [41]. In the present work, we investigated the effect of hesperidin, a citrus flavonoid, on bone metabolism in rats, focusing primarily on bone acquisition but also on skeletal impairment (induced by estrogen deficiency) because maintenance of skeletal health and development determines the individual risk of osteoporosis [42]. Indeed, the structural basis of bone fragility takes root during growth and gains full expression during aging [43].

As expected with this experimental model [34], castration (validated by uterine weight, Fig. 1B) induced a significant decrease in trabecular femoral BMD (Fig. 2A,B), as indicated by total and metaphyseal BMD, while no effect was elicited on diaphyseal BMD (Fig. 2C). This last observation can be correlated with measurement of femoral failure load (Table II), which also remained unchanged in TOVX versus TSH rats, as already observed in a previous study [25]. Both D-BMD and femoral failure load are related to the cortical compartment, which is less sensitive to estrogen deficiency than cancellous bone; in fact, increased bone loss after menopause is associated with a higher periosteal apposition rate, which partially preserves bone strength [44]. Moreover, bone biomechanical strength depends on both microarchitecture quality and mineral density [45,46]. Finally, osteopenia, as in humans [47], probably resulted from an increased bone turnover, as indicated by a higher urinary DPD excretion in OVX rats [34] than in SH (Fig. 3B) on day 90.

At the end of the experiment, no difference in fat mass content was observed between groups (Fig. 1A). As hypothesized, the rats fed the diet containing hesperidin, although devoid of any uterotrophic effect, experienced both an improvement of BMD at the three regions in intact rats and a lower cancellous bone loss rate following ovariectomy, as shown by HpOVX femoral mineral density (Fig. 2). Furthermore, the BMD sparing effect in HpOVX rats was associated with a significant greater femoral failure load (Table II). Actually, OVX rats might be more sensitive than SH animals, as femurs in intact rats are already protected by steroid hormone. Recently, Chiba *et al.* [33] clearly demonstrated that hesperidin consumption, given at the same level as that in our experiment (0.5% in the diet), was able to inhibit ovariectomy-induced trabecular bone loss in mice (2 months old). Nevertheless, in this work, no data concerning intact animals were reported; moreover, bone turnover was not assessed. In fact, in our experimental conditions, urinary DPD excretion was significantly reduced by hesperidin consumption, while osteocalcin was enhanced, but only in OVX rats (Fig. 3). We can thus hypothesize that such a prevention of osteopenia may have resulted from slowing down bone resorption, coupled with an anabolic effect (stimulation of osteoblastic cells activity) in OVX rats and from a reduced catabolism in HpSH animals. Anyway, our results on bone resorption are in accordance with the findings of Chiba *et al.* [33] indicating that hesperidin is effective in preventing trabecular bone loss by reducing the osteoclasts number at the femoral metaphysis of OVX mice. Nevertheless, our work strongly suggests that hesperidin can have both properties: stimulating bone mass acquisition in intact growing rats and protecting skeletal impairment following gonadal failure.

Several mechanism could account for such an effect, even if they are still unclear. Hesperidin is a flavanone belonging to the flavonoid family. It is actually a hesperetin-7-O-rutinoside that is not absorbed as such but must be hydrolyzed by intestinal bacteria [48] into aglycones recovered in plasma (as shown in Fig. 4), urine, and bile as glucuronides and sulfoglucuronides [49]. Flavonoids are typical phenolics compounds and, therefore, act as potent metal chelators and free-radical scavengers [50]. Concerning a possible involvement in oxidative processes, first it is important to remember that it is now well established that antioxidant defenses are markedly decreased in osteoporotic women, thus osteoporosis is characterized by increased oxidative stress [51]. Although flavanones do not exhibit the most potent antioxidant activity among polyphenols [52], hesperidin has been shown to be able to suppress *in vivo* oxidative stress in diabetics rats [53]. Furthermore, flavonoids and tocopherols share a common structure, and hesperidin found in orange juice exhibits the same antioxidant activity as that of vitamin E [54]. Moreover, it has been shown that naringenin, another flavanone, can replace alpha-tocopherol as a chain-breaking antioxidant against lipid peroxidation in liver microsomal membranes [55]. Vitamin E, which is an antioxidant, is able to stimulate trabecular bone formation [56], and supplementation has been shown to prevent bone impairment caused by oxidizing agents [57]. Moreover, vitamin E maintains bone mineral density in ovariectomized rats [58], and it has been observed that lower dietary intakes of vitamins C and E may increase the risk of hip fracture induced by oxidative stress in those who smoke [59]. Thus, hesperidin, might act as a free-radical scavenger in preventing bone loss in OVX rats (Fig. 2). Because it is evident that the decline in ovarian function with menopause induces increases in proinflammatory cytokines [3], we cannot exclude a possible antiinflammatory effect of hesperidin, as previously reported in rats where inflammatory conditions were elicited [60], to explain the bone sparing effect in our OVX rats. Indeed, hesperidin and diosmin are able to prevent colonic inflammation induced by trinitrobenzenesulfonic acid (TNBS) in colitis rats [61]. Nevertheless, no inflammatory parameter has been assessed in our experiment.

On the other hand, the anabolic effect of hesperidin could be due in part to a osteoblastic proliferation-stimulating activity, as previously demonstrated in the UMR106 cell line cultured in vitro with flavonoids of fruits extract [62]. Moreover, a positive effect on osteoblast differentiation and, thus, on calcium deposition after inducing the activity of alkaline phosphate (ALP) has been demonstrated by other flavonoids (such as kaempferol) [27]. We can thus hypothesize that, in our experimental conditions, hesperidin might have influenced osteoblastic proliferation and differentiation which led to stimulated bone accretion, as shown by the increased BMD and plasma OC concentrations (Figs. 2 and 3). Finally, it has also been reported that orange juice consumption in animals [63] and humans [64] results in reduced plasma cholesterol and triglycerides levels, as well as HMG-CoA activity, this effect being in part due to hesperidin content [65,66]. Recently, it has been reported that statins, which are cholesterol-lowering agents (through inhibition of hepatic HMG-CoA reductase), can inhibit bone resorption and also stimulate formation by activation of bone morphogenic protein (BMP) production [67]. We can thus suppose that hesperidin is also able to interact on bone, as statins, through the BMP pathway to stimulate bone formation even if the molecular mechanism must be further investigated.

In conclusion, hesperidin demonstrated a capacity to inhibit bone resorption and to reduce estrogen-dependent bone loss without uterine stimulation. Thus, this flavanone may have potential as a new approach in treating and preventing postmenopausal osteoporosis. Moreover, a stimulation of bone acquisition was elicited, indicating a possible role in peak bone mass achievement. Nevertheless, if the hesperidin molecule is one of the active compounds in citrus fruits for bone improvement or protection, whole fruit consumption must be emphasized. Through overlapping or complementary effects, the complex mixture of phytochemicals in fruits and vegetables provides a better protective effect on health than a single phytochemical [68].

REFERENCES

1. New, S.A. (2001). Exercise, bone and nutrition. *Proc. Nutr. Soc.* 60: 265–274.
2. Riggs, B.L., Khosla, S., Melton, L.J., 3rd (2002). Sex steroids and the construction and conservation of the adult skeleton. *Endocr. Rev.* 23: 279–302.
3. Pfeilschifter, J., Koditz, R., Pfohl, M., and Schatz, H. (2002). Changes in proinflammatory cytokine activity after menopause. *Endocr. Rev.* 23: 90–119.
4. Cuzzocrea, S., Mazzon, E., Dugo, L., Genovese, T., Di Paola, R., Ruggeri, Z., Vegeto, E., Caputi, A.P., Van De Loo, F.A., Puzzolo, D., and Maggi, A. (2003). Inducible nitric oxide synthase mediates bone loss in ovariectomized mice. *Endocrinology* 144: 1098–1107.
5. Garrett, I.R., Boyce, B.F., Oreffo, R.O., Bonewald, L., Poser, J., Mundy, G.R. (1990). Oxygen-derived free radicals stimulate osteoclastic bone resorption in rodent bone *in vitro* and *in vivo*. *J. Clin. Invest.* 85: 632–639.
6. Fraser, J.H., Helfrich, M.H., Wallace, H.M., and Ralston, S.H. (1996). Hydrogen peroxide, but not superoxide, stimulates bone resorption in mouse calvariae. *Bone* 19: 223–226.
7. Mody, N., Parhami, F., Sarafian, T.A., and Demer, L.L. (2001). Oxidative stress modulates osteoblastic differentiation of vascular and bone cells. *Free Radic. Biol. Med.* 31: 509–519.
8. Lean, J.M., Davies, J.T., Fuller, K., Jagger, C.J., Kirstein, B., Partington, G.A., Urry, Z.L., and Chambers, T.J. (2003). A crucial role for thiol antioxidants in estrogen-deficiency bone loss. *J. Clin. Invest.* 112: 915–923.
9. Basu, S., Michaelsson, K., Olofsson, H., Johansson, S., and Melhus, H., (2001). Association between oxidative stress and bone mineral density. *Biochem. Biophys. Res. Commun.* 288: 275–279.
10. Liu, R.H. (2003). Health benefits of fruit and vegetables are from additive and synergistic combinations of phytochemicals. *Am. J. Clin. Nutr.* 78: 517S–520S.
11. Lampe, J.W. (1999). Health effects of vegetables and fruit: assessing mechanisms of action in human experimental studies. *Am. J. Clin. Nutr.* 70: 475S–490S.
12. van't Veer, P., Jansen, M.C., Klerk, M., and Kok, F.J. (2000). Fruits and vegetables in the prevention of cancer and cardiovascular disease. *Public Health Nutr.* 3: 103–107.
13. Halliwell, B. (1996). Antioxidants in human health and disease. *Ann. Rev. Nutr.* 16: 33–50.
14. Collins, A.R. (1999). Oxidative DNA damage, antioxidants, and cancer. *Bioassays* 21: 238–246.
15. Miller, H.E., Rigelhof, F., Marquart, L., Prakash, A., and Kanter, M. (2000). Antioxidant content of whole grain breakfast cereals, fruits and vegetables. *J. Am. Coll. Nutr.* 19: 312S–319S.
16. Szeto, Y.T., Tomlinson, B., and Benzie, I.F. (2002). Total antioxidant and ascorbic acid content of fresh fruits and vegetables: implications for dietary planning and food preservation. *Br. J. Nutr.* 87: 55–59.
17. New, S.A., Robins, S.P., Campbell, M.K., Martin, J.C., Garton, M.J., BoltonSmith, C., Grubb, D.A., Lee, S.J., and Reid, D.M. (2000). Dietary influences on bone mass and bone

metabolism: further evidence of a positive link between fruit and vegetable consumption and bone health? *Am. J. Clin. Nutr.* 71: 142–151.

18. New, S.A. and Millward, D.J. (2003). Calcium, protein, and fruit and vegetables as dietary determinants of bone health. *Am. J. Clin. Nutr.* 77: 1340–1341.

19. Benavente-Garcia, O., Castillo, J., Marin, F.R., Ortuno, A., and del Rio, J.A. (1997). Uses and properties of citrus flavonoids. *J. Agric. Food Chem.* 45: 4505–4515.

20. Setchell, K.D. and Lydeking-Olsen, E. (2003). Dietary phytoestrogens and their effect on bone: evidence from *in vitro* and *in vivo*, human observational, and dietary intervention studies. *Am. J. Clin. Nutr.* 78: 593S–609S.

21. Wu, C.H., Yang, Y.C., Yao, W.J., Lu, F.H., Wu, J.S., and Chang, C.J, (2002). Epidemiological evidence of increased bone mineral density in habitual tea drinkers. *Arch. Intern. Med.* 162: 1001–1006.

22. Hegarty, V.M., May, H.M., and Khaw, K.T. (2000). Tea drinking and bone mineral density in older women. *Am. J. Clin. Nutr.* 71, 1003–1007.

23. Mühlbauer, R.C., Lozano, A., and Reinli, A. (2002). Onion and a mixture of vegetables, salads, and herbs affect bone resorption in the rat by a mechanism independent of their base excess. *J. Bone Mineral Res.* 17: 1230–1236.

24. Mühlbauer, R.C. and Li, F. (1999). Effect of vegetables on bone metabolism. *Nature* 401: 343–344.

25. Horcajada-Molteni, M.N., Crespy, V., Coxam, V., Davicco, M.J., Remesy, C., and Barlet, J.P. (2000). Rutin inhibits ovariectomy-induced osteopenia in rats. *J. Bone Mineral Res.* 15: 2251–2258.

26. Wattel, A., Kamel, S., Mentaverri, R., Lorget, F., Prouillet, C., Petit, J.P., Fardelonne, P., and Brazier, M. (2003). Potent inhibitory effect of naturally occurring flavonoids quercetin and kaempferol on *in vitro* osteoclastic bone resorption. *Biochem. Pharmacol.* 65: 35–42.

27. Miyake, M., Arai, N., Ushio, S., Iwaki, K., Ikeda, M., and Kurimoto, M. (2003). Promoting effect of kaempferol on the differentiation and mineralization of murine pre-osteoblastic cell line MC3T3–E1. *Biosci. Biotechnol. Biochem.* 67, 1199–1205.

28. Kumpulainen, J.T. (2001). Intake of flavonoids, phenolic acids and lignans in various populations, in *Proc. 3rd International Conference on Natural Antioxidants and Anticarcinogens in Food, Health and Disease*, Voutilainen, S. and Salonen, J.T., Eds., Kuopion University Publications D. Medical Sciences, Helsinki, p. 24.

29. Tomas-Barberan, F.A. and Clifford, M.N. (2000). Flavanones, chalcones and dihydrochalcones: nature, occurrence and dietary burden. *J. Sci. Food Agric.* 80: 1073–1080.

30. Garg, A., Garg, S., Zaneveld, L.J., and Singla, A.K. (2001). Chemistry and pharmacology of the citrus bioflavonoid hesperidin. *Phytother. Res.* 15: 655–669.

31. Bok, S.H., Lee, S.H., Park, Y.B., Bae, K.H., Son, K.H., Jeong, T.S., and Choi, M.S. (1999). Plasma and hepatic cholesterol and hepatic activities of 3-hydroxy-3-methyl-glutaryl-CoA reductase and acyl CoA: cholesterol transferases are lower in rats fed citrus peel extract or a mixture of citrus bioflavonoids. *J. Nutr.* 129: 1182–1185.

32. Edwards, C.J., Hart, D.J., and Spector, T.D. (2000). Oral statins and increased bone-mineral density in postmenopausal women. *Lancet* 355: 2218–2219.

33. Chiba, H., Uehara, M., Wu, J., Wang, X., Masuyama, R., Suzuki, K., Kanazawa, K., and Ishimi, Y. (2003). Hesperidin, a citrus flavonoid, inhibits bone loss and decreases serum and hepatic lipids in ovariectomized mice. *J. Nutr.* 133: 1892–1897.

34. Kalu, D.N. (1991). The ovariectomized rat model of postmenopausal bone loss. *Bone Minerals* 15: 175–191.

35. Bertin, E., Ruiz, J.C., Mourot, J., Peiniau, P., and Portha, B. (1998). Evaluation of dual-energy x-ray absorptiometry for body-composition assessment in rats. *J. Nutr.* 128: 1550–1554.

36. Pastoureau, P., Chomel, A., and Bonnet, J. (1995). Specific evaluation of localized bone mass and bone loss in the rat using dual-energy x-ray absorptiometry subregional analysis. *Osteoporosis Int.* 5: 143–149.
37. Turner, C.H. and Burr, D.B. (1993). Basic biomechanical measurements of bone: a tutorial. *Bone* 14: 595–608.
38. Robins, S.P. (1994). Biochemical markers for assessing skeletal growth. *Eur. J. Clin. Nutr.* 48: S199–209.
39. Manach, C., Morand, C., Gil-Izquierdo, A., Bouteloup-Demange, C., and Remesy, C. (2003). Bioavailability in humans of the flavanones hesperidin and narirutin after the ingestion of two doses of orange juice. *Eur. J. Clin. Nutr.* 57: 235–242.
40. Willett, W.C. (1994). Diet and health: what should we eat? *Science* 264: 532–537
41. Horcajada-Molteni, M.N., Crespy, V., Coxam, V., Davicco, M.J., Remesy, C., and Barlet, J.P. (2000). Rutin inhibits ovariectomy-induced osteopenia in rats. *J. Bone Mineral Res.* 15: 2251–2258
42. Hallworth, R.B. (1998). Prevention and treatment of postmenopausal osteoporosis. *Pharm. World Sci.* 20: 198–205.
43. Seeman, E. (2002). Pathogenesis of bone fragility in women and men. *Lancet* 359: 1841–1850.
44. Ahlborg, H.G., Johnell, O., Turner, C.H., Rannevik, G., and Karlsson, M.K. (2003). Bone loss and bone size after menopause. *N. Engl. J. Med.* 349: 327–334.
45. Recker, R.R. (1989). Low bone mass may not be the only cause of skeletal fragility in osteoporosis. *Proc. Soc. Exp. Biol. Med.* 191: 272–274.
46. Uchiyama, T., Tanizawa, T., Muramatsu, H., Endo, N., Takahashi, H.E., and Hara, T. (1999). Three-dimensional microstructural analysis of human trabecular bone in relation to its mechanical properties. *Bone* 25: 487–491.
47. Riggs, B.L., Khosla, S., Atkinson, E.J., Dunstan, C.R., and Melton, L.J., 3rd (2003). Evidence that type I osteoporosis results from enhanced responsiveness of bone to estrogen deficiency. *Osteoporosis Int.* 18: 18.
48. Rasmussen, S.E. and Breinholt, V.M. (2003). Non-nutritive bioactive food constituents of plants: bioavailability of flavonoids. *Int. J. Vitamin Nutr. Res.* 73: 101–111.
49. Felgines, C., Texier, O., Morand, C., Manach, C., Scalbert, A., Regerat, F., and Remesy, C. (2000). Bioavailability of the flavanone naringenin and its glycosides in rats. *Am. J. Physiol. Gastrointest. Liver Physiol.* 279: G1148–G1154.
50. Middleton, E., Kandaswami, C., and Theoharides, T.C. (2000). The effects of plant flavonoids on mammalian cells: implications for inflammation, heart disease, and cancer. *Pharmacol. Rev.* 52: 673–751.
51. Maggio, D., Barabani, M., Pierandrei, M., Polidori, M.C., Catani, M., Mecocci, P., Senin, U., Pacifici, R., and Cherubini, A. (2003). Marked decrease in plasma antioxidants in aged osteoporotic women: results of a cross-sectional study. *J. Clin. Endocrinol. Metab.* 88: 1523–1527.
52. Rice-Evans, C.A., Miller, N.J., and Paganga, G. (1996). Structure-antioxidant activity relationships of flavonoids and phenolic acids. *Free Rad. Biol. Med.* 20: 933–956.
53. Miyake, Y., Yamamoto, K., Tsujihara, N., and Osawa, T. (1998). Protective effects of lemon flavonoids on oxidative stress in diabetic rats. *Lipids* 33: 689–695.
54. Rice-Evans, C.A., Miller, N.J., and Paganga, G. (1997). Antioxidant properties of phenolic compounds. *Trends Plant Sci.* 2: 152–159.
55. Van Acker, F.A., Schouten, O., Haenen, G.R., Van der Vijgh, W.J., and Bast, A. (2000). Flavonoids can replace alpha-tocopherol as an antioxidant. *FEBS Lett.* 473: 145–148.
56. Xu, H., Watkins, B.A., and Seifert, M.F. (1995). Vitamin E stimulates trabecular bone formation and alters epiphyseal cartilage morphometry. *Calcif. Tissue Int.* 57: 293–300.

57. Yee, J.K. and Ima-Nirwana, S. (1998). Palm vitamin E protects against ferric-nitrilotriacetate-induced impairment on bone calcification. *Asia Pacific J. Pharmacol.* 13: 1–7.
58. Norazlina, M., Ima-Nirwana, S., Gapor, M.T., and Khalid, B.A. (2000). Palm vitamin E is comparable to alpha-tocopherol in maintaining bone mineral density in ovariectomised female rats. *Exp. Clin. Endocrinol. Diabetes* 108: 305–310.
59. Melhus, H., Michaelsson, K., Holmberg, L., Wolk, A., and Ljunghall, S. (1999). Smoking, antioxidant vitamins, and the risk of hip fracture. *J. Bone Mineral Res.* 14: 129–135.
60. Galati, E.M., Monforte, M.T., Kirjavainen, S., Forestieri, A.M., Trovato, A., and Tripodo, M.M. (1994). Biological effects of hesperidin, a citrus flavonoid. Note I. Antiinflammatory and analgesic activity. *Farmaco* 40: 709–712.
61. Crespo, M.E., Galvez, J., Cruz, T., Ocete, M.A., and Zarzuelo, A. (1999). Anti-inflammatory activity of diosmin and hesperidin in rat colitis induced by TNBS. *Planta Med.* 65: 651–653.
62. Wang, D. Li, F., and Jiang, Z. (2001). Osteoblastic proliferation stimulating activity of *Psoralea corylifolia* extracts and two of its flavonoids. *Planta Med.* 67: 748–749.
63. Kurowska, E.M., Borradaile, N.M., Spence, J.D., and Carroll, K.K. (2000). Hypocholesterolemic effects of dietary citrus juices in rabbits. *Nutr. Res.* 20: 121–129.
64. Kurowska, E.M., Spence, J.D., Jordan, J., Wetmore, S., Freeman, D.J., Piche, L.A., and Serratore, P. (2000). HDL-cholesterol-raising effect of orange juice in subjects with hypercholesterolemia. *Am. J. Clin. Nutr.* 72: 1095–1100.
65. Bok, S.H. Shin, Y.W., Bae, K.H., Jeong, T.S., Kwon, Y.K., Park, Y.B., and Choi, M.S. (2000). Effects of naringin and lovastatin on plasma and hepatic lipids in high-fat and high-cholesterol fed rats. *Nutr. Res.* 20: 1007–1015.
66. Kim, H.K., Jeong, T.S., Lee, M.K., Park, Y.B., and Choi, M.S. (2003). Lipid-lowering efficacy of hesperetin metabolites in high-cholesterol fed rats. *Clin. Chim. Acta.* 327: 129–137.
67. Mundy, G., Garrett, R., Harris, S., Chan, J., Chen, D., Rossini, G., Boyce, B., Zhao, M., and Gutierrez, G. (1999). Stimulation of bone formation *in vitro* and in rodents by statins. *Science* 286: 1946–1949.
68. Eberhardt, M.V., Lee, C.Y., and Liu, R.H, (2000). Antioxidant activity of fresh apples. *Nature* 405: 903–904.

CHAPTER 10

Vitamin B-Complex, Methylenetetrahydrofolate Reductase Polymorphism and Bone: Potential for Gene–Nutrient Interaction

H.M. MACDONALD and D.M. REID

Osteoporosis Research Unit, Department of Medicine and Therapeutics, University of Aberdeen, Aberdeen, United Kingdom

ABSTRACT

A polymorphism (C to T) of methylenetetrahydrofolate reductase (MTHFR) producing a heat-labile, less-active enzyme has been associated with low bone mineral density (BMD) in postmenopausal Japanese women. The MTHFR polymorphism has been found to be associated with a number of disease states, including heart disease and neural tube defects. The MTHFR enzyme is required, with vitamin B12 and folate, for clearing circulating homocysteine. The homocysteine-lowering effect of MTHFR may also depend on riboflavin status. Homocystinuria, a rare condition characterized by very high levels of homocysteine, is associated with early-onset osteoporosis, but whether moderately raised homocysteine levels are a risk factor for osteoporosis is not yet known. Homocysteine metabolites inhibit lysyl oxidase, the enzyme that produces collagen cross-links. Preliminary work from a subset of the Aberdeen Prospective Osteoporosis Screening Study (APOSS) showed no significant difference in BMD or BMD loss between MTHFR genotypes; however, for women who were TT homozygotes for MTHFR, there was a

Nutritional Aspects of Osteoporosis, Second Edition

127

positive relationship between energy-adjusted riboflavin intake and femoral neck BMD. Riboflavin has been shown to be a key nutrient in normalizing homocysteine levels for subjects with the heat-labile enzyme in Northern Ireland. Vitamins of the B-complex may provide a simple and cost-effective means of positively influencing bone health for women who are TT homozygotes for the MTHFR enzyme.

INTRODUCTION

Although the general consensus is that osteoporosis risk is governed primarily by genetic factors, accounting for up to 75% of the variation in fracture risk, no single gene or combination of genes has yet been identified as being responsible for the development of this distressing and debilitating disease [1]. The most extensively studied gene in relation to bone health has been the vitamin D receptor site, with a variety of polymorphisms being investigated. However, although there appears to be a suitable mechanism to explain how this might be a functional gene and influence bone health, namely through control of calcium uptake, the numerous studies carried out have only succeeded in producing mixed results [2]. One suggestion, for this gene at least, is that dietary factors may be responsible for the differences in results between different studies. Many other candidate genes have been identified, including the gene coding for methylenetetrahydrofolate reductase (MTHFR), which could also be influenced by dietary factors. The MTHFR enzyme is required for clearing circulating homocysteine. A relatively common polymorphism of the gene coding for MTHFR produces a less active enzyme that results in elevated homocysteine levels [3]. It is known that homocystinuria, a rare condition characterized by very high levels of homocysteine, is associated with early-onset osteoporosis [4], but whether moderately raised homocysteine levels are a risk factor for osteoporosis is not known.

WHAT IS THE ROLE OF METHYLENE
TETRAHYDROFOLATE REDUCTASE
(MTHFR) ENZYME?

The enzyme methylenetetrahydrofolate reductase (MTHFR; EC 1.5.1.20) removes homocysteine from the circulation. The requirement for two B vitamins, folate and vitamin B12, is well known [5]. More recently, it has been found that, compared to the normal enzyme, the heat-labile form of the enzyme is ten times as likely to disassociate from its prosthetic group flavin adenine dinucleotide (FAD) [6]. Riboflavin is essential for the production of

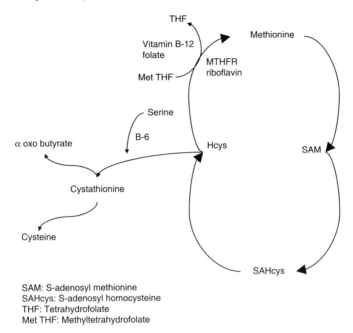

SAM: S-adenosyl methionine
SAHcys: S-adenosyl homocysteine
THF: Tetrahydrofolate
Met THF: Methyltetrahydrofolate

FIGURE 1   Homocysteine (Hcys) metabolism (MTHFR, methyltetrahydrofolate reductase).

FAD, so it would now appear that this vitamin of the B complex is also required for optimal MTHFR activity [7]. Another enzyme pathway can remove homocysteine — namely, cystathionine beta-synthase, which functions when methionine is plentiful (whereas the MTHFR pathway dominates in the fasted state). Cystathionine beta-synthase requires vitamin B6. Both pathways are regulated via *S*-adenosyl methionine (SAM) (Fig. 1) so that a defect in one pathway automatically leads to impairment in the other [8]. SAM is a donor for many important cellular methylation reactions, including the methylation of cytosine in DNA.

MTHFR POLYMORPHISM

DISTRIBUTION OF MTHFR 677CT POLYMORPHISM

The polymorphism of the MTHFR gene, at locus 1p36.3, involves a genetic change from C to T at nucleotide 677 that causes an amino acid change (alanine to valine) in the variant. The mutant form of the enzyme is more heat labile and less active compared to the wild type. Fasting levels of

TABLE I   Distribution of MTHFR Genotypes in a Selection of Different Populations

Study	CC	CT	TT	%T	%TT	Ref.
Aberdeen Prospective Osteoporosis Screening study	499	617	125	35	10	MacDonald et al. (2003) submitted
European Concerted Action Project	352	314	81	32	11	Meleady et al. (2003) [42]
U.K. population	345	337	72	32	10	Dekou et al. (2001) [43]
Portugese population	51	54	12	33	10	Castro et al. (2003) [44]
Review of 1995–1998 pooled data:						Botto and Yang Q. (2000) [45]
United Kingdom	443	465	138	35	13	
Ireland	600	568	141	33	11	
Italy	626	1057	370	44	18	
Norway	209	145	37	28	10	
Japan	1017	1171	284	35	12	
U.S. whites	499	512	136	34	12	
U.S. blacks	163	127	6	14	1	
Africa	263	38	0	6	0	

homocysteine in individuals with two copies of the variant gene can be more than twice those seen in the heterozygote and homozygote wild type [3]. The distribution of the MTHFR genotype varies with population. It is very low in African populations, whereas in Europe and North America the prevalence of T homozygotes ranges between 5 and 15%. In Italy, an even higher prevalence has been reported in some regions (Table I) [9]. The frequency of the T gene (i.e., including the gene frequency in the heterozygote population) in Europe tends to be around a third but is higher in the south and lower in the Baltic countries [10].

THE ROLE OF MTHFR GENOTYPE IN CHRONIC DISEASE

Evidence suggests that homocysteine levels are associated with increased risk of heart disease [11], stroke [12,13], cognitive decline in the elderly, and Alzheimer's disease [14,15]. The MTHFR genotype has been linked with neural tube defects [16] and vascular disease [17] but is also associated with reduced leukemia and breast cancer risk (Table II) [18,19]. The decreased risk of colorectal cancer associated with the MTHFR T genotype appears to be dependent on dietary folate intake [20]. The

TABLE II   Homocysteine Levels or MTHFR Genotype Involvement in Chronic Multifactorial Diseases

Disease	Homocysteine or MTHFR	Risk	Study
Coronary heart disease	Homocysteine	Increased	Numerous; for summary, see Refsum and Ueland (1998) [46]; Eikelboom et al. (1999) [47]
Stroke	Homocysteine	Increased	Matsui et al. (2001) [13]; Bostom et al. (1999) [12]
Neural tube defect	MTHFR	Increased	Shields et al. (1999) [16]
Alzheimer's disease	Homocysteine	Increased	Clarke et al. (1998) [15]
Cognitive function	Homocysteine	Increased	Duthie et al. (2002) [14]
Late onset depression	MTHFR	Increased	Hickie et al. (2001) [48]
Leukaemia	MTHFR	Reduced	Robien and Ulrich (2003) [18]
Breast cancer	MTHFR	Reduced	Sharp et al. (2002) [19]
Colorectal cancer	MTHFR	Mixed	Reduced: Ma et al. (1997) [25] Increased: Ryan and Weir (2001) [49]

mechanism is thought to be through homocysteine accumulation (homocysteine being toxic) and/ or the ability to carry out cellular methylation reactions. A suggested mechanism for the protective effect of MTHFR genotype in relation to cancer is through the less-active enzyme causing increased 5,10-methylenetetrahydrofolate levels for DNA synthesis, thus reducing the chance of uracil misincorporation. To add to the complexity of possible causative mechanisms, homocysteine can induce DNA damage [21]. There has been recent controversy as to whether the role of homocysteine in cardiovascular risk is causative or whether it simply reflects other established risk factors (e.g., age, sex, smoking, blood pressure, cholesterol, physical activity) and impaired renal function in particular [22–24].

THE ROLE OF MTHFR IN BONE HEALTH

It is known that the MTHFR polymorphism is associated with increased levels of homocysteine, and there is a link between homocystinuria and osteoporosis occurring at an early age, with 50% risk of developing osteoporosis before the age of 16 years [25]. Although collagen synthesis for patients with homocystinuria was comparable to matched controls, there was a significant reduction in cross-link production [26]. More recently, in vitro experiments showed that homocysteine metabolites inhibit lysyl oxidase, the enzyme that produces collagen cross-links [27], providing a plausible reason why elevated homocysteine levels may influence bone health. The MTHFR polymorphism was found to be associated with low bone mineral density in postmenopausal Japanese women [28]; however, we have not found an association between MTHFR genotype and BMD in our Scottish population of early postmenopausal women (Macdonald *et al.*, submitted). One explanation for the difference in results is the mixed menopausal status and hormone replacement therapy (HRT) usage of our population, as the influence of hormones dominates bone loss around the time of the menopause [29]. Also, it is likely that there will be differences in dietary intake of B-complex vitamins between the two populations.

VITAMIN B-COMPLEX

ROLE OF B VITAMINS IN REDUCING CIRCULATING HOMOCYSTEINE

It was found that inadequate plasma concentrations of one or more B vitamins contributed to 67% of the cases of high homocysteine in a study of the Framingham elderly [30], and dietary intakes of B vitamins were inversely related to homocysteine levels. The effect of the MTHFR genotype on homocysteine levels is more pronounced at low folate intakes, suggesting the existence of gene nutrient interaction [31]. An intervention trial using healthy subjects ages 20 to 63 years found that T homozygotes required higher folate intakes than individuals with the CT or CC genotype to achieve similarly low homocysteine concentrations, although homocysteine levels were still lower with folate intervention than without [32]. Similarly, in a study of healthy young women ages 19 to 39 years, there were differences in response to folate according to genotype [33].

VITAMINS OF THE B-COMPLEX IN RELATION TO BONE HEALTH

Very few studies have examined whether there is a relationship between B-complex vitamins and markers of bone health. To our knowledge, the only study reporting a relationship between dietary B vitamin intake and a marker of bone health was published in 1986. This longitudinal study of postmenopausal women reported that dietary folate intake was associated with less bone loss at the radius [34]. Most studies on diet and bone health have tended to concentrate on calcium and vitamin D, and only recently have other nutrients started to receive more attention (e.g., protein, salt, vitamin K). Interestingly, erythrocyte folate was found to be a factor associated with greater BMD in postmenopausal Mexican-American women [35]. There is also some evidence to show that hip fracture patients may be vitamin B6 deficient [36]. Although we have investigated dietary folate, riboflavin, vitamin B6, and vitamin B12 in relation to bone health, we could find no association between any vitamin of the B-complex and BMD in postmenopausal women. However, there was a relationship between riboflavin intake and BMD in women who were homozygote for the heat-labile variant of the MTHFR enzyme, suggesting the presence of gene–nutrient interaction (Macdonald et al., submitted).

NORMAL DIETARY INTAKES OF B VITAMINS

In our population of postmenopausal women, the dietary intake of B-complex vitamins appeared to be adequate by U.K. standards (Table III). With the exception of folate, less than 5% of women had intakes of B vitamins below the reference nutrient intake (RNI). Also, most women (89%) had sufficient levels of folate in their diet (exceeding the RNI of 200 µg per day). Intakes were similar or slightly greater than those found for women ages 50 to 64 years in the National Diet and Nutrition Survey of the United Kingdom [37]. However, it may be relevant that a supplementation study of an elderly population, carried out in Aberdeen, found that homocysteine was reduced only with daily supplementation at 400 or 600 µg [38]. This would mean that 86% and 99%, respectively, of our population could be deficient in folate even without taking into account the background contribution from dietary folate in their study (300 µg).

Important food sources of B-complex vitamins for women ages 50 to 64 years are shown in Table IV. Milk and milk products are the main source of riboflavin. In the United Kingdom, milk can be delivered to the home, which is a traditional and important means of obtaining milk for the elderly who may not find it easy to get outside. However, because it is provided in glass bottles and riboflavin is sensitive to light, much of this nutrient could be lost if the bottles are left on the doorstep and exposed to sunlight for any period of time. For vitamin B12, milk and milk products again feature as important sources followed by meat and fish; however, in comparison, for the Framingham study, vitamin B12 supplements, fortified cereal, and milk were the major contributors to intake for this vitamin [39]. Although foods are not supplemented with folate to the same extent in the United Kingdom as in the United States, nevertheless fortified cereals do

TABLE III   B Vitamin Complex Intakes in APOSS Population (Ages 50 to 59 Years) Compared to National Population of Women Ages 51 to 64 Years

B-Complex Vitamin	Intake (Mean ± SD)	U.K. RNI	% Women <RNI	U.K. LRNI	% Women <LRNI	U.K. NDNS (Women 51–64 years)	U.K. NDNS (% Women <LRNI)
Riboflavin (mg/day)	2.0 ± 0.6	1.1	3.8	0.8	1.5	1.8 ± 0.7	6
Folate (µg/day)	304 ± 102	200	11	100	0.3	268 ± 96	2
Vitamin B12 (µg/day)	6.8 ± 3.7	1.5	0.8	1.0	0.4	5.7 ± 3.2	0
Vitamin B6 (mg/day)	2.1 ± 0.6	1.2	3.5	0.8	0.2	2.1 ± 0.7	2

Note: RNI = reference nutrient intake; LRNI = Lower Reference Nutrient Intake; NDNS = National Diet and Nutrition Survey.
Source: Henderson, L. et al. (2003) National Diet and Nutrition Survey: Adults Aged 19 to 64 Years. Social Survey Division of the Office of Population Censuses and Surveys (OPCS) and Medical Research Council Human Nutrition Research, on behalf of the Food Standards Agency and Department of Health, TSO, London.

TABLE IV   Food Sources of B-Complex Vitamins for Women Ages 50 to 64 Years

Vitamin	Important Dietary Sources	Contribution (%)
Vitamin B6	Cereal and cereal products	23
	Potatoes and savory snacks	19
	Meat and meat products	18
	Milk and milk products	10
	Fruit and nuts	10
	Other foods	20
Vitamin B12	Milk and milk products	36
	Fish and fish dishes	26
	Meat and meat products	25
	Other foods	13
Folate	Cereal and cereal products	33
	Vegetables (excluding potatoes)	17
	Potatoes and savory snacks	12
	Fruit and nuts	4
	Other foods	34
Riboflavin (B2)	Milk and milk products	36
	Cereal and cereal products	25
	Meat and meat products	13
	Other foods	26

Source: Henderson, L. et al. (2003) National Diet and Nutrition Survey: Adults Aged 19 to 64 Years. Social Survey Division of the Office of Population Censuses and Surveys (OPCS) and Medical Research Council Human Nutrition Research, on behalf of the Food Standards Agency and Department of Health, TSO, London.

provide an important source of B vitamins, with fruit and vegetables contributing only 4% to the folate intake of middle-aged women (Table IV).

Because homocysteine levels are known to increase with age [40], the MTHFR polymorphism may have a greater influence in older populations. Actual intakes of vitamin B are lower in the elderly and may be deficient. A total of 49% free-living elderly in Northern Ireland were found to have suboptimal intakes of riboflavin [41]. Also, there may be greater demand for folic acid in the elderly. Intakes of 900 µg per day were suggested to be necessary to protect the elderly against heart disease caused by insufficient folate [38]. It is unlikely that this level of intake would be achieved by the majority of people through diet alone because of the large amounts of fruit and vegetables that would need to be consumed, indicating that supplementation or food fortification with folate would be required.

CONCLUSIONS

An association between MTHFR genotype and BMD has been observed in a population of Japanese women, but this finding has not yet been confirmed in another population. It is known that B vitamins influence homocysteine levels, which affect other disease outcomes such as heart disease risk and neural tube defects. There are plausible reasons for why homocysteine may influence bone health. MTHFR requires vitamin B12 and folate to degrade homocysteine, and there is a greater requirement of folate for the heat-labile form of the enzyme. It appears that there may also be a greater requirement for riboflavin. Because homocysteine levels increase with age and B vitamin intake is low in the elderly, MTHFR genotype may play a role in the bone health of the elderly. Further work is required to establish whether homocysteine is a risk factor for osteoporosis, particularly in the elderly population. It is important that future studies with the MTHFR genotype take into account dietary B vitamin intake due to the potential for gene–nutrient interaction. If homocysteine is found to be a risk factor for osteoporosis, supplementation with B vitamins would provide a simple and effective means of reducing the risk and would have the added benefit of reducing the risk of other common chronic diseases such as coronary heart disease, stroke, and Alzheimer's disease.

REFERENCES

1. Ralston, S.H. (2002). Genetic control of susceptibility to osteoporosis. *J. Clin. Endocrinol. Metab.* 87: 2460–2466.

2. Uitterlinden, A.G., Fang, Y., Bergink, A.P., van Meurs, J.B., van Leeuwen, H.P., and Pols, H.A. (2002). The role of vitamin D receptor gene polymorphisms in bone biology. *Mol. Cell. Endocrinol.* 197: 15–21.

3. Frosst, P., Blom, H.J., Milos R., Goyette P., Sheppard C.A., Matthews R.G. *et al.* (1995). A candidate genetic risk factor for vascular disease: a common mutation in methylene-tetrahydrofolate reductase. *Nature Genet.* 10: 111–113.

4. Mudd, S.H., Skovby, F., Levy, H.L., Pettigrew, K.D., Wilcken, B., Pyeritz, R.E., Andria, G., Boers, G.H., Bromberg, I.L., Cerone, R. *et al.* (1985). The natural history of homocystinuria due to cystathionine beta-synthase deficiency. *Am. J. Hum. Genet.* 37: 1–31.

5. Linder, M.C. (1991). *Nutritional Biochemistry and Metabolism with Clinical Applications,* 2nd ed., Elsevier, New York.

6. Guenther, B.D., Sheppard, C.A., Tran, P., Rozen, R., Matthews, R.G., and Ludwig, M.L. (1999). The structure and properties of methylenetetrahydrofolate reductase from *Escherichia coli* suggest how folate ameliorates human hyperhomocysteinemia. *Nature Struct. Biol.* 6: 359–365.

7. McNulty, H., McKinley, M.C., Wilson, B., McPartlin, J., Strain, J.J., Weir, D.G., and Scott, J.M. (2002). Impaired functioning of thermolabile methylenetetrahydrofolate reductase is dependent on riboflavin status: implications for riboflavin requirements. *Am. J. Clin. Nutr.* 76: 436–441.

8. Selhub, J.M.J.W. (1992). The pathogenesis of homocysteinemia: interruption of the coordinate regulation by S-adenosylmethionine of the remethylation and transsulfuration of homocysteine. *Am. J. Clin. Nutr.* 55: 131–138.

9. Cortese, C. and Motti, C. (2001). MTHFR gene polymorphism, homocysteine and cardiovascular disease. *Public Health Nutr.* 4: 493–497.

10. Gudnason, V., Stansbie, D., Scott, J., Bowron, A., Nicaud, V., and Humphries, S. (1998). C677T (thermolabile alanine/valine) polymorphism in methylenetetrahydrofolate reductase (MTHFR): its frequency and impact on plasma homocysteine concentration in different European populations, EARS group. *Atherosclerosis* 136: 347–354.

11. Clarke, R., Daly, L., Robinson, K., Naughten, E., Cahalane, S., and Fowler, B. (1991). Hyperhomocysteinemia: an independent risk factor for vascular disease. *N. Engl. J. Med.* 324: 1149–1155.

12. Bostom, A.G., Rosenberg, I.H., Silbershatz, H., Jacques, P.F., Selhub, J., D'Agostino, R.B., Wilson, P.W., and Wolf, P.A. (1999). Nonfasting plasma total homocysteine levels and stroke incidence in elderly persons: the Framingham study. *Ann. Intern. Med.* 131: 352–355.

13. Matsui, T., Arai, H., Yuzuriha, T., Yao, H., Miura, M., Hashimoto, S., Higuchi, S., Matsushita, S., Morikawa, M., Kato, A., and Sasaki, H. (2001). Elevated plasma homocysteine levels and risk of silent brain infarction in elderly people. *Stroke* 32: 1116–1169.

14. Duthie, S.J., Whalley, L.J., Collins, A.R., Leaper, S., Berger, K., and Deary, I.J. (2002). Homocysteine, B vitamin status, and cognitive function in the elderly. *Am. J. Clin. Nutr.* 75: 908–913.

15. Clarke, R., Smith, A.D., Jobst, K.A., Refsum, H., Sutton, L., and Ueland, P.M. (1998). Folate, vitamin B12, and serum total homocysteine levels in confirmed Alzheimer disease. *Arch. Neurol.* 55: 1449–1455.

16. Shields, D.C., Kirke, P.N., Mills, J.L., Ramsbottom, D., Molloy, A.M., Burke, H., Weir, D.G., Scott, J.M., and Whitehead, A.S. (1999). The "thermolabile" variant of methylenetetrahy-drofolate reductase and neural tube defects: an evaluation of genetic risk and the relative importance of the genotypes of the embryo and the mother. *Am. J. Hum. Genet.* 64: 1045–1055.

17. Tsai, M.Y., Welge, B.G., Hanson, N.Q., Bignell, M.K., Vessey, J., Schwichtenberg, K., Yang, F., Bullemer, F.E., Rasmussen, R., and Graham, K.J. (1999). Genetic causes of mild

hyperhomocysteinemia in patients with premature occlusive coronary artery diseases. *Atherosclerosis* 143: 163–170.

18. Robien, K. and Ulrich, C.M. (2003). 5,10-Methylenetetrahydrofolate reductase polymorphisms and leukemia risk: a HUGE minireview. *Am. J. Epidemiol.* 157: 571–182.

19. Sharp, L., Little, J., Schofield, A.C., Pavlidou, E., Cotton, S.C., Miedzybrodzka, Z., Baird, J.O., Haites, N.E., Heys, S.D., and Grubb, D.A. (2002). Folate and breast cancer: the role of polymorphisms in methylenetetrahydrofolate reductase (MTHFR). *Cancer Lett.* 181: 65–71.

20. Ma, J., Stampfer, M.J., Giovannucci, E., Artigas, C., Hunter, D.J., Fuchs, C., Willett, W.C., Selhub, J., Hennekens, C.H., and Rozen, R. (1997). Methylenetetrahydrofolate reductase polymorphism, dietary interactions and risk of colon cancer. *Cancer Res.* 57: 1098–1102.

21. Huang, R.F., Huang, S.M., Lin, B.S., Wei, J.S., and Liu, T.Z. (2001). Homocysteine thiolactone induces apoptotic DNA damage mediated by increased intracellular hydrogen peroxide and caspase 3 activation in Hl-60 cells. *Life Sci.* 68: 2799–2811.

22. Brattstrom, L., Wilcken, D.E., Ohrvik, J., and Brudin, L. (1998). Common methylenetetrahydrofolate reductase gene mutation leads to hyperhomocysteinemia but not to vascular disease: the result of a meta-analysis. *Circulation* 98: 2520–2526.

23. Brattstrom, L. and Wilcken, D.E. (2000). Homocysteine and cardiovascular disease: cause or effect? *Am. J. Clin. Nutr.* 72: 315–323.

24. Ueland, P.M., Refsum, H., Beresford, S.A., and Vollset, S.E. (2000). The controversy over homocysteine and cardiovascular risk. *Am. J. Clin. Nutr.* 72: 324–332.

25. Ma, J., Stampfer, M.J., Giovannucci, E., Artigas, C., Hunter, D.J., Fuchs, C., Willett, W.C., Selhub, J., Hennekens, C.H., and Rozen, R. (1997). Methylenetetrahydrofolate reductase polymorphism, dietary interactions, and risk of colorectal cancer. *Cancer Res.* 57: 1098–1102.

26. Lubec, B., Fang-Kircher, S., Lubec, T., Blom, H.J., and Boers, G.H.J. (1996). Evidence for McKuisik's hypothesis of deficient collagen cross–linking in patients with homocystinuria. *Biochim Biophys Acta* 1315: 159–162.

27. Liu, G., Nellaiappan, K., and Kagan, H.M. (1997). Irreversible inhibition of lysyl oxidase by homocysteine thiolactone and its selenium and oxygen analogues. *J. Biol. Chem.* 51: 32370–32377.

28. Miyao, M., Morita, H., Hosoi, T., Kurihara, H., Inoue, S., Hoshino, S., Shiraki, M., Yazaki, Y., and Ouchi, Y. (2000). Association of methylenetetrahydrofolate reductase (MHTFR) polymorphism with bone mineral density in postmenopausal Japanese women. *Calcif. Tissue Int.* 66: 190–194.

29. Macdonald, H.M., New, S.A., Golden, M.H.N., Campbell, M.K., and Reid, D.M. (2004). Nutritional associations with bone loss during the menopausal transition: evidence of a beneficial effect for calcium, alcohol, and fruit and vegetable nutrients and a detrimental effect for fatty acids. *Am. J. Clin. Nutr.* 79: 155–165.

30. Selhub, J., Jacques, P.F., Wilson, P.W., Rush, D., and Rosenberg, I.H. (1993). Vitamin status and intake as primary determinants of homocysteinemia in an elderly population. *JAMA* 270: 2693–2698.

31. Ma, J., Stampfer, M.J., Hennekens, C.H., Frosst, P., Selhub, J., Horsford, J., Malinow, M.R., Willett, W.C., and Rozen, R. (1996). Methylenetetrahydrofolate reductase polymorphism, plasma folate, homocysteine, and risk of myocardial infarction in U.S. physicians. *Circulation* 94: 2410–2416.

32. Ashfield-Watt, P.A., Pullin, C.H., Whiting, J.M., Clark, Z.E., Moat, S.J., Newcombe, R.G., Burr, M.L., Lewis, M.J., Powers, H.J., and McDowell, I.F. (2002). Methylenetetrahydrofolate reductase 677C ⇒ T genotype modulates homocysteine responses to a folate-rich diet or a low-dose folic acid supplement: a randomized controlled trial. *Am. J. Clin. Nutr.* 76: 180–186.

33. Fohr, I.P., Prinz-Langenohl, R., Bronstrup, A., Bohlmann, A.M., Nau, H., Berthold, H.K., and Pietrzik, K. (2002). 5,10-Methylenetetrahydrofolate reductase genotype determines the

plasma homocysteine-lowering effect of supplementation with 5-methyltetrahydrofolate or folic acid in healthy young women. *Am. J. Clin. Nutr.* 75: 275–282.

34. Freudenheim, J.L., Johnson, N.E., and Smith, E.L. (1986). Relationships between usual nutrient intake and bone mineral content of women 35–65 years of age: longitudinal and cross-sectional analysis. *Am. J. Clin. Nutr.* 44: 863–876.

35. Villa, M.L., Marcus, R., Ramirez-Delay, R., and Kelsey, J.L. (1995). Factors contributing to skeletal health of postmenopausal Mexican-American women. *J. Bone Mineral Res.* 10: 1233–1242.

36. Reynolds, T.M., Marshall, P.D., and Brain, A.M. (1992). Hip fracture patients may be vitamin B6 deficient. *Acta Orthop. Scand.* 63: 635–638.

37. Henderson, L., Irving, K., Gregory, J., Bates, C.J., Prentice, A., Perks, J., Swan, G., and Farron, M. (2003). *National Diet and Nutrition Survey: Adults Aged 19 to 64 Years.* Social Survey Division of the Office of Population Censuses and Surveys (OPCS) and Medical Research Council Human Nutrition Research, on behalf of the Food Standards Agency and Department of Health, TSO, London.

38. Rydlewicz, A., Simpson, J.A., Taylor, R.J., Bond, C.M., and Golden, M.H. (2002). The effect of folic acid supplementation on plasma homocysteine in an elderly population. *QJM* 95: 27–35.

39. Tucker, K.L., Rich, S., Rosenberg, I., Jacques, P., Dallal, G., Wilson, P.W., Selhub, J. (2000). Plasma vitamin B-12 concentrations relate to intake source in the Framingham Offspring study. *Am. J. Clin. Nutr.* 71: 514–522.

40. Jacques, P.F., Bostom, A.G., Wilson, P.W., Rich, S., Rosenberg, I.H., and Selhub, J. (2001). Determinants of plasma total homocysteine concentration in the Framingham Offspring cohort. *Am. J. Clin. Nutr.* 73: 613–621.

41. Madigan, S.M., Tracey, F., McNulty, H., Eaton-Evans, J., Coulter J., McCartney, H., and Strain, J.J. (1998). Riboflavin and vitamin B-6 intakes and status and biochemical response to riboflavin supplementation in free-living elderly people. *Am. J. Clin. Nutr.* 68: 389–395.

42. Meleady, R., Ueland, P.M., Blom, H., Whitehead, A.S., Refsum, H., Daly, L.E., Vollset, S.E., Donohue, C., Giesendorf, B., Graham, I.M., Ulvik, A., Zhang, Y., Bjorke Monsen, A.L., and the European Concerted Action Project: Homocysteine and Vascular Disease. (2003). Thermolabile methylenetetrahydrofolate reductase, homocysteine, and cardiovascular disease risk: the European Concerted Action Project. *Am. J. Clin. Nutr.* 77: 63–70.

43. Dekou, V., Gudnason, V., Hawe, E., Miller, G.J., Stansbie, D., and Humphries, S.E. (2001). Gene–environment and gene–gene interaction in the determination of plasma homocysteine levels in healthy middle-aged men. *Thrombosis Haemostasis* 85: 67–74.

44. Castro, R., Rivera, I., Ravasco, P., Jakobs, C., Blom, H.J., Camilo, M.E., and de Almeida, I.T. (2003). 5,10-Methylenetetrahydrofolate reductase 677C $\Rightarrow$ T and 1298A $\Rightarrow$ C mutations are genetic determinants of elevated homocysteine. *QJM* 96: 297–303.

45. Botto, L.D. and Yang Q. (2000). 5,10-Methylenetetrahydrofolate reductase gene variants and congenital anomalies: a HUGE review. *Am. J. Epidemiol.* 151: 862–877.

46. Refsum, H., Ueland, P.M., Nygard, O., and Vollset, S.E. (1998). Homocysteine and cardiovascular disease. *Annu. Rev. Med.* 49: 31–62.

47. Eikelboom, J.W., Lonn, E., Genest, J., Jr., Hankey, G., and Yusuf, S. (1999). Homocyst(e)ine and cardiovascular disease: a critical review of the epidemiologic evidence. *Ann. Intern. Med.* 131: 363–375.

48. Hickie, I., Scott, E., Naismith, S., Ward, P.B., Turner, K., Parker, G., Mitchell, P., and Wilhelm, K. (2001). Late-onset depression: genetic, vascular and clinical contributions. *Psychol. Med.* 31: 1403–1412.

49. Ryan, B.M. and Weir, D.G. (2001). Relevance of folate metabolism in the pathogenesis of colorectal cancer. *J. Lab. Clin. Med.* 138: 164–176.

PART IV

Nutrition and Bone Health Miscellaneous

A Placebo Controlled Randomized Trial of Chromium Picolinate Supplementation on Indices of Bone and Calcium Metabolism in Healthy Women

MONICA ADHIKARI,[1] BRIAN W. MORRIS,[2] RICHARD EASTELL,[3] and AUBREY BLUMSOHN[3]

[1]Human Nutrition Unit; [2]Clinical Biochemistry; [3]Bone Metabolism Group, University of Sheffield, Northern General Hospital, Sheffield, United Kingdom

ABSTRACT

BACKGROUND

It has been suggested that the trace element chromium may be required for bone health. Chromium supplementation has been shown to reduce excretion of hydroxyproline in one study. This hypothesis has not otherwise been tested in humans but is promoted in the health-food literature. It does have a possible biochemical rationale, because chromium may enhance the anabolic-effect action of insulin on bone or modulate parathyroid hormone (PTH) action.

OBJECTIVE

We examined the effect of chromium picolinate supplementation ($n = 18$; 300 μg daily for 8 weeks) or matched placebo ($n = 8$) on indices of skeletal metabolism in apparently healthy premenopausal or postmenopausal women.

Nutritional Aspects of Osteoporosis, Second Edition
Copyright © 2004 by Elsevier Science (USA)

Design

Second-void urine samples were collected on three consecutive days prior to supplementation, following 4 weeks of supplementation, and at the end of the supplementation period. Blood samples were collected before and after supplementation. Measurements included serum β C-terminal telopeptide of type I collagen (sβCTX) and urinary N-telopeptide as markers of bone resorption, serum procollagen type I N-terminal propeptide, and bone-specific alkaline phosphatase as markers of bone formation, PTH, fasting insulin and glucose, and urinary chromium.

Results

There was no significant effect of chromium supplementation on any measurement (all $P > 0.05$, paired t-test), apart from urinary chromium. Urinary chromium increased about 20-fold with supplementation (0.23 ± 0.04 SEM to 4.6 ± 1.0 µmol/mol creatinine; $P < 0.001$). sβCTX was 0.292 ± 0.04 ng/mL and 0.305 ± 0.04 ng/mL before and after supplementation, respectively ($P = 0.992$, paired t-test).

Conclusions

We have found no evidence to support the assertion that chromium supplementation influences bone metabolism in healthy women.

INTRODUCTION

It has been estimated that 10 million Americans take supplemental chromium [1]. The role of this trace element in human metabolism has not been clearly defined. Isolated overt chromium deficiency is associated with impaired glucose tolerance and elevated plasma lipids in both animals and humans [2,3], and these changes are reversed by chromium supplementation. We and others have provided evidence supporting a possible role for chromium supplementation in patients with type II diabetes mellitus [1,4–6] and have shown that chromium supplementation may improve diabetic control and insulin sensitivity in patients with type II diabetes [7] and corticosteroid-induced diabetes [8].

The benefits of chromium supplementation in the general population, however, are less certain. Estimated dietary chromium intake in most populations is of the order of about 30 μg/day [9]. Several small studies conducted by ourselves [10] and others (see Gunton et al. [11] and Anderson [9] for review) have found that chromium supplementation may lower fasting serum glucose and fasting serum insulin, increase insulin sensitivity, and lower plasma lipids in apparently healthy adults. We have also found that circadian changes in plasma chromium and urine chromium excretion appear to relate to plasma insulin in healthy volunteers [12]. Plasma glucose and insulin in healthy individuals declined in one study when these individuals were maintained on a diet containing levels of chromium found in the lowest quartile of normal intake[9]. Albeit controversial, these studies suggest that chromium "deficiency" might, in some sense be common.

Clinicians treating patients with diabetes mellitus have been reluctant to explore the possible clinical benefits of chromium supplementation in larger studies, despite ample evidence suggesting they should do this. Paradoxically however, the widespread use of chromium supplements in the population appears to have more to do with the perceived ability of supplementation to alter body composition by enhancing weight loss, increasing lean body mass, and increasing bone mineral density. The evidence underlying the widespread promotion of chromium supplements to alter body composition is far more problematical. Chromium supplementation has been reported to increase muscle bulk and growth in some animal studies [13–15]. Evans [16] reported that chromium supplementation in humans resulted in greater increments in muscle bulk during resistance training in comparison with no supplementation. Similar results were reported by Crawford et al. [17] in a study in African-American women. Almost all other investigators, however, have failed to show any significant benefit (for collated data, see [18] and also [17,19–21]).

It has also been hypothesized that chromium is required for bone health and preservation of bone mineral content[22,23]. One study reported by Evans et al. [24] (only in abstract form) showed that urinary excretion of hydroxyproline (a non-specific indicator biochemical marker of bone collagen resorption) as well as calcium excretion decrease following chromium supplementation in healthy women. This hypothesis has not otherwise been tested at all in humans but is nevertheless widely cited in health-food literature and on the Internet.

The hypothesis that chromium supplementation might benefit bone does have a possible biochemical rationale. Insulin receptors are present on osteoblasts, and insulin modulates bone collagen synthesis [25]. Insulin sensitivity may be associated with bone mineral density in non-diabetic men [26]. It is also possible that chromium might influence the skeletal action of parathyroid hormone, at least in theory [22]. Chromium is incorporated into bone [27] and might alter the assembly of collagen in bone [28]. In contrast to these hypothetical benefits, relatively high concentrations of chromium have been shown to suppress osteoblast production of alkaline phosphatase, osteocalcin, and type I collagen *in vitro* [29,30], suggesting a possible deleterious effect on bone metabolism. At least in the Japanese quail, chromium supplementation does not appear to have a major effect on femur fracture force or calcium content [31]. Slightly higher bone breaking strength was observed in broilers fed chromium supplements in one study [32], but this finding was not statistically significant.

The aim of this study was to investigate whether chromium supplementation has any effect on bone metabolism in healthy women.

SUBJECTS

A total of 26 apparently healthy women were randomly assigned to one of two treatment groups using unbalanced randomization (18 participants received chromium, 8 received placebo). Participants were recruited through posters and advertisements. Exclusion criteria included use of any drugs known to influence bone metabolism within the previous 6 months, any previous use of a bisphosphonate, any disease known to influence calcium metabolism, a fracture within the previous year, or use of a chromium-containing multivitamin supplement. Signed informed consent was obtained from participants, and the study was approved by the North Sheffield Research Ethics Committee.

METHODS

STUDY DESIGN

The study was a double-blind, placebo, controlled, randomized trial of chromium picolinate supplementation (300 µg elemental chromium per day). Chromium picolinate (Chromax supplied by Nutrition 21, New York; http://www.ambiinc.com/) and placebo were compounded using a matched excipient and were supplied in identical gelatin capsules. Supplement or placebo were taken between 08:00 hr and 11:00 hr daily for a period of 8 weeks and 3 days. Compliance was assessed by tablet count and assay of urinary chromium.

Second-morning-void urine samples were collected on 3 consecutive days prior to supplementation and on the same 3 days of the week at the end of the supplementation period. Second-morning-void urine samples were also collected on 2 consecutive days after 4 weeks of supplementation. Fasting blood samples were collected between 09:00 hr and 09:30 hr prior to and on the last day of supplementation. Aliquots of serum and urine were stored at $-80°C$ until assayed.

BIOCHEMICAL METHODS

Urinary chromium was determined by electrothermal atomic absorption spectrophotometry (Perkin-Elmer SIMAA 6000 Zeeman; Perkin-Elmer, Ltd., Norwalk, CT) as previously described [33]. Plasma insulin was measured using a two-site immunometric assay which has negligible cross-reactivity with intact proinsulin (Roche Elecsys; Roche Diagnostics, Mannheim, Germany). Biochemical markers of bone resorption included serum β C-terminal telopeptide fragment of type I collagen (sβCTX, Roche Elecsys; Roche Diagnostics, Mannheim, Germany) and urinary N-terminal telopeptide of type I collagen (uNTX; Ortho-Clinical Diagnostics, Rochester, USA). Biochemical markers of bone formation included serum procollagen type I N-terminal propeptide (sPINP; Roche Elecsys; Roche Diagnostics, Mannheim, Germany) and serum bone-specific alkaline phosphatase (bone ALP, Alkphase B; Metra Biosystems, Inc., Mountain View, CA). Serum parathyroid hormone (PTH) was measured by immunoassay (Roche Elecsys; Roche Diagnostics, Mannheim, Germany). Urinary creatinine and plasma glucose were measured using dry slide technology (Vitros 250; Ortho-Clinical Diagnostics, Rochester, NY) and urinary results were expressed as a ratio to creatinine excretion. The intra-assay analytical imprecision was less than 4% (coefficient of variation) for all assays over the reference interval with the exception of sβCTX, which was 8.1%.

STATISTICAL ANALYSIS

Analyses were performed using *Statistical Package for the Social Sciences* (SPSS). All tests were two-tailed, and $P < 0.05$ was regarded as being statistically significant. Simple paired t-tests were used to compare measurements before and after supplementation. Study power calculated *a priori* showed that there was 95% power to detect a 15% change in bone turnover using uNTX as the primary response variable based on triplicate urine collection and the known standard deviation of change in healthy untreated women.

RESULTS

There were no significant differences between baseline characteristics of participants randomized to receive chromium picolinate or placebo (Table I). Compliance was assessed by direct questioning at interview by tablet count and measurement of urinary chromium (Fig. 1). One participant appeared to have omitted 3 doses of supplement based on tablet count, but other participants omitted 2 doses or fewer. Baseline urinary chromium excretion was not significantly different between placebo and supplemented groups, and there was a highly significant increase (approximately 20-fold, $P < 0.001$) in urinary chromium excretion in participants randomized to receive chromium (Fig. 1). There were no reported adverse events in participants receiving chromium. One participant randomized to placebo reported pain in the right metacarpo-phalangeal joint following 6 weeks of supplementation.

Change in other analytes in response to chromium picolinate or placebo are shown in Table II. There was no significant change in any analyte apart from urinary chromium in response to either chromium supplementation or placebo. Results for one serum marker of bone resorption

TABLE I Baseline Characteristics of Study Participants

	Randomization		
	Placebo (mean ± SEM)	Chromium (mean ± SEM)	P
Number	8 (4 postmenopausal)	18 (9 postmenopausal)	—
Age	45.0 ± 7.0	46.2 ± 3.1	NS
Weight (kg)	63.4 ± 2.6	66.9 ± 2.8	NS
Height (m)	1.65 ± 0.02	1.65 ± 0.02	NS
uChromium (μmol/mmol)	0.22 ± 0.06	0.23 ± 0.04	NS
Fasting glucose (mmol/L)	5.3 ± 1.3	5.4 ± 1.1	NS
Plasma insulin (pmol/L)	6.8 ± 1.1	7.8 ± 1.3	NS
sβCTX (ng/mL)	0.288 ± 0.04	0.292 ± 0.04	NS
uNTX (nmol/mmol)	46.7 ± 7.1	45.5 ± 6.4	NS
sPINP (ng/mL)	42.4 ± 4.4	47.30 ± 2.9	NS
Bone ALP	17.3 ± 1.2	19.3 ± 1.1	NS
PTH (pg/mL)	30.0 ± 2.7	31.8 ± 3.1	NS

Note: Urinary data are expressed as a ratio to creatinine excretion. NS: not significant.

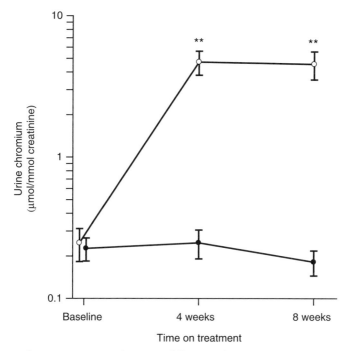

FIGURE 1   Change in urinary chromium following chromium supplementation (○) or placebo (●). **$P < 0.001$ versus both placebo (t-test) or baseline chromium excretion (paired t-test).

(sβCTX) in individual participants receiving chromium picolinate are shown in Fig. 2. There was also no significant relationship between urinary chromium excretion prior to supplementation and the change in any marker of bone turnover in response to chromium supplementation (Pearson correlation: all $P > 0.52$, all $R^2 < 4\%$).

DISCUSSION

Despite clear evidence that chromium does play an important biological role [2,3], relatively little is known about the exact biological form of "active" chromium or its biological action. Chromium is believed to act physiologically as a low-molecular-weight Cr–nicotinic acid complex named glucose tolerance factor (GTF). Simonoff *et al.* [34] found that the GTF activity of yeast might not be dependent on its chromium content. A naturally occurring low-molecular-weight chromium-binding substance (LMWCr) has been

TABLE II   Percentage Change in Biochemical Measurements Following 8 Week
Supplementation Period

	Randomization		
	Placebo (mean ± SEM)	Chromium (mean ± SEM)	P^a
Number	8	18	—
Urine chromium	2.1 ± 31.6	5188 ± 1727**	0.008
Fasting glucose	0.3 ± 4.1	−4.9 ± 2.5	0.273
Plasma insulin	ND	4.9 ± 11	—
sβCTX	−1.2 ± 6.9	2.3 ± 5.2	0.70
UNTX	0.07 ± 10.6	−7.4 ± 8.3	0.61
sPINP	3.9 ± 7.5	−3.1 ± 2.1	0.24
Bone ALP	0.88 ± 5.6	−5.5 ± 2.8	0.27
PTH	−4.4 ± 12.3	−7.4 ± 10.0	0.86

[a]Significance of difference in change in treated versus placebo arms (unpaired t-test assuming
unequal variance).
**$P < 0.001$, significance of change from baseline in chromium supplemented group (paired
t-test). ND: not determined; two specimens in placebo arm hemolyzed

identified and purified, and it appears that this substance binds to the insulin
receptor, potentiating insulin action [35].

Chromium is incorporated into bone [27] and might alter the assembly of
collagen in bone [28]. There is hypothetical evidence that chromium might
influence the action of insulin or parathyroid hormone on bone [22], and it is
known that insulin sensitivity may be associated with bone mineral density in
non-diabetic men [26]; however, we have been unable to confirm the
assertion [22–24] that chromium picolinate supplementation has any effect
on skeletal metabolism in healthy women.

One study reported by Evans et al. [24] showed that urinary excretion of
hydroxyproline as well as calcium excretion decrease following chromium
supplementation in healthy women. Urinary hydroxyproline lacks specificity
as a marker of bone resorption due to contributions from non-osseous
sources, dietary absorption, and extensive metabolism. Other recently
developed methodologies are much more specific and are highly responsive
to changes in turnover [36]. Markers of bone turnover are sensitive and
specific indicators of the skeletal response to other nutrients thought to
influence bone health, such as calcium [37,38].

The exact dose of chromium likely to be beneficial is unknown. In one
study, supplementation with 1000 μg of chromium as chromium picolinate
appeared to have a somewhat greater effect on postprandial insulin and
glucose than did a 200 μg dose [39]. We employed the commonly
recommended dose of 300 μg of chromium as chromium picolinate.

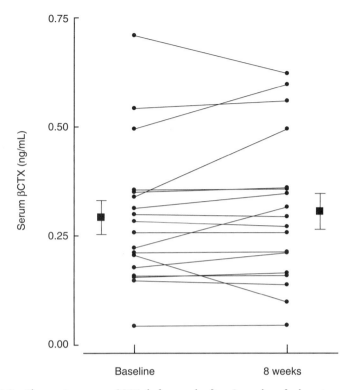

FIGURE 2   Change in serum βCTX before and after 8 weeks of chromium picolinate supplementation. Results for individual participants (●) with mean ±SEM before and after supplementation (■). Paired *t*-test, $P = 0.36$.

The type of supplement may be important. It has been suggested that the failure of many studies to show other beneficial effects of chromium supplementation may relate to the use of supplements other than chromium picolinate [11]. Chromium picolinate is a commercially licensed supplement that appears to be more efficiently absorbed. The quality of reports are variable, however, and the impact of publication and commercial bias is difficult to assess. More importantly, the long-term clinical impact of these observed physiological responses to chromium are not known.

Any possible beneficial effects of chromium supplementation has to be weighed against the possibility of adverse side effects. Concerns have been raised about potential for chromium toxicity, but in general the risk of obvious adverse effects with generally obtainable trivalent chromium supplements appears small [9,40]. There are isolated case reports of renal failure [41,42], rhabdomyolysis [43], and acute pustular dermatitis [44] following ingestion of over-the-counter chromium supplements. It is also suggested picolinic acid may induce psychiatric disorders in susceptible individuals, and theoretical concerns have been raised that chromium picolinate might cleave DNA and have a mutagenic effect [45] *in vitro*.

In conclusion, we have found no evidence to support the assertion that chromium supplementation influences bone metabolism in healthy women. Possible effects of chromium on body composition are controversial. There is currently no evidence to support the use of chromium supplements for management of skeletal risk in unselected women.

ACKNOWLEDGMENTS

We thank Roche Diagnostics GmbH, Mannheim, Germany, for supply of reagents, AMBI, Inc./Nutrition 21 for supply of chromium picolinate. None of the authors has any competing interests.

REFERENCES

1. Hellerstein, M.K. (1998). Is chromium supplementation effective in managing type II diabetes? *Nutr. Rev.* 56: 302–306.
2. Jeejeebhoy, K.N., Chu, R.C., Marliss, E.B., Greenberg, G.R., and Bruce-Robertson, A. (1977). Chromium deficiency, glucose intolerance, and neuropathy reversed by chromium supplementation, in a patient receiving long-term total parenteral nutrition. *Am. J. Clin. Nutr.* 30: 531–538.
3. Brown, R.O., Forloines-Lynn, S., Cross, R.E., and Heizer, W.D. (1986). Chromium deficiency after long-term total parenteral nutrition. *Dig. Dis. Sci.* 31: 661–664.
4. Morris, B.W., Kemp, G.J., and Hardisty, C.A. (1985). Plasma chromium and chromium excretion in diabetes. *Clin. Chem.* 31: 334–335.
5. Morris, B.W., MacNeil, S., Hardisty, C.A., Heller, S., Burgin, C., and Gray, T.A. (1999). Chromium homeostasis in patients with type II (NIDDM) diabetes. *J. Trace Elem. Med. Biol.* 13: 57–61.
6. Morris, B.W. (1999). Chromium action and glucose homeostasis. *J. Trace Elements Exp. Med.* 12: 61–70.
7. Morris, B.W., Kouta, S., Robinson, R., MacNeil, S., and Heller, S. (2000). Chromium supplementation improves insulin resistance in patients with type 2 diabetes mellitus. *Diabet. Med.* 17: 684–685.
8. Ravina, A., Slezak, L., Mirsky, N., Bryden, N.A., and Anderson, R.A. (1999). Reversal of corticosteroid-induced diabetes mellitus with supplemental chromium. *Diabet. Med.* 16: 164–167.
9. Anderson, R.A. (1997). Chromium as an essential nutrient for humans. *Regul. Toxicol. Pharmacol.* 26: S35–S41.
10. Morris, B., Peacey, S.R., MacNeil, S., Gray, T. (1998). Enhancement in insulin sensitivity in healthy volunteers following supplementation with chromium picolinate. *Med. Biochem.* 1: 65–72.

11. Gunton, J.E., Hams, G., Hitchman, R., and McElduff, A. (2001). Serum chromium does not predict glucose tolerance in late pregnancy. *Am. J. Clin. Nutr.* 73: 99–104.
12. Morris, B.W., Blumsohn, A., Mac, N.S., and Gray, T.A. (1992). The trace element chromium—a role in glucose homeostasis. *Am. J. Clin. Nutr.* 55: 989–991.
13. Boleman, S.L., Boleman, S.J., Bidner, T.D., Southern, L.L., Ward, T.L., Pontif, J.E., and Pike, M.M. (1995). Effect of chromium picolinate on growth, body composition, and tissue accretion in pigs. *J. Anim. Sci.* 73: 2033–2042.
14. Mooney, K.W. and Cromwell, G.L. (1997). Efficacy of chromium picolinate and chromium chloride as potential carcass modifiers in swine. *J. Anim. Sci.* 75: 2661–2671.
15. Kornegay, E.T., Wang, Z., Wood, C.M., and Lindemann, M.D. (1997). Supplemental chromium picolinate influences nitrogen balance, dry matter digestibility, and carcass traits in growing-finishing pigs. *J. Anim. Sci.* 75: 1319–1323.
16. Evans, G.W. (1989). The effect of chromium picolinate on insulin controlled parameters in humans. *J. Biosoc. Med. Res.* 11: 163–180.
17. Crawford, V., Scheckenbach, R., and Preuss, H.G. (1999). Effects of niacin-bound chromium supplementation on body composition in overweight African-American women. *Diabetes Obes. Metab.* 1: 331–337.
18. Trent, L.K. and Thieding-Cancel, D. (1995). Effects of chromium picolinate on body composition. *J. Sports Med. Phys. Fitness* 35: 273–280.
19. Lukaski, H.C. (2000). Magnesium, zinc, and chromium nutriture and physical activity. *Am. J. Clin. Nutr.* 72: 585S–593S.
20. Clarkson, P.M. and Rawson, E.S. (1999). Nutritional supplements to increase muscle mass. *Crit. Rev. Food Sci. Nutr.* 39: 317–328.
21. Kobla, H.V. and Volpe, S.L. (2000). Chromium, exercise, and body composition. *Crit. Rev. Food Sci. Nutr.* 40: 291–308.
22. McCarty, M.F. (1995). Anabolic effects of insulin on bone suggest a role for chromium picolinate in preservation of bone density. *Med. Hypoth.* 45: 241–246.
23. McCarty, M.F. (1997). Insulin and bone: speculations and future prospects. *Endocrinol. Metab.* 4: 1–3.
24. Evans, G.W., Swenson, G., and Walters, K. (1995). Chromium picolinate decreases calcium excretion and increases dehydroepiandrosterone (DHEA) in post menopausal women. *FASEB J.* 9: A449.
25. Pun, K.K., Lau, P., and Ho, P.W. (1989). The characterization, regulation, and function of insulin receptors on osteoblast-like clonal osteosarcoma cell line. *J. Bone Mineral Res.* 4: 853–862.
26. Abrahamsen, B., Rohold, A., Henriksen, J.E., and Beck-Nielsen, H. (2000). Correlations between insulin sensitivity and bone mineral density in non-diabetic men. *Diabet. Med.* 17: 124–129.
27. O'Flaherty, E.J., Kerger, B.D., Hays, S.M., and Paustenbach, D.J. (2001). A physiologically based model for the ingestion of chromium(III) and chromium(VI) by humans. *Toxicol. Sci.* 60: 196–213.
28. Gayatri, R., Sharma, A.K., Rajaram, R., and Ramasami, T. (2001). Chromium(III)-induced structural changes and self-assembly of collagen. *Biochem. Biophys. Res. Commun.* 283: 229–235.
29. Wang, J.Y., Wicklund, B.H., Gustilo, R.B., and Tsukayama, D.T. (1997). Prosthetic metals interfere with the functions of human osteoblast cells in vitro. *Clin. Orthop.* 339: 216–226.
30. Allen, M.J., Myer, B.J., Millett, P.J., and Rushton, N. (1997). The effects of particulate cobalt, chromium and cobalt–chromium alloy on human osteoblast-like cells *in vitro*. *J. Bone Joint Surg. Br.* 79: 475–482.

31. Hermann, J., Goad, C., Stoecker, B., Arquitt, A., Porter, R., Adeleye, B., Claypool, P.L., and Brusewitz, G. (1997). Effects of dietary chromium, copper and zinc on femur fracture force and femur calcium concentration in male Japanese quail. *Nutr. Res.* 17: 1529–1540.

32. Lee, D.N., Wu, F.Y., Cheng, Y.H., Lin, R.S., and Wu, P.C. (2003). Effects of dietary chromium picolinate supplementation on growth performance and immune responses of broilers. *Asian–Austr. J. Anim. Sci.* 16: 227–233.

33. Lagarda, M.J., Alonso, D.A., and Farre, R. (1991). The use of direct determination of chromium in human urine by electrothermal atomic absorption spectrometry in diabetic patients. *J. Pharm. Biomed. Anal.* 9: 191–194.

34. Simonoff, M., Shapcott, D., Alameddine, S., Sutter-Dub, M.T., and Simonoff, G. (1992). The isolation of glucose tolerance factors from brewer's yeast and their relation to chromium. *Biol. Trace Elem. Res.* 32: 25–38.

35. Vincent, J.B. (1999). Mechanisms of chromium action: low-molecular-weight chromium-binding substance. *J. Am. Coll. Nutr.* 18: 6–12.

36. Blumsohn, A. and Eastell, R. (1997). The performance and utility of biochemical markers of bone turnover: do we know enough to use them in clinical practice? *Ann. Clin. Biochem.* 34(pt. 5): 449–459.

37. Blumsohn, A., Herrington, K., Hannon, R.A., Shao, P., Eyre, D.R., and Eastell, R. (1994). The effect of calcium supplementation on the circadian rhythm of bone resorption. *J. Clin. Endocrinol. Metab* 79: 730–735.

38. Rubinacci, A., Divieti, P., Polo, R.M., Zampino, M., Resmini, G., and Tenni, R. (1996). Effect of an oral calcium load on urinary markers of collagen breakdown. *J. Endocrinol. Invest* 19: 719–726.

39. Anderson, R.A., Cheng, N., Bryden, N.A., Polansky, M.M., Cheng, N., Chi, J., and Feng, J. (1997). Elevated intakes of supplemental chromium improve glucose and insulin variables in individuals with type 2 diabetes. *Diabetes* 46: 1786–1791.

40. Anderson, R.A., Bryden, N.A., and Polansky, M.M. (1997). Lack of toxicity of chromium chloride and chromium picolinate in rats. *J. Am. Coll. Nutr.* 16: 273–279.

41. Wasser, W.G., Feldman, N.S., and D'Agati, V.D. (1997). Chronic renal failure after ingestion of over-the-counter chromium picolinate. *Ann. Intern. Med.* 126: 410.

42. Cerulli, J., Grabe, D.W., Gauthier, I., Malone, M., and McGoldrick, M.D. (1998). Chromium picolinate toxicity. *Ann. Pharmacother.* 32: 428–431.

43. Martin, W.R. and Fuller, R.E. (1998). Suspected chromium picolinate-induced rhabdomyolysis. *Pharmacotherapy* 18: 860–862.

44. Young, P.C., Turiansky, G.W., Bonner, M.W., and Benson, P.M. (1999). Acute generalized exanthematous pustulosis induced by chromium picolinate. *J. Am. Acad. Dermatol.* 41: 820–823.

45. Speetjens, J.K., Collins, R.A., Vincent, J.B., and Woski, S.A. (1999). The nutritional supplement chromium(III) *tris*(picolinate) cleaves DNA. *Chem. Res. Toxicol.* 12: 483–487.

CHAPTER 12

Nutrition and Teeth

ELIZABETH A. KRALL

*Department of Health Policy and Health Services Research, Boston University
School of Dental Medicine, Boston, Massachusetts*

ABSTRACT

Loss of the tooth-supporting alveolar bone is a key diagnostic feature of
periodontal disease and a risk factor for tooth loss. Individuals with
osteopenia or osteoporosis appear to be at greater risk of periodontal disease
and tooth loss. Nutritional factors related to bone development and turnover
elsewhere in the body, particularly calcium, vitamin D, and phosphorus,
may have roles in maintaining oral bone, but their clinical importance is
controversial. Relationships of intakes of calcium, vitamin D, and phosphorus
to alveolar bone loss (ABL), clinical attachment loss (CAL), and tooth loss
were examined in a prospective study of oral health in men ages 43 to
86 years at the initial study examination. Over an average of 12 years, usual
calcium intakes of approximately 1 g or more per day were associated with
23% less alveolar bone loss, 25% less clinical attachment loss, and 31%
fewer teeth lost compared to intakes below 1 g. These findings support the
concept that nutritional factors that are important in preventing osteoporosis,

Nutritional Aspects of Osteoporosis, Second Edition
Copyright © 2004 by Elsevier Science (USA)
All rights of reproduction in any form reserved.

particularly calcium, also have roles in maintaining oral bone and teeth in older adults.

INTRODUCTION

The cancellous alveolar process of the jawbone surrounds and anchors the teeth in sockets lined with a plate of compact bone called *alveolar bone*. Thus, alveolar bone provides physical support and protection for the teeth and tooth roots. These functions provide a rationale for examining the relationships of systemic bone status with periodontal disease and tooth loss, because excess bone resorption is implicated in both of these prevalent oral conditions. Throughout the lifespan, many nutrients have important roles in the development and maintenance of bone, but key nutrients are calcium, phosphorus, and vitamin D. Calcium and phosphorus are quantitatively the major mineral components of hydroxyapatite in tooth enamel and bone. Vitamin D promotes the absorption of calcium from the intestinal tract. In contrast to the many studies of the effects of calcium and vitamin D intakes on bone mass and bone turnover at skeletal sites such as the spine, hip, and radius [1], there have been relatively few that have focused on the effects of these nutrients on oral bone loss.

ORAL BONE LOSS AND SYSTEMIC BONE MINERAL DENSITY

In adults, two distinct diseases of excess bone resorption affect the oral cavity and are prevalent in the middle-aged and elderly population: osteoporosis and periodontal disease. The most common cause of oral bone loss in adults is periodontal disease. The tooth root is enclosed in the tooth socket and attached to the alveolar bone layer by bundles of collagenous fibers called the *periodontal ligament*. The root and alveolar process are further protected by gingival tissue that attaches to the tooth near the cemento-enamel junction (CEJ), a slight indentation that delineates the crown from the root of the tooth. Bacteria can invade and collect in subgingival pockets around the tooth root and produce inflammatory factors that increase bone resorption, decrease bone formation, and destroy periodontal ligament. As the supporting bone and ligament are lost, the gingival tissue pulls away from the CEJ, causing deeper pockets and loss of attachment. Inflammation is reversible; however, the cumulative damage to the bone and periodontal ligament is not, and as the support for the tooth declines the risk of tooth loss increases. In the elderly, more than 25% of missing teeth were extracted because of periodontal disease [2].

More than half of all most adults in developed countries have some form of periodontal disease [3–6], and the prevalence increases with age [7]. In most individuals, the disease is mild or limited to a few teeth. It is estimated that 10 to 25% of adults have the moderate to severe forms of periodontal disease [3–6] that place the affected teeth at an increased risk of tooth loss.

Common periodontal disease measures include probing pocket depth, alveolar bone loss, and clinical attachment loss. Probing pocket depth is the distance from the gingival margin to the bottom of the pocket and is an indicator of the current extent of periodontal inflammation. As the disease progresses, the cumulative damage is detected on clinical examination by attachment loss (the total distance from the CEJ to the bottom of the pocket, which includes both probing pocket depth and gum recession), and on dental radiographs by measuring the height of the alveolar bone (expressed as a percentage of the distance from the CEJ to the tip of the root). In examining the relationship of systemic bone status to periodontal disease, the most useful measures are clinical attachment loss and alveolar bone loss. Periodontal bone loss is known to be a direct consequence of bacterial inflammation, but it has also been hypothesized that oral bone that has been compromised by osteopenia is more likely than denser bone to exhibit rapid bone loss upon exposure to resorptive factors [8].

Approximately 40% of women and 15% of men worldwide can expect to suffer an osteoporotic fracture during their lifetime [9]. A review of the literature by Wactawski-Wende [8] describes generally consistent positive associations between osteoporosis or low bone mineral density (BMD) at various skeletal sites and oral outcomes, including low BMD of the jaw, greater alveolar bone loss, and fewer teeth retained. Results of recently published studies are mixed, with one reporting an association of periodontal disease with metacarpal BMD in postmenopausal but not premenopausal women [10] and another reporting weak correlations between alveolar bone and spine or femoral BMD [11]. The most consistent relationships of systemic and oral bone in cross-sectional studies appear to be found in populations of older adults when tooth loss is the outcome measurement [10,12–16].

The few prospective studies that exist to date also suggest that alveolar bone loss is more extensive in women with osteoporosis [17], and greater rates of bone loss at systemic sites are related to risk of tooth loss [18]. A 2-year prospective study of 38 postmenopausal women by Payne et al. [17] compared changes in alveolar bone height between women with spinal osteoporosis and those with normal BMD and found that the osteoporotic group developed more sites with significant alveolar bone loss than the normal BMD group. In a prospective, 7-year observational study of 329 postmenopausal women, rates of bone loss at the hip, spine, and total body were approximately 3 times faster in women who lost any teeth than in women who lost no teeth [18]. The risk of tooth loss increased by at least 50% for each 1% per year increment in the rate of systemic bone loss; however, a limitation of that study was that no information was provided on other oral factors, such as caries burden, that cause tooth loss.

Like most studies of BMD and oral bone loss or tooth loss, the majority of studies of systemic BMD and clinical measures of periodontal disease have also been cross-sectional in design. The overall findings have been equivocal [8], although recent cross-sectional studies support a positive relationship. Postmenopausal Japanese women with osteoporosis tended to have deeper pockets on average than women with normal BMD [10]. In an analysis of the third National Health and Examination Survey (NHANES III) adult population, Ronderos et al. [19] reported greater levels of clinical attachment loss in women with low BMD who also had high levels of calculus (an irritant that exacerbates attachment loss). Findings were similar in men but not statistically significant. No associations were seen in subjects with low or moderate levels of calculus. A prospective study of 135 patients reported that greater BMD was consistently associated with less clinical attachment loss, although the correlations were relatively weak [20].

In summary, it is not known if generalized low bone density in the jaw directly influences the risks of periodontal disease and tooth loss or what biological mechanisms lead to the associations. Many studies support the existence of a relationship, but, because the majority are cross-sectional studies, it is not possible to determine the temporality of changes in systemic BMD, oral BMD, clinical periodontal changes, and tooth loss. The few prospective studies that exist tend to support the relationship, but more research is needed for confirmation.

NUTRITION, PERIODONTAL DISEASE AND TOOTH LOSS

Older individuals with low BMD appear to be at an increased risk of periodontal disease and tooth loss. Whether osteopenic oral bone is more susceptible to destruction by bacterial inflammatory factors or periodontal disease and osteoporosis simply occur together as a result of common risk factors, calcium and vitamin D nutrition may be important in either scenario. Although a large number of studies confirm the need for adequate calcium and vitamin D intakes to maintain bone mass in other parts of the body, relatively little attention has been paid to these nutrients and their role in periodontal disease and tooth loss. Osteoporotic changes in the jawbones and alveolar crest of animals can be produced experimentally by feeding a diet with a low calcium content or low calcium-to-phosphorus ratio [21–24], but changes in periodontal status or number of teeth as a result of manipulation of nutrient content were reported by only one group of investigators [25,26].

In humans, a cross-sectional analysis of data from more than 12,000 adults who participated in NHANES III suggested that higher intakes of calcium are associated with lower risk of periodontal disease [27]. Intake of calcium from food sources was categorized as 800 mg or more, 500 to 800 mg, or less than 500 mg. Periodontal disease was defined as average clinical attachment loss of 1.5 mm or more, and the prevalence was 25% in the total population. Controlling for smoking, age, and gingival bleeding, individuals with calcium intake between 500 and 800 mg had 30% higher odds of periodontal disease compared to the reference group with at least 800 mg per day. The odds of disease were 30% higher (in men) to 60% higher (in women) with calcium intakes below 500 mg /day.

These findings are supported by a prospective analysis of alveolar bone loss in relation to usual calcium intakes in 552 older men [28]. Progression of alveolar bone loss at each tooth was defined as a change from low bone loss (80% or more of alveolar bone remaining around the tooth) to high bone loss (less than 80% of bone remaining), and the number of teeth with progression was summed for each participant. During the average follow-up period of 4 years, men whose calcium intakes were below 1000 mg per day had 30% more teeth exhibiting rapid progression of alveolar bone loss compared to men with calcium intakes above this level (2.6 ± 2.0 teeth versus 2.0 ± 2.5 teeth, $P = 0.04$). These estimates were controlled for age, initial number of teeth, smoking status, vitamin D intake, caries status, and periodontal disease status.

Estimates of usual dietary intakes obtained from food frequency questionnaires and other self-report instruments are subject to measurement error and recall bias, limitations that are reduced in controlled supplement trials. Several supplement trials have been conducted to examine the effect of calcium [29,30] or calcium plus vitamin D supplementation [31,32] on oral outcomes. Two studies in patients with periodontal disease [29,31] suggested that supplemental calcium (at levels of 750 to 1000 mg/day) could reduce tooth mobility and pocket depth and prevent periodontal bone loss, but these studies also had serious limitations such as small sample size, short follow-up periods (6 months to 1 year), and, in one study, lack of a control group [29]. A third 6-month study failed to find any differences in average probing depth or tooth mobility between the supplemented and placebo groups [30].

Longer follow-up times may be needed to detect a difference in tooth loss rates by intake level. Calcium intake and tooth loss were examined in 145 healthy elderly men and women during a series of two studies that spanned 5 years [32]. The first study, a 3-year randomized controlled clinical trial, assigned subjects to either placebos or supplements containing 500 mg of calcium and 700 IU of vitamin D per day. The second study, years 4 and 5, was an observational study during which total calcium and vitamin D intakes were self-selected. During the randomized trial, the odds of losing any teeth were significantly reduced in the supplemented group to 0.4 (confidence interval, 0.2 to 0.9) compared to the placebo group. During the 2-year follow-up of the same individuals, the odds of tooth loss were also significantly lower (OR = 0.5) in subjects whose total calcium intake was at least 1000 mg per day compared to those who consumed less than 1000 mg. There were no radiographic measurements of oral bone, and clinical periodontal disease measures were made only once, at the end of the follow-up period.

These larger, recent studies [27,28,32] individually suggest that higher calcium intakes are beneficial to oral bone, periodontal attachment loss, or prevention of tooth loss, but none has demonstrated an effect on all three outcomes, which are progressively linked: Alveolar bone loss leads to clinical attachment loss and eventually may lead to tooth loss.

RELATIONSHIP OF CALCIUM, VITAMIN D, AND PHOSPHORUS TO PERIODONTAL DISEASE AND TOOTH LOSS

The Veterans Administration Dental Longitudinal Study (DLS) has information on multiple oral outcomes and more than 30 years of total follow-up. The DLS is a prospective, observational study of aging and oral health in men that began in 1968 with 1231 healthy males [33] and continues to conduct examinations every 3 years. We examined the relationships of intakes of calcium, vitamin D, and phosphorus to alveolar bone loss, clinical attachment loss, and tooth loss in this study cohort. Based on earlier findings, we expected that men whose usual intakes of calcium were approximately 800 to 1000 mg/day or more had not only a slower progression of alveolar bone loss but also fewer consequences of bone loss (i.e., less clinical attachment loss and a lower incidence of tooth loss).

METHODS

This analysis of calcium intake and alveolar bone loss was conducted in 482 DLS participants who had contemporaneous dietary data (collected only since 1985) and at least two dental examinations between 1985 and 2002. The majority of subjects are white, and all are community-dwelling men who receive their medical and dental care in the private sector. Subjects give informed consent as approved by the Human Subjects Subcommittee of the Veterans Administration Boston Healthcare System.

Dietary surveys were conducted with a semiquantitative food frequency questionnaire [34]. Total calcium and vitamin D intakes were computed from foods, supplements, and multivitamins. Total calcium intakes estimated from repeated questionnaires were correlated at $r = 0.64$ in this group of men.

A single examiner conducted dental examinations. At each examination, data collected include a count of the number of teeth remaining, evaluation of each tooth surface for restorations and caries, and clinical attachment loss. Clinical attachment loss was measured with a probe and recorded in millimeters; these measurements were then grouped into categories of 0, 1–2, or 3 or more mm. Alveolar bone loss was measured at the distal and mesial sites of each tooth on periapical radiographs using a modified Schei ruler method [35], which measures bone loss on a 6-point scale, where 0 indicates no bone loss and each 1-point increment represents 20% loss of bone height between the cemento–enamel junction and root tip. Progression of clinical attachment loss was defined as the number of teeth that advanced to a higher CAL score from the first examination (in 1985) to the most recent examination. Progression of alveolar bone loss was defined as the number of teeth that advanced to a higher Schei score from the first to the most recent dental examination. Tooth loss was defined as the number of teeth lost between examinations. Clinical attachment loss, alveolar bone loss, and tooth loss were standardized to a 10-year period.

STATISTICAL METHODS

The distributions of total calcium, vitamin D, and phosphorus intakes per day from dietary and supplemental sources were divided into quartiles. Characteristics in the four intake groups were compared with F-test or chi-square statistics. Analysis of covariance was performed to compare the mean number of teeth lost and mean changes in number of teeth showing progression of alveolar bone loss and clinical attachment loss among the calcium intake quartiles. Means in each quartile were adjusted for the following characteristics present at the beginning of the observation period: age, total number of teeth remaining, smoking status, socioeconomic status, and mean vitamin D and phosphorus intakes. Furthermore, different models contained additional variables: The model evaluating tooth loss included percent of teeth at baseline with ABL of 20% or more and percent of teeth with caries and restorations; the model evaluating ABL included percent of teeth at baseline with ABL of 20% or more; and the model evaluating CAL included percent of teeth at baseline with CAL of 3 mm or more. If the main effect for calcium quartile in the analysis of covariance was significant at $P < 0.10$, two comparisons were performed; the mean in quartile 4 was compared to the combined mean of the lower 3 quartiles, and the means in the 4 quartiles were tested for linear trend.

RESULTS

The mean follow-up period was 12 years and ranged from 2 to 17 years. Characteristics of the men at the beginning of the observation period are shown in Table I. Mean total intakes during the follow-up period were 830 ± 344 mg of calcium, 374 ± 240 IU of vitamin D, and 1352 ± 478 mg of phosphorus. When the distribution of calcium intakes was divided into quartiles, the intake ranges were ≤ 590 mg in quartile 1, 591–782 mg in quartile 2, 783–990 mg in quartile 3, and ≥ 990 mg in quartile 4. There were no significant differences in baseline age, smoking status, socioeconomic status, or oral status among the quartiles.

The number of teeth lost averaged 2.4 teeth per decade in the study group. Tooth loss differed significantly by calcium intake quartile, as shown in Table II. Men in the highest quartile of calcium intake (quartile 4) lost approximately 31% fewer teeth than men with lower calcium levels. The number of teeth that exhibited progression of alveolar bone loss averaged 7.4 overall. Progression of ABL in calcium intake quartile 4 was approximately

TABLE I Characteristics of Study Group of 482 Men at Beginning of the Observation Period

Characteristic	Mean ± SD
Age (years)	62 ± 8
Number of teeth remaining	23 ± 6
Percent of teeth with caries and/or restorations	67 ± 19
Percent of teeth with <80% alveolar bone remaining	22 ± 25
Percent of teeth with clinical attachment loss (CAL) of 3 mm or more	24 ± 27

TABLE II   Adjusted Mean Number of Teeth Lost and Number of Teeth with Progression of Periodontal Disease by Quartile of Calcium Intake

Calcium Intake Quartile	Calcium Intake Range (mg/day)	Number of Teeth Lost per Decade (mean ± SE)[a]	Number of Teeth/Decade with ABL Progression (mean ± SE)[b]	Number of Teeth/Decade with CAL Progression (mean ± SE)[c]
1	≤590	2.4 ± 0.3	8.1 ± 0.6	8.0 ± 0.6
2	591–782	2.8 ± 0.2	7.5 ± 0.6	6.6 ± 0.5
3	783–990	2.7 ± 0.2	8.5 ± 0.6	6.5 ± 0.5
4	≥990	1.8 ± 0.3	6.2 ± 0.7	5.3 ± 0.6

[a]Means are adjusted by analysis of covariance for baseline age, smoking status, socioeconomic status, number of teeth remaining, percentage of teeth with alveolar bone loss (ABL) of 20% or more, percentage of teeth with caries and/or restorations, and mean intakes of vitamin D and phosphorus during follow-up. Quartile 4 versus all others, $P <0.03$.

[b]Means are adjusted by analysis of covariance for baseline age, smoking status, socioeconomic status, number of teeth remaining, percentage of teeth with alveolar bone loss (ABL) of 20% or more, and mean intakes of vitamin D and phosphorus during follow-up. Quartile 4 versus all others, $P < 0.02$; test for linear trend, $P < 0.01$.

[c]Means are adjusted by analysis of covariance for baseline age, smoking status, socioeconomic status, number of teeth remaining, percentage of teeth with clinical attachment loss (CAL) of 3 mm or more, and mean intakes of vitamin D and phosphorus during follow-up. Quartile 4 versus all others, $P < 0.02$.

23% less than in the lower intake levels (Table II). The number of teeth that exhibited progression of CAL averaged 6.6 overall. Progression of CAL in calcium intake quartile 4 was approximately 25% less than in the lower intake levels, and there was a significant, inverse linear relationship between calcium quartile and number of teeth with CAL progression (Table II). There were no significant associations of tooth loss, ABL progression, or CAL progression with vitamin D intake or phosphorus intakes.

CONCLUSIONS

The interpretation of these data may be limited by the fact that the study cohort includes only middle-aged and elderly men. Also, progression of alveolar bone loss could not be determined for teeth that were lost between study examinations, but because periodontal disease is a major cause of tooth loss, the data for progression of ABL shown in this study may underestimate the true level. Overall, approximately 40% of the teeth present did not have detectable alveolar bone loss at the beginning of the observation period; therefore, the influence of a high calcium intake on alveolar bone loss in subjects with generalized periodontal disease is unknown. Finally, it is possible that the relationship is not specific to calcium but that calcium is merely a marker for a healthy diet; however, analysis of vitamin D intake levels and phosphorus intake levels did not reveal any relationships of ABL, CAL, or tooth loss with these nutrients. These findings from a prospective study provide further support for the hypothesis that calcium intake has a role in the progression of periodontal bone loss.

SUMMARY

Periodontal disease is a complex, multifactorial disease. While the presence of bacteria is necessary to initiate an inflammatory response, many other factors affect susceptibility to disease and its rate of progression. The literature suggests systemic bone status may be one of these factors. Tooth loss is also determined by multiple factors, ranging from biologic to economic and esthetic. In maintaining oral bone and the support for the teeth that it provides, a plausible role exists for calcium and vitamin D intakes because of their importance to bone mineral metabolism. The few previous studies of calcium and vitamin D intake levels or supplements have reached contra-dictory conclusions. But, more recent, large studies that control for potential confounding factors consistently support the hypothesis that calcium and vitamin D nutritional status influence the progression of periodontal disease and the risk of tooth loss to some degree. These findings need to be replicated in other populations and with randomized clinical trials.

REFERENCES

1. Reid, I.R. (1998). The roles of calcium and vitamin D in the prevention of osteoporosis. *Endocrinol. Metab. Clin. N. Amer.* 27: 389–398.
2. Brown, L.J, Brunelle, J.A., and Kingman, A. (1996). Periodontal status in the United States, 1988-1991: prevalence, extent, and demographic variation. *J. Dent. Res.* 75(Spec. No.): 672–683.
3. Schurch, E., Jr., Minder, C.E., Lang, N.P., and Geering, A.H. (1988). Periodontal conditions in a randomly selected population in Switzerland. *Commun. Dent. Oral Epidemiol.* 16: 181–186.
4. Benigeri, M., Brodeur, J.M., Payette, M., Charbonneau, A., and Ismail, A.I. (2000). Community periodontal index of treatment needs and prevalence of periodontal conditions. *J. Clin. Periodontol.* 27: 308–312.
5. Bourgeois, D., Hescot, P., and Doury, J. (1997). Periodontal conditions in 35–44-yr-old adults in France, 1993. *J. Periodont. Res.* 32: 570–574.
6. Anagnou-Vareltzides, A., Diamanti-Kipioti, A., Afentoulidis, N., Moraitaki-Tsami, A., Lindhe, J., Mitsis, F., and Papapanou, P.N. (1996). A clinical survey of periodontal conditions in Greece. *J. Clin. Periodontol.* 23: 758–763.

7. Albandar, J.M., Brunelle, J.A., and Kingman, A. (1999). Destructive periodontal disease in adults 30 years of age and older in the United States, 1988–1994. *J. Periodontol.* 70: 13–29.
8. Wactawski-Wende, J. (2001). Periodontal diseases and osteoporosis: association and mechanisms. *Ann. Periodontol.* 6: 197–208.
9. International Osteoporosis Foundation, *The Facts About Osteoporosis and Its Impact* (http://www.osteofound.org/press_centre/fact_sheet.html).
10. Inagaki, K., Kurosu, Y., Kamiya, T., Kondo, F., Yoshinari, N., Noguchi, T., Krall, E.A., and Garcia, R.I. (2001). Low metacarpal bone density tooth loss, and periodontal disease in Japanese women. *J. Dent. Res.* 80: 1818–1822.
11. Shrout, M.K., Hildebolt, C.F., Potter, B.J., Brunsden, T.K.B., Pilgram, T.K., Dotson, M., Yokoyama-Crothers, N., Hauser, J., Cohen, S., Kardaris, E., Civitelli, R., and Hanes, P. (2000). Comparison of morphological measurements extracted from digitized dental radiographs with lumbar and femoral bone mineral density measurements in postmenopausal women. *J. Periodontol.* 71: 335–340.
12. May, H., Reader, R., Murphy, S., and Khaw, K.T. (1995). Self-reported tooth loss and bone mineral density in older men and women. *Age Ageing* 24: 217–221.
13. Krall, E.A., Dawson-Hughes, B., Papas, A., and Garcia, R.I. (1994). Tooth loss and skeletal bone density in healthy postmenopausal women. *Osteoporosis Int.* 4: 104–109.
14. Daniell, H.W. (1983). Postmenopausal tooth loss: contributions to edentulism by osteoporosis and cigarette smoking. *Arch. Intern. Med.* 143: 1678–1682.
15. Taguchi, A., Suei, Y., Ohtsuka, M., Otani, K., Tanimoto, K., and Hollender, L.G. (1999). Relationship between bone mineral density and tooth loss in elderly Japanese women. *Dento-Maxillo-Facial Radiol.* 28: 219–223.
16. Kribbs, P.J. (1990). Comparison of mandibular bone in normal and osteoporotic women. *J. Prosthet. Dent.* 63: 218–222.
17. Payne, J.B., Reinhardt, R.A., Nummikoski, P.V., and Patil, K.D. (1999). Longitudinal alveolar bone loss in postmenopausal osteoporotic/osteopenic women. *Osteoporosis Int.* 10: 34–40.
18. Krall, E.A., Garcia, R.I., and Dawson-Hughes, B. (1996). Increased risk of tooth loss is related to bone loss at the whole body, hip, and spine. *Calc. Tiss. Int.* 9: 433–437.
19. Ronderos, M., Jacobs, D.R., Himes, J.H., and Pihlstrom, B.L. (2000). Associations of periodontal disease with femoral bone mineral density and estrogen replacement therapy: cross-sectional evaluation of U.S. adults from NHANES III. *J. Clin. Periodontol.* 27: 778–786.
20. Pilgram, T.K., Hildebolt, C.F., Dotson, M., Cohen, S.C., Hauser, J.F., Kardaris, E., and Civitelli, R. (2002). Relationships between clinical attachment level and spine and hip bone mineral density: data from healthy postmenopausal women. *J. Periodontol.* 73: 298–301.
21. Bissada, N.F. and DeMarco, T.J. (1974). The effect of a hypocalcemic diet on the periodontal structures of the adult rat. *J. Periodontol.* 45: 739–745.
22. Oliver, W.M. (1969). The effect of deficiencies of calcium, vitamin D or calcium and vitamin D and of variations in the source of dietary protein on the supporting tissues of the rat molar. *J. Periodont. Res.* 4: 56–69.
23. Ferguson, H.W. and Hartles, R.L. (1964). The effects of diets deficient in calcium or phosphorus in the presence and absence of supplements of vitamin D on the secondary cementum and alveolar bone of young rats. *Arch. Oral Biol.* 9: 647–658.
24. Svanberg, G., Lindhe, J., Hugoson, A., and Grondahl, H.G. (1973). Effect of nutritional hyperparathyroidism on experimental periodontitis in the dog. *Scand. J. Dent. Res.* 81: 1551–1562.
25. Henrikson, P.A. (1968). Periodontal disease and calcium deficiency: an experimental study in the dog. *Acta Odontol. Scand.* 26(suppl. 50): 1–132.

26. Krook, L., Lutwak, L., Henrikson, P.A., Kallfelz, F., Hirsch, C., Romanus, B., Marier, J.R., and Sheffey, B.E. (1971). Reversibility of nutritional osteoporosis; physicochemical data on bones from and experimental study in dogs. *J. Nutr.* 101: 233–246.
27. Nishida, M., Grossi, S.G., Dunford, R.G., Ho, A.W., Trevisan, M., and Genco, R.J. (2000). Calcium and the risk for periodontal disease. *J. Periodontol.* 71: 1057–1066.
28. Krall, E.A. (2001). The periodontal–systemic connection: implications for treatment of patients with osteoporosis and periodontal disease. *Ann. Periodontol.* 6: 209–213.
29. Krook, L., Lutwak, L., Whalen, J.P., Henrikson, P.A., Lesser, G.V., and Uris, R. (1972). Human periodontal disease: morphology and response to calcium therapy. *Cornell Vet.* 62: 32–53.
30. Uhrbom, E. and Jacobson, L. (1984). Calcium and periodontitis: clinical effect of calcium medication. *J. Clin. Periodontol.* 11: 230–241.
31. Spiller, W.F. (1971). A clinical evaluation of calcium therapy for periodontal disease. *Dental Dig.* 77: 522–526.
32. Krall, E.A., Wehler, C., Harris, S.S., Garcia, R.I., and Dawson-Hughes, B. (2001). Calcium and vitamin D supplements reduce tooth loss in the elderly. *Am. J. Med.* 111: 452–456.
33. Kapur, K.K., Glass, R.L., Loftus, E.R., Alman, J.E., and Feller, R.P. (1972). The Veterans Administration longitudinal study of oral health and disease. *Aging Hum. Devel.* 3: 125–137.
34. Willett, W.C., Sampson, L., Stampfer, M.J., Rosner, B., Bain, C., Witschi, J., Hennekens, C.H., and Speizer, F.E. (1985). Reproducibility and validity of a semiquantitative food frequency questionnaire. *Am. J. Epidemiol.* 122: 51–65.
35. Schei, O., Waerhaug, J., Lovdal, A., and Arno, A. (1959). Alveolar bone loss as related to oral hygiene and age. *J. Periodontol.* 30: 7–16.

CHAPTER 13

Cognitive Dietary Restraint, Cortisol and Bone Density in Normal-Weight Women: Is There a Relationship?

SUSAN I. BARR

Department of Agricultural Sciences, University of British Columbia, Vancouver, British Columbia, Canada

ABSTRACT

Clinical eating disorders such as anorexia nervosa are known to adversely affect bone but are relatively rare. In contrast, subtle disturbances of eating attitudes, such as high levels of cognitive dietary restraint, are much more prevalent, as many normal-weight young women consciously monitor and attempt to limit their food intake in an effort to conform to societal ideals for body weight and shape. Whether high levels of cognitive dietary restraint are negatively associated with bone density is largely unexplored. This article proposes that high levels of dietary restraint act as a subtle stressor, activating the hypothalamic–pituitary–adrenal (HPA) axis and leading to increased cortisol release. Activation of the HPA axis can suppress the hypothalamic–pituitary–gonadal (HPG) axis, and women with high dietary restraint appear to experience more subclinical ovulatory disturbances and irregular menstrual cycles. Both of these hormonal alterations (increased cortisol and lower reproductive hormones) are known to have adverse effects on bone. Although data are limited, available

Nutritional Aspects of Osteoporosis, Second Edition

evidence comparing healthy women with high and low levels of cognitive dietary restraint suggests that high dietary restraint is associated with increased cortisol release and lower values for bone mineral density or content. Additional prospective research monitoring change in bone density over time in women with high and low levels of cognitive dietary restraint is warranted to assess the clinical importance of these findings.

INTRODUCTION

The negative effect on bone density of the clinical eating disorder, anorexia nervosa, has been recognized for almost two decades [1,2]. Bone loss in this condition is undoubtedly multifactorial and is contributed to by low body weight, altered status of reproductive and other hormones, and inadequate intakes of calcium and other nutrients required for bone formation and maintenance [3]. Clinical anorexia, however, is rare, with an estimated lifetime prevalence of approximately 0.5% [4]. In contrast, body weight and shape dissatisfaction is so prevalent among Western women that it is almost normative, even among women who are not overweight. This dissatisfaction is in turn associated with efforts to monitor or limit food intake in an attempt to control body weight. For example, 37% of Canadian women with a body mass index (BMI) in the healthy range of 20 to 25 kg/m^2 reported that they were currently trying to lose weight [5]. Other women may not "diet" in the sense of reducing their energy intake over a relatively short period of time but instead are always aware of what and how much they are eating. This continuous monitoring and attempt to limit food intake is known as *cognitive dietary restraint*, or more simply, dietary restraint [6].

Whether subtle disturbances of eating attitudes, such as high levels of cognitive dietary restraint, are negatively associated with bone mineral density (BMD) in normal-weight women is largely unknown and is examined in this article. First, a possible mechanism that could underlie such an association is presented. This is followed by a brief discussion of the assessment of dietary restraint. Next, associations between cognitive dietary restraint and the menstrual cycle are examined, as are studies that have attempted to determine whether subclinical disturbances of the menstrual cycle are associated with bone loss. This is followed by an examination of whether women with high levels of dietary restraint have elevated cortisol levels. Finally, the limited data on associations between cognitive dietary restraint and bone mass in normal-weight women are discussed, and directions for future research are outlined.

POSSIBLE MECHANISM

A possible mechanism underlying an association between high levels of cognitive dietary restraint and bone loss is shown in Fig. 1. High levels of cognitive dietary restraint may represent a subtle stressor and, as such, would activate the hypothalamic–pituitary–adrenal (HPA) axis, leading to increased release of corticotropin-releasing hormone (CRH), adrenocorticotropic hormone (ACTH), and ultimately, cortisol. Cortisol is known to have negative effects on the skeleton: It affects bone formation, bone resorption, intestinal calcium absorption, and renal calcium excretion [7]. Furthermore, chronic activation of the HPA axis is associated with inhibition of the hypothalamic-pituitary-gonadal (HPG) axis [8]. Elevated levels of CRH appear to inhibit release of gonadotropin-releasing hormone (GnRH). This, in turn, would lead to reductions in the release of follicle-stimulating hormone (FSH) and luteinizing hormone (LH), which are responsible for the cyclic release of estradiol and progesterone from the ovary during the menstrual cycle. Accordingly, reproductive hormone levels would be reduced. And in women, suppression of reproductive hormones is generally associated with bone loss [1,9,10].

ASSESSMENT OF DIETARY RESTRAINT

Several instruments are currently used to assess dietary restraint, including the Restraint Scale (RS) [11], the restraint subscale of the Three Factor Eating Questionnaire (TFEQ-R) [6], and the restrained eating subscale of the Dutch Eating Behavior Questionnaire (DEBQ-R) [12]. Each of these instruments, however, reflects a somewhat different construct, and scores cannot be used interchangeably [13]. The RS, for example, includes items that reflect both weight fluctuation and a concern for dieting, but the scoring system provides only a total score. Thus, it is difficult to determine which aspect of the RS (i.e., weight fluctuation or concern for dieting) contributes to associations with other variables of interest. In contrast, the TFEQ contains separate subscales for cognitive dietary restraint, disinhibition, and hunger, allowing one to distinguish among associations more clearly. Similarly, the DEBQ contains subscales for restrained eating, emotional eating, and external eating. Most studies assessing relationships among dietary restraint, the menstrual cycle, cortisol, and bone have used the TFEQ-R.

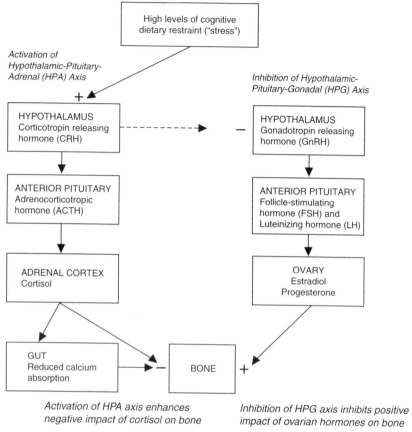

FIGURE 1   Simplified possible mechanism for an association between high levels of dietary restraint and bone in women. High levels of restraint act as a stressor that (1) activates the HPA axis and leads to increased cortisol release, and (2) inhibits the HPG axis and leads to reduced ovarian hormone release. The increase in cortisol and the reduction in reproductive hormones both have adverse effects on bone.

ASSOCIATIONS BETWEEN DIETARY RESTRAINT AND MENSTRUAL DISTURBANCES

THE NORMAL MENSTRUAL CYCLE AND MENSTRUAL DISTURBANCES

Before describing studies that have assessed associations between dietary restraint and disturbances of the menstrual cycle, it is important to review normal human ovarian function [14]. The menstrual cycle typically lasts 28 days and is divided into two phases: the first half constitutes the follicular phase, which culminates in ovulation on day 14, and the second half is known as the luteal phase. By convention, day 1 of the cycle begins with menstrual flow, during which time circulating levels of both estrogen and progesterone are low. Gonadotropin-releasing hormone is released from the hypothalamus in a pulsatile manner, and stimulates release of FSH and LH from the pituitary. FSH stimulates the growth of a number of ovarian follicles, one of which becomes the dominant follicle and begins to synthesize estrogen. Increasing levels of estrogen are a prerequisite for the mid-cycle surge in LH, which in turn triggers ovulation. After ovulation, the ruptured follicle is transformed into the corpus luteum, which releases estrogen, progesterone, and inhibin A. If fertilization does not occur, the corpus luteum undergoes luteolysis, and estrogen, progesterone, and inhibin A secretions fall, leading to the shedding of the endometrial lining as menstrual flow and the onset of another cycle.

The regular ovulatory cycle described above does not occur invariably between menarche and menopause. Although deviations from the normal pattern are most common during the years following menarche and preceding menopause, they can occur at any age, and include secondary amenorrhea (absence of menses for at least 6 months in a non-pregnant woman), oligomenorrhea (irregular cycles lasting from 36 to 180 days), anovulatory cycles (cycles of regular length in which ovulation does not occur), and short-luteal-phase cycles (cycles of regular length in which the luteal phase lasts less than 10 days). Although amenorrhea and oligomenorrhea are readily apparent to women who experience them, anovulatory and short luteal phase cycles are clinically silent, as they can occur within cycles of normal length. They can be detected through serial blood or salivary hormone measurements; for example, a cycle in which progesterone concentrations did not increase during the second half would be classified as anovulatory, while a cycle in which progesterone concentrations were above baseline for fewer than 10 days would be classified as having a short luteal phase. Subclinical ovulatory disturbances can also be detected by using basal body temperature measurements [15]. The hypothalamus has a thermic response to progesterone, such that basal body temperature in the luteal phase of the cycle (when progesterone levels are high) averages approximately $0.3°C$ higher than during the follicular phase (when progesterone levels are very low). Computerized analysis of daily basal temperature records can determine whether or not a cycle is ovulatory (indicated by a biphasic temperature curve) and provides an index of the luteal phase length (indicated by the number of days that temperature is elevated) [15].

MENSTRUAL CHARACTERISTICS OF WOMEN WITH
HIGH COGNITIVE DIETARY RESTRAINT

The first study to report an association between cognitive dietary restraint and menstrual characteristics was that of Schweiger and colleagues [16], who compared young German women with scores above the 75th percentiles for dietary restraint on the TFEQ-R and the DEBQ-R to those with scores below the 50th percentile. All women reported regular menstrual cycles of normal length, had not lost weight recently, did not use oral contraceptives, and did not participate in endurance exercise or avoid major food groups. Menstrual cycles were monitored by serial serum hormone measurements and compared to pre-established criteria for a normal cycle. The two groups were similar in terms of age, BMI, and activity level, but mean cycle length, luteal phase length, and progesterone concentrations were all significantly lower among the women with high dietary restraint. Furthermore, only two of nine women with high dietary restraint scores had cycles that met the standard criteria for a normally ovulatory cycle, compared to 11 of 13 women with low scores for restraint.

Both exercise and vegetarianism have been associated with an increased likelihood of menstrual disturbances [17–20]; however, these observations may have been confounded by other variables (e.g., weight loss) or a recruitment bias in which women with irregular cycles may have been more likely to volunteer for study participation. To further explore these areas and to avoid a recruitment bias, Barr and colleagues [21,22] studied *subclinical* menstrual disturbances among women who reported regular menstrual cycles of normal length, did not use oral contraceptives, and were weight stable. Among other variables, cognitive dietary restraint was assessed in these studies. In one study, 27 women with a wide range of physical activity completed the TFEQ-R and kept daily physical activity and basal body temperature records for at least three menstrual cycles (mean $= 12.8 \pm 2.7$ cycles) [21]. Physical activity level was not related to menstrual cycle characteristics, so associations with cognitive dietary restraint were assessed. Compared to those in the upper tertile of dietary restraint scores (mean TFEQ-R score $= 15.1 \pm 2.4$), those in the lower tertile (mean TFEQ-R score $= 3.9 \pm 1.8$) were similar in age, BMI, percent body fat, waist-to-hip ratio, and physical activity. Mean menstrual cycle length was similar between groups, but the women with high scores for dietary restraint had a significantly shorter mean luteal phase length (8.6 ± 2.7 days versus 10.5 ± 1.5 days, $P < 0.05$) [21].

In a subsequent study, Barr and colleagues [22] assessed menstrual characteristics of healthy vegetarian and omnivorous women. Vegetarians had excluded all meat, fish, and poultry for at least 2 years, and omnivores consumed meat (beef or pork) at least three times weekly. Women kept basal body temperature records for six consecutive menstrual cycles, completed three sets of 3-day diet records, and completed the TFEQ. In the primary analysis, vegetarians and omnivores were found to have similar menstrual cycle and follicular phase lengths. However, in contrast to what had been suggested in earlier, less well-controlled studies, vegetarians had a significantly *lower* proportion of anovulatory cycles and a *longer* mean luteal phase length [22]. Because vegetarians also had significantly lower dietary restraint scores than omnivores (6.4 ± 4.4 versus 9.5 ± 3.7; $P = 0.015$), additional analyses were conducted to assess whether the difference in dietary restraint was associated with the menstrual cycle observations. Women in both diet groups were combined, and those with TFEQ-R scores below the median of 7 were compared to those with scores above 13. Age, gynecologic age, exercise, height, weight, and dietary intakes did not differ between these two groups, but the high dietary restraint group had fewer ovulatory cycles (3.6 ± 2.3 versus 5.0 ± 1.4, $P < 0.05$) and a shorter mean luteal phase length (7.4 ± 4.1 days versus 10.7 ± 3.1 days, $P < 0.05$) [22].

Lebenstedt and colleagues [23] studied subclinical menstrual disturbances in women athletes. Participants were weight stable, had a BMI between 18 and 25 kg/m^2, did not use oral contraceptives, reported at least 9 menstrual cycles within the past year, and completed at least 30 minutes of endurance training every other day. They measured basal body temperature daily and collected saliva samples every other day over the course of one menstrual cycle, and also completed a 7-day food record and the TFEQ. Of the 33 participants, 21 had salivary progesterone levels consistent with a normally ovulatory cycle, and 12 were characterized as having cycle disturbances. The two groups were similar in age, gynecologic age, BMI, sports activity, and reported dietary intake, but the athletes with disturbed cycles had a significantly higher mean TFEQ-R score than those with normally ovulatory cycles (9.9 ± 4 versus 5.5 ± 5; $P < 0.05$) [23].

Finally, McLean and colleagues [24] assessed the prevalence of self-reported irregular menstrual cycles in a group of 424 university women who did not use oral contraceptives. Based on scores on the TFEQ-R, they were categorized as having low dietary restraint (a score of ≤ 5), medium dietary restraint (a score of 6–12), or high dietary restraint (a score of ≥ 13). Women with low, medium, and high dietary restraint were similar in age and BMI. The proportion of women reporting irregular menstrual cycles was similar in those with low and medium dietary restraint, at 17.6 and 16.6% respectively, but it was essentially twice as high (34%) in those with high dietary restraint [24].

In summary, studies that have explored menstrual characteristics of normal-weight women with high levels of cognitive dietary restraint have consistently reported that they are more likely to experience subclinical menstrual disturbances and irregular cycles, as compared to otherwise similar women with low dietary restraint scores.

ASSOCIATIONS BETWEEN SUBCLINICAL MENSTRUAL DISTURBANCES AND BONE LOSS

Although it is well-established that hypothalamic amenorrhea is associated with bone loss in women [1], little research has been conducted to assess the impact on bone of more subtle disturbances of the menstrual cycle. Prior and colleagues [25] conducted a 1-year prospective study of 66 women who were prescreened as having normally ovulatory cycles. Participants kept basal body temperature records throughout the study, and spinal cancellous BMD was measured at baseline and 1 year using quantitative computed tomography. Over the year, 29% of cycles had a short luteal phase length or were anovulatory, and spinal bone loss was strongly related to these disturbances: Women who maintained normal ovulatory cycles throughout the year maintained BMD, while the 13 who experienced one or more anovulatory cycles had a mean decrease in spinal BMD of 4.2% over the year [25]. Thus, these data suggest that bone is also affected by subclinical menstrual disturbances.

ASSOCIATIONS BETWEEN DIETARY RESTRAINT AND CORTISOL

The proposed mechanism underlying a possible association between cognitive dietary restraint and bone is that high levels of dietary restraint represent a subtle stressor that activates the HPA axis. If true, one would expect that cortisol levels would be elevated in those with high dietary restraint. To date, three studies have explored this hypothesis.

The first study was that of Pirke and colleagues [26], who studied 22 healthy, normal-weight young women. Nine were classified as restrained (a score above the 75th percentile on the TFEQ-R) and 13 as unrestrained (a score below the median). Blood was sampled at 30-minute intervals from an indwelling venous catheter during an overnight study period. The results showed that cortisol did not differ between groups; however, the overnight study period may have precluded the detection of a difference.

Presumably, stress associated with dietary restraint would likely occur with food intake and decisions around food-related behavior, which take place during the daytime rather than while asleep.

McLean and colleagues [27] compared 24-hour urinary cortisol excretion between women with high and low scores for dietary restraint (≥ 13 and ≤ 5 on the TFEQ-R, respectively). Participants had a stable body weight with BMI between 18 and 25 kg/m^2, did not use oral contraceptives, and had self-reported normal menstrual cycle intervals. Women with high and low scores for dietary restraint were similar in age and BMI, but urinary cortisol excretion was significantly higher in the high dietary restraint group (418.8 ± 134.6 nmol/24 hr versus 354.7 ± 83.7 nmol/24 hr; $P < 0.05$).

Anderson and colleagues [28] studied 85 college-age women who completed both the TFEQ-R and the RS and provided a saliva sample for cortisol analysis. They found that both measures of dietary restraint were correlated with salivary cortisol concentrations, but that the TFEQ-R was more strongly associated than the RS. Those who scored above the median on the TFEQ-R had significantly higher salivary cortisol than those with scores below the median (0.32 ± 0.51 µg/dL versus 0.15 ± 0.12 µg/dL; $P < 0.05$).

Although the elevations in cortisol reported in women with high dietary restraint are still well within the normal range, there is evidence that even modest increases in cortisol are associated with adverse effects on bone. For example, free-living older adults with higher baseline urinary cortisol excretion were at higher risk of fracture during follow-up [29].

ASSOCIATION BETWEEN DIETARY RESTRAINT AND BONE

The preceding discussion has established that mechanisms exist whereby high levels of cognitive dietary restraint have the potential to impact negatively on bone mineral density. To date, only two studies have examined whether this does occur. Van Loan and Keim [30] studied 185 women ages 18 to 45 years who were between 90 and 150% of ideal weight. All women completed the TFEQ, and total body BMD and bone mineral content (BMC) were measured using dual-energy x-ray absorptiometry (DEXA). Women with TFEQ-R scores < 9 (mean $= 4.7 \pm 2.0$) were compared to those with scores ≥ 9 (mean $= 13.4 \pm 3.0$), and the two groups did not differ in terms of age or BMI. When they divided their sample into four weight quartiles, women with high restraint in the three lowest weight quartiles

(≤ 71 kg) had lower total body BMC than those with low restraint. In the highest weight quartile, however, high restraint was not associated with lower BMC. Restraint score also entered a regression equation for prediction of BMC, along with height, fat-free mass, and percentage body fat. No associations were observed with BMD.

McLean and colleagues [31] assessed total body and lumbar spine BMD and BMC using DEXA in 62 women, 29 with low scores for cognitive dietary restraint (≤ 5 on the TFEQ-R) and 33 with high scores (≥ 13). Enrolment criteria included age 20 to 35 years, stable body weight with a BMI of 18 to 25 kg/m^2, self-reported normal-length menstrual cycles, exercise ≤ 7 hr/wk, and nulliparity, while exclusion criteria included oral contraceptive or bone active medication use, cigarette smoking, hirsutism, and a history of having been diagnosed with or treated for an eating disorder. The low and high dietary restraint groups were similar in age (22.2 ± 3.1 yr and 2.12 ± 1.7 yr for low and high restraint, respectively), fat mass (14.9 ± 5.6 kg and 15.1 ± 3.8 kg for low and high restraint, respectively), and bone-free lean mass (40.7 ± 5.2 kg and 41.0 ± 4.7 kg for low and high restraint, respectively). Women with high dietary restraint, however, reported more hours of exercise per week (3.4 ± 1.7 hr/wk versus 2.2 ± 1.8 hr/wk; $P = 0.01$). Analysis of covariance, with exercise as a covariate, found that total body BMC was significantly lower among women in the high dietary restraint group, and that the difference in spinal BMD approached significance ($P = 0.062$). Multiple regression analysis was also used to assess the independent effect of dietary restraint. For both total body BMD and BMC, TFEQ-R score was a significant negative predictor, and weekly hours of exercise were a significant positive predictor. For lumbar spine BMD, exercise entered the equation, and the TFEQ-R score was narrowly excluded ($P = 0.07$).

Although it did not assess dietary restraint *per se*, one other study provides some insight into the association between eating attitudes and bone. Barr and colleagues [32] conducted a 2-year prospective study in 45 girls initially 10.5 ± 0.6 years of age. They monitored nutrient intakes, physical activity, growth, and sexual maturation. Eating attitudes were assessed using the children's Eating Attitudes Test [33], which contains subscales for oral control, dieting, and bulimia. Although the oral control subscale is not synonymous with dietary restraint, there may be some parallels, as subscale scores reflect the individual's perception that they can limit or control their food intake. Body composition and BMC at the spine and total body were assessed at baseline and annually thereafter using DEXA. Girls with high and low oral control scores had similar body composition, dietary intake, physical activity, and sexual maturation at baseline and 2 years, but girls with high scores had significantly lower total body BMC at baseline and 2 years, and lower spinal BMC at 2 years. In multiple regression analysis, oral control score negatively predicted baseline, 2-year, and 2-year change in total body and spinal BMC [32].

SUMMARY

In an effort to conform to societal ideals for body weight and shape, many young women consciously monitor and attempt to limit their food intake, which is known as cognitive dietary restraint. High levels of dietary restraint appear to act as a subtle stressor and, as such, activate the HPA axis and lead to increased release of cortisol. Furthermore, activation of the HPA axis can suppress the HPG axis, and women with high dietary restraint have consistently been found to experience more subclinical ovulatory disturbances, as well as irregular menstrual cycles. Both of these hormonal alterations (increased cortisol and lower reproductive hormones) are known to have adverse effects on bone. And, although few data exist, available evidence comparing healthy women with high and low levels of cognitive dietary restraint does suggest that high dietary restraint is associated with lower values for bone mineral density or content. Additional prospective research evaluating change in bone density over time in women with high and low levels of cognitive dietary restraint is warranted to assess the clinical importance of these findings. Studies designed to reduce the stress associated with eating and/or body weight and shape in women with high dietary restraint, using cortisol excretion and ovulatory function as endpoints, will help determine whether management strategies can be identified that would reduce potential adverse effects.

ACKNOWLEDGMENTS

The British Columbia Health Care Research Foundation, the British Columbia Medical Services Foundation, and the British Columbia Children's Hospital Foundation supported portions of the research reported herein. I would also like to thank my graduate students and colleagues, including Ms. Christina Janelle, Dr. Judy McLean, Dr. Moira Petit, Dr. Jerilynn Prior, and Ms. Yvette Vigna.

REFERENCES

1. Cann, C.E., Martin, M.C., Genant, H.K., and Jaffe, R.B. (1984). Decreased spinal mineral content in amenorrheic women. *JAMA* 251: 626–629.
2. Rigotti, N.A., Nussbaum, S.R., Herzog, D.B., and Neer, R.M. (1984). Osteoporosis in women with anorexia nervosa. *N. Engl. J. Med.* 311: 1601–1606.

3. Rideout, C.A., Barr, S.I., and Prior, J.C. (2003). Clinical eating disorders and subclinical disordered eating: implications for bone health, in *Nutritional Aspects of Bone Health*, New, S.A. and Bonjour, J.P., Eds., Royal Society of Chemistry, Cambridge, U.K.

4. APA. (2000). *Diagnostic and Statistical Manual of Mental Disorders*, 4th ed. American Psychiatric Association, Washington, D.C.

5. Health and Welfare Canada. (1993). *Canada's Health Promotion Survey 1990: Technical Report*. Minister of Supply and Services, Ottawa.

6. Stunkard, A.J. and Messick, S. (1985). The three-factor eating questionnaire to measure dietary restraint, disinhibition and hunger. *J. Psychosom. Res.* 29: 71–83.

7. Reid, I.R. (1997). Glucocorticoid osteoporosis: mechanisms and management. *Eur. J. Endocrinol.* 137: 209–217.

8. Tsigos, C. and Chrousos, G.P. (2002). Hypothalamic–pituitary–adrenal axis, neuroendocrine factors and stress. *J. Psychosom. Res.* 53: 865–871.

9. Heaney, R.P., Recker, R.R., and Saville, P.D. (1978). Menopausal changes in calcium balance performance. *J. Lab. Clin. Med.* 92: 953–963.

10. Hadjidakis, D., Kokkinakis, E., Sfakianakis, M., and Raptis, S.A. (1999). The type and time of menopause as decisive factors for bone mass changes. *Eur. J. Clin. Invest.* 29: 877–885.

11. Herman, C.P. and Polivy, J. (1980). Restrained eating, in *Obesity*, Stunkard, A.J., Ed., Saunders, Philadelphia, PA, pp. 208–225.

12. Van Strien, T., Fritjers, J.E.R., Bergers, G.P.A., and Degares, P.B. (1986). The Dutch Eating Behavior Questionnaire (DEBQ) for assessment of restrained, emotional, and external eating behavior. *Int. J. Eating Disord.* 5: 295–315.

13. Gorman, B.S. and Allison, D.B. (1995). Measures of restrained eating, in *Handbook of Assessment Methods for Eating Behaviors and Weight-Related Problems. Measures, Theory, and Research*, Allison, D.B., Ed., Sage, Thousand Oaks, CA, pp. 149–184.

14. Buffet, N.C., Djakoure, C., Maitre, S.C., and Bouchard, P. (1998). Regulation of the human menstrual cycle. *Fron. Neuroendocrinol.* 19: 151–186.

15. Prior, J.C., Vigna, Y.M., Schulzer, M., Hall, J.E., and Bonen, A. (1990). Determination of luteal phase length by quantitative basal temperature methods: validation against the midcycle LH peak. *Clin. Invest. Med.* 13: 123–131.

16. Schweiger, U., Tuschl, R.J., Platte, P., Broocks, A., Laessle, R.G., and Pirke, K.M. (1992). Everyday eating behavior and menstrual function in young women. *Fertil. Steril.* 57: 771–775.

17. Highet, R. (1989). Athletic amenorrhoea: an update on aetiology, complications and management. *Sports Med.* 7: 82–108.

18. Brooks, S.M., Sanborn, C.F., Albrecht, B.H., and Wagner, W.W., Jr. (1984). Diet in athletic amenorrhoea. *Lancet* 1: 559–560.

19. Slavin, J., Lutter, J., and Cushman, S. (1984). Amenorrhoea in vegetarian athletes. *Lancet* 1: 1474–1475.

20. Pedersen, A.B., Bartholomew, M.J., Dolence, L.A., Aljadir, L.P., Netteburg, K.L., and Lloyd, T. (1991). Menstrual differences due to vegetarian and non-vegetarian diets. *Am. J. Clin. Nutr.* 53: 879–885.

21. Barr, S.I., Prior, J.C., and Vigna, Y.M. (1994). Restrained eating and ovulatory disturbances: possible implications for bone health. *Am. J. Clin. Nutr.* 59: 92–97.

22. Barr, S.I., Janelle, K.C., and Prior, J.C. (1994). Vegetarian vs. nonvegetarian diets, dietary restraint, and subclinical ovulatory disturbances: prospective 6-mo study. *Am. J. Clin. Nutr.* 60: 887–894.

23. Lebenstedt, M., Platte, P., and Pirke, K.M. (1999). Reduced resting metabolic rate in athletes with menstrual disorders. *Med. Sci. Sports Exerc.* 31: 1250–1256.

24. McLean, J.A. and Barr, S.I. (2003). Cognitive dietary restraint is associated with eating behaviors, lifestyle practices, personality characteristics and menstrual irregularity in college women. *Appetite* 40: 185–192.
25. Prior, J.C., Vigna, Y.M., Schechter, M.T., and Burgess, A.E. (1990). Spinal bone loss and ovulatory disturbances. *N. Engl. J. Med.* 323: 1221–1227.
26. Pirke, K.M., Tuschl, R.J., Spyra, B., Laessle, R.G., Schweiger, U., Broocks, A., Sambauer, S., and Zitzelsberger, G. (1990). Endocrine findings in restrained eaters. *Physiol. Behav.* 47: 903–906.
27. McLean, J.A., Barr, S.I., and Prior, J.C. (2001). Cognitive dietary restraint is associated with higher urinary cortisol excretion in healthy premenopausal women. *Am. J. Clin. Nutr.* 73: 7–12.
28. Anderson, D.A., Shapiro, J.R., Lundgren, J.D., Spataro, L.E., and Frye, C.A. (2002). Self-reported dietary restraint is associated with elevated levels of salivary cortisol. *Appetite* 38: 13–17.
29. Greendale, G.A., Unger, J.B., Rowe, J.W., and Seeman, T.E. (1999). The relation between cortisol excretion and fractures in healthy older people: results from the MacArthur studies. *J. Am. Ger. Soc.* 47: 799–803.
30. Van Loan, M.D. and Keim, N.L. (2000). Influence of cognitive eating restraint on total-body measurements of bone mineral density and bone mineral content in premenopausal women aged 18–45 y: a cross-sectional study. *Am. J. Clin. Nutr.* 72: 837–843.
31. McLean, J.A., Barr, S.I., and Prior, J.C. (2001). Dietary restraint, exercise and bone density in young women: are they related? *Med. Sci. Sports Exerc.* 33: 1292–1296.
32. Barr, S.I., Petit, M.A., Vigna, Y.M., and Prior, J.C. (2001). Eating attitudes and habitual calcium intake in peripubertal girls are associated with initial bone mineral content and its change over 2 years. *J. Bone Miner. Res.* 16, 940–947.
33. Maloney, M.J., McGuire, J., and Daniels, S.R. (1988). Reliability testing of a children's version of the Eating Attitudes Test. *J. Am. Acad. Clin. Adolesc. Psychiatr.* 25: 541–543.

PART V

Vitamin D—First Part

Functions of Vitamin D: Importance for Prevention of Common Cancers, Type 1 Diabetes and Heart Disease

MICHAEL F. HOLICK

Department of Endocrinology, Boston University School of Medicine, Boston, Massachusetts

EVOLUTION OF VITAMIN D

Little is known about when vitamin D was first photosynthesized in living organisms. It had long been speculated that the reason why cod liver oil, salmon, and other oily fish have high concentrations of vitamin D was because of the concentrating ability of the food chain. This is well demonstrated in a fish that consumes approximately 1.2% of its body weight every 24 hours. Approximately 1/2 ton of diatoms eaten by sea creatures and ultimately eaten by seals equals 1 pound of killer whale, which eat seals, require 5 tons of diatoms per pound [1]. To further investigate this, at Wood's Hole Marine Research Facility our laboratory grew a phytoplankton species that has been living in the Sargasso Sea unchanged for more than 750 million years. When this organism was grown in culture and exposed to simulated sunlight, it was found that *Emiliania huxlei* Bt-6 had approximately 1 μg of ergosterol (provitamin D_2) per gram weight and that it was converted to previtamin D_2 when exposed to ultraviolet radiation [1].

Nutritional Aspects of Osteoporosis, Second Edition

181

Approximately 350 million years ago, when aquatic organisms began venturing onto land, they were confronted with a major nutritional problem: The plentiful calcium in their ocean environment was absent on land. The calcium was stored in the soils, and these organisms had to evolve an efficient method to digest plants that absorbed the calcium into their leaves. For reasons that are not at all understood, it was the exposure of skin of early land vertebrates to sunlight that resulted in the production of vitamin D and played an essential role in guaranteeing that the calcium in the plants was bioavailable to the animals [2]. Most vertebrate organisms, including amphibians, reptiles, birds, and non-human primates, take advantage of sunlight to produce vitamin D in their skin [1,3].

PHOTOSYNTHESIS AND REGULATION OF PREVITAMIN D_3

The ozone layer is very efficient in absorbing all of the high-energy ultraviolet radiation up to 290 nm. Solar ultraviolet radiation with energies between 290 and 315 nm (UVB) that are able to reach the surface of the Earth are responsible for converting 7-dehydrocholesterol (provitamin D_3) to previtamin D_3 in the skin [4]. Once previtamin D_3 is formed in the plasma membrane of the epidermal and dermal cells, it is rapidly converted to vitamin D_3 by a membrane-enhanced process [5]. Vitamin D_3, which is structurally less rigid, is ejected out of the skin cell into the extracellular space, where it enters into the circulation (Fig. 1).

Approximately 0.1% of the solar UVB photons reaches the surface of the Earth. Thus, a small change in the zenith angle of the sun has a dramatic influence on the cutaneous production of vitamin D_3. When the rays of the sun are more oblique, the UVB photons have a longer path of ozone to traverse and thus are efficiently absorbed by the ozone layer; therefore, few, if any, UVB photons reach the surface of the Earth. This is the explanation for why time of day, season, and latitude have a dramatic influence on the cutaneous production of vitamin D_3 (Fig. 2) [6,7]. People who live at higher latitudes cannot make vitamin D_3 in their skin during the winter. In Boston and Edmonton, Canada, exposure to sunlight from November through February and from October through March results in little, if any, production of vitamin D_3 in the skin [6]. Skin pigment (melanin) efficiently absorbs UVB radiation and therefore markedly reduces the cutaneous production of vitamin D_3 [8]. Typically, African-Americans with skin types 5 or 6 (exposure to sunlight will never cause them to burn) require 10 to 50 times more sun exposure than a Caucasian with skin type 2 (always burns, sometimes tans) to make enough vitamin D_3 in their skin [8]. Aging can also influence the cutaneous production of vitamin D_3 (Fig. 2) [2].

Clothing absorbs most, if not all, UVB radiation, similar to a sunscreen [9,10]. Thus, wearing clothing on sun-exposed areas or wearing a sunscreen will essentially eliminate the cutaneous production of vitamin D_3. A sunscreen with an SPF of 15 will reduce the production of vitamin D_3 by as much as 99% (Fig. 2).

VITAMIN D AND BONE HEALTH

It is estimated that 10 million households have a reptile as a pet. Reptiles, like humans, are vertebrates and require a source of calcium and vitamin D. Often, reptiles are housed in glass enclosures and are exposed to incandescent lighting. Without an adequate source of calcium and vitamin D, they develop severe osteoporosis and osteomalacia that results in spinal and long-bone fractures that ultimately result in death. The reptile pet trade has become aware of the problem and, as a result, various fluorescent and other types of lamps have been developed that provide a source of UVB radiation. When reptiles are exposed to these lamps, they make enough vitamin D_3 to satisfy their requirement [11].

Vitamin D is solely responsible for regulating the efficiency of intestinal calcium absorption (Fig. 1). Typically, in a vitamin-D-deficient state, the intestine can absorb no more than 10 to 15% of dietary calcium; however, in vitamin D sufficiency, the small intestine absorbs approximately 30% of dietary calcium [12,13]. During growth spurts and during lactation and pregnancy, this is enhanced to more than 50% [13]. The major physiologic function of vitamin D is to maintain the serum calcium within a physiologically acceptable range. When dietary calcium is not sufficient to satisfy the body's requirement, then vitamin D mobilizes calcium stores from the skeleton (Fig. 1).

METABOLISM AND BIOLOGIC FUNCTIONS OF VITAMIN D

Before vitamin D (either vitamin D_2 or vitamin D_3) can carry out its biologic functions, it requires a hydroxylation on carbon-25 in the liver to form 25-hydroxyvitamin D [25(OH)D]. 25(OH)D is the major circulating

184

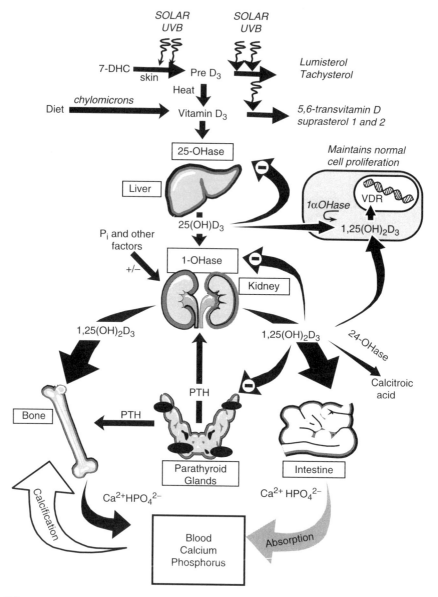

FIGURE 1   Schematic representation for cutaneous production of vitamin D and its metabolism
and regulation for calcium homeostasis and cellular growth. During exposure to sunlight,
7-dehydrocholesterol (7-DHC) in the skin absorbs solar ultraviolet B (UVB) radiation and
is converted to previtamin D_3 (preD$_3$). Once formed, D$_3$ undergoes thermally induced
transformation to vitamin D$_3$. Further exposure to sunlight converts preD$_3$ and vitamin D$_3$ to
biologically inert photoproducts. Vitamin D coming from the diet or from the skin enters the

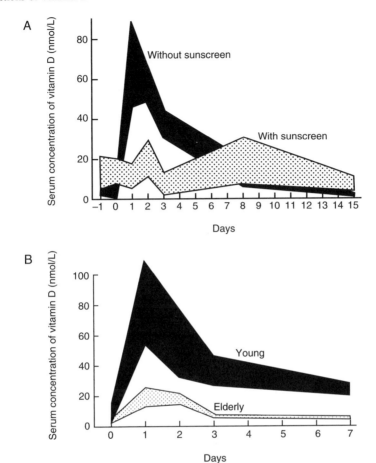

FIGURE 2 (A) Circulating concentrations of vitamin D_3 after a single exposure to one minimal erythemal dose of simulated sunlight with a sunscreen, with a sun protection factor of 8 (SPF-8), or with a topical placebo cream. (B) Circulating concentrations of vitamin D in response to a whole-body exposure to one minimal erythemal dose in healthy young and elderly subjects. (From Holick, M.F., *Am. J. Clin. Nutr.*, 60, 619–630, 1994. With permission.)

circulation and is metabolized in the liver by the vitamin D-25-hydroxylase (25-OHase) to 25-hydroxyvitamin D_3 [25(OH)D_3]. 25(OH)D_3 re-enters the circulation and is converted in the kidney by the 25-hydroxyvitamin D_3-1α-hydroxylase (1-OHase) to 1,25-dihydroxyvitamin D_3 [1,25(OH)$_2D_3$]. A variety of factors, including serum phosphorus (P_i) and parathyroid hormone (PTH), regulate the renal production of 1,25(OH)$_2$D. 1,25(OH)$_2$D regulates calcium metabolism through its interaction with its major target tissues, the bone and the intestine. 1,25(OH)$_2D_3$ also induces its own destruction by enhancing the expression of the 25-hydroxyvitamin D-24-hydroxylase (24-OHase). 25(OH)D is metabolized in other tissues for the purpose of regulation of cellular growth. (© Michael F. Holick, 2003. Used with permission.)

form of vitamin D that is measured to determine vitamin D status
[13]; however, 25(OH)D is biologically inert and requires an additional
hydroxylation on carbon-1 to form 1,25-dihydroxyvitamin D [1,25(OH)$_2$D]
(Fig. 1). 1,25(OH)$_2$D carries out many of its biologic functions on calcium
metabolism by interacting with its specific nuclear vitamin D receptor
(VDR) [14]. This complex combines with the retinoic acid X receptor and
migrates to sites on the DNA that specifically recognize this complex (vitamin
D responsive element, or VDRE).

In the intestine, 1,25(OH)$_2$D stimulates the production of calbindin$_{9k}$
(calcium-binding protein) and the epithelial calcium channel. This results in
an increase in the efficiency of intestinal calcium absorption. When calcium
from the diet is inadequate to maintain serum calcium levels, the decrease
in ionized calcium is recognized by the calcium sensor in the parathyroid
gland, which in turn induces a cascade of events resulting in an increase
in the production and secretion of parathyroid hormone (PTH) (Fig. 1)
[3,13]. PTH is the major hormonal factor that enhances the renal production
of 1,25(OH)$_2$D; it also increases tubular reabsorption of calcium in the
kidney. In addition, PTH interacts with its PTH-1 receptor and 1,25(OH)$_2$D
interacts with its VDR in osteoblasts in the bone. This causes an increase
in the expression of RANKL (receptor activator of NFκB ligand). The
RANKL interacts with its receptor RANK on the pre-osteoclast. This results
in a signal transduction to the pre-osteoclast to initiate it to become a
mature osteoclast. The mature osteoclasts secrete hydrochloric acid to
dissolve bone and various proteases and collagenases to dissolve the matrix.
The result is to release precious calcium stores into the circulation to
maintain serum calcium levels within a physiologically acceptable range
(Fig. 1). Once 1,25(OH)$_2$D performs its function, it is sequentially metabolized on the side chain on carbons 24 and 23 by the 25-hydroxyvitamin
D-24-hydroxylase(24-OHase), which leads to oxidative cleavage between
carbons 23 and 24 to yield the biologically inactive water soluble calcitroic
acid (Fig. 1) [13,14].

PREVALENCE AND CONSEQUENCES OF
VITAMIN D DEFICIENCY ON BONE HEALTH

Vitamin D deficiency in children is synonymous with rickets. Rickets is
considered to be a disease like the plague; that is, it is no longer a significant
medical problem for the 21st century. However, vitamin D deficiency is
an unrecognized epidemic throughout the industrialized world. This is
especially true in northern Europe and the United States. Upwards of 50%

of adults over the age of 65 years have been reported to be vitamin D deficient [16–20]. We observed that 32% of Caucasians, 42% Hispanics, and 84% of African-Americans over the age of 65 years were vitamin D deficient [25(OH)D < 20 ng/mL] at the end of the summer [13]. Rickets is making a resurgence in young African-American children who receive their total nutrition from breastfeeding [21]. Young and middle-aged adults who work indoors and always wear sun protection when outside are also at increased risk of vitamin D deficiency [22]. This is especially true during the winter when little, if any, vitamin D_3 can be produced in the skin at latitudes above 37° [6,13]. A survey of women of child-bearing age in the United States revealed that, at the end of the winter, 42% of African-American women ages 15 to 49 years and 4% of Caucasian women at the end of the summer were vitamin D deficient [23]. In Boston, we observed that 32% of medical personnel ages 18 to 29 years were vitamin D deficient at the end of the winter, and 4% remained vitamin D deficient at the end of the summer [22]. Most alarming, we observed in 49 mother–infant pairs that 76% were severely vitamin D deficient (J. Lee, B. Phillip, and M.F. Holick, unpublished results).

Vitamin D deficiency causes a disruption of chondrocyte maturation in the growing bones of children. This leads to a widening of the epiphyseal plates that is typically seen as widening at the end of the long bones, especially the wrists and the costochondral junctions at the rib cage (known as rachitic rosary). In addition, vitamin D deficiency causes a mineralization defect, and the combination of poor chondrocyte maturation and inadequate mineralization of the "rubbery" collagen matrix results in an inward or outward bowing of the legs due to the influence of gravity when the child begins to stand and walk (Fig. 3).

The effect of vitamin D deficiency on the adult skeleton is much more subtle. The epiphyseal plates have closed and there is enough mineral in the skeleton to prevent any skeletal deformities typically seen with rickets. Vitamin D deficiency causes secondary hyperparathyroidism. As a result, there is an increase in osteoclastic activity that results in the destruction of mineralized bone, which can precipitate or exacerbate osteoporosis.

Vitamin D deficiency also causes a mineralization defect in the adult's skeleton that results in osteomalacia. It is often erroneously thought that in vitamin D deficiency the serum calcium is low, which leads to a poor skeletal mineralization. In fact, the serum calcium is usually normal in a vitamin-D-deficient patient. This is in part due to secondary hyperparathyroidism and the PTH action on mobilizing calcium from the skeleton. PTH also causes phosphate wasting in the kidney which results in a low normal or low serum phosphorus. This results in an inadequate calcium × phosphorus product and an inability for hydroxyapatite to crystallize in the collagen matrix.

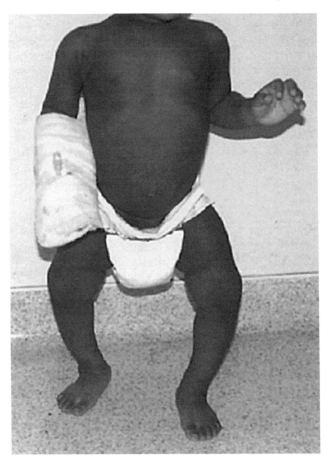

FIGURE 3   African-American 2-year-old child who presented to our hospital with severe vitamin D deficiency and rickets. (© Michael F. Holick, 2003. Used with permission.)

Unlike osteoporosis, which is a silent disease until a fracture occurs, osteomalacia often causes a throbbing pain in the bones. In addition, vitamin D deficiency causes muscle weakness and muscle aches [24–26]. Symptoms of bone discomfort and muscle aches and pains in patients with a normal sedimentation rate often are ignored as just being part of the aches and pains of aging. In some cases, patients often go undiagnosed or are misdiagnosed as some type of collagen vascular disease or are given the diagnosis of fibromyalgia. It has been estimated that 40 to 80% of patients with this diagnosis have vitamin-D-deficiency osteomalacia [24,25].

OTHER HEALTH CONSEQUENCES OF VITAMIN D DEFICIENCY: INCREASED RISK OF AUTOIMMUNE DISEASES, SOLID TUMORS, AND CARDIOVASCULAR HEART DISEASE

In 1941, Apperley [27] noted that people living at higher latitudes are at increased risk of dying of cancer and suggested that sunlight exposure imparted some type of immunity to solid tumors. He further suggested that the observation of increased risk of skin cancer at lower latitudes was of little consequence in light of the seriousness of the consequences of solid tumors, such as prostate, colon, and breast cancer. It is also recognized that living at higher latitudes increases the risk of autoimmune diseases, including multiple sclerosis and type 1 diabetes, as well as hypertension and congestive heart failure [28–30].

The β-islet cells in the pancreas possess a VDR. In NOD mice, which typically develop type 1 diabetes within 200 days of life when pretreated with $1,25(OH)_2D_3$ after birth, the risk of getting type 1 diabetes was reduced by 80% [31]. This observation has been mirrored in humans by Hypponnen et al. [32], who reported that children in Finland who received 2000 IU of vitamin D a day throughout their childhood reduced their risk of developing type 1 diabetes by 80%.

In two mouse models that developed multiple sclerosis and rheumatoid-like arthritis [31], pretreatment with $1,25(OH)_2D_3$ essentially eradicated the risk of developing both of these debilitating diseases [33]. Rotstand [29] reported that hypertension was more common for people living at higher latitudes worldwide. To evaluate the role of sunlight and hypertension, adults with moderate hypertension were randomized and exposed to a tanning bed that either irradiated the patient with UVB and UVA or just UVA radiation. The patients who were exposed to UVA radiation did not experience a rise in their blood levels of 25(OH)D, and after 3 months of therapy they showed no change in their blood pressure. However, the patients who were exposed to the tanning bed that transmitted both UVB and UVA radiation increased their circulating concentrations of 25(OH)D by 80%. Furthermore, after 3 months their hypertension was completely resolved (Fig. 4) [34]. The blood pressure decreased on average by 6 mmHg for both systolic and diastolic blood pressures. It is now recognized that $1,25(OH)_2D_3$ is a potent downregulator of the renal production of renin [35]. This may also be the explanation for why patients with coronary artery disease are more likely to develop congestive heart failure if they are vitamin D deficient [30].

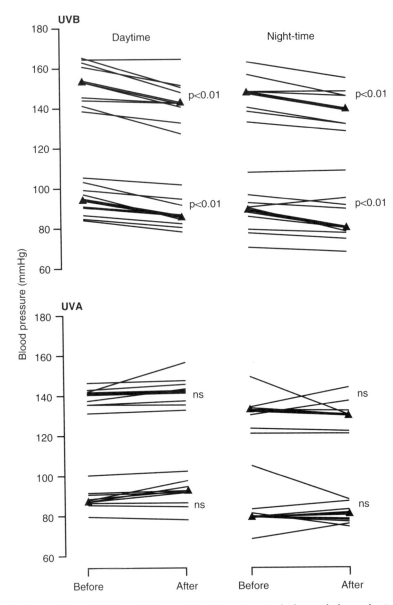

FIGURE 4 Effect of UV-B and UV-A irradiation from a tanning bed on ambulatory daytime and nighttime blood pressure in hypertensive adults before and after exposure to the tanning bed radiation three times a week for 3 months (ns, not significant; thick line, mean). (From Krause, R. et al., *Lancet*, 352, 709–710, 1998. With permission.)

In the 1990s, several epidemiologic studies and a few prospective studies suggested that increasing vitamin D intake or exposure to sunlight could decrease risk of colon, prostate, and breast cancer [36–38]. A more recent evaluation of latitude and cancer incidence by Grant suggests that many common cancers are due to lack of UVB exposure. Both white males and females are at higher risk of dying of cancer in general if they have minimum exposure to sunlight (Fig. 5) [39,40]. In a prospective study, Garland et al. [41] reported that adults who had a 25(OH)D of at least 20 ng/mL (50 nmol/L) lowered their risk of getting colon cancer by 50%.

It is well known that most tissues and cells in the body, including brain, heart, stomach, pancreas, prostate, breast, monocytes, activated T and B lymphocytes, and the skin, all possessed a VDR [13,14]. The observation that $1,25(OH)_2D_3$ was a potent inhibitor of cellular proliferation of tumor cells and normal cells that have a VDR suggested the possibility that living at lower latitudes, which increases the production of vitamin D_3 in the skin, ultimately increased circulating concentrations of $1,25(OH)_2D$. The higher $1,25(OH)_2D$ levels, in turn, would downregulate cellular proliferation and keep cell growth in check. However, it was also known that the renal production of $1,25(OH)_2D$ was tightly regulated by PTH, calcium, and phosphorus and that increasing exposure to sunlight or increasing vitamin D intake would not result in the increased renal production of $1,25(OH)_2D$ [13]. Indeed, in vitamin D intoxication, $1,25(OH)_2D$ levels are often low rather than elevated [42]. Thus, there needed to be another explanation for how exposure to sunlight at lower latitudes might be related to the vitamin D–cancer connection.

In 1998, it was reported that normal prostate cells expressed 25-hydroxyvitamin D-1α-hydroxylase (1-OHase) that was identical to the enzyme present in the kidney [43]. Furthermore, it was demonstrated that normal cultured prostate cells and prostate cancer cells that had the 1-OHase converted $25(OH)D_3$ to $1,25(OH)_2D_3$ [43,44]. This observation suggested that it was possible that many tissues in the body have the enzymatic machinery to produce $1,25(OH)_2D_3$ for the purpose of keeping cellular proliferation and differentiation in a normative state. Once $1,25(OH)_2D$ carries out this function, it induces the 24-OHase, which causes its destruction to calcitroic acid (Fig. 1).

This was a major revelation that suggested that many tissues in the body, including skin, lung, prostate, breast, and mononuclear cells, have the enzymatic machinery to produce $1,25(OH)_2D$ locally for the purpose of autocrine and paracrine regulation of cellular growth. This may help explain why living at lower latitudes or having an increased exposure to sunlight decreases the risk of a wide variety of chronic diseases.

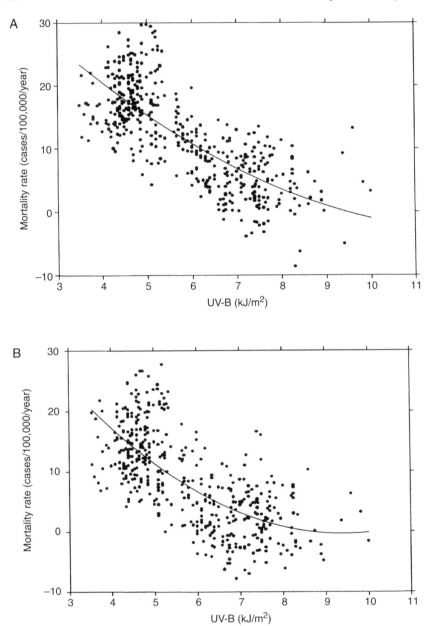

FIGURE 5   (A) Premature mortality due to cancer: white females versus total ozone mapping spectrometer (TOMS), July 1992, DNA-weighted UV-B. (B) Premature mortality due to cancer: U.S. white males with insufficient UV-B, 1970–1994 versus July 1992, DNA-weighted UV-B radiation. (© William B. Grant, 2003. Used with permission.)

To test the hypothesis that the endogenous local production of $1,25(OH)_2D_3$ was important for inhibiting cancer cell growth, a prostate cancer cell line (LNCaP) that does not express or have any 1-OHase activity was transfected either with a plasmid that contained the 1-OHase cDNA or a plasmid that had an empty vector. The transfected cells were incubated with $25(OH)D_3$. The cells transfected with the 1-OHase plasmid showed a marked inhibition of proliferation, whereas cells transfected with an empty vector had no significant effect except at very high concentrations (10^{-6} M). It was also demonstrated that the LNCaP cells transfected with the 1-OHase plasmid converted ^{3}H-$25(OH)D_3$ to ^{3}H-$1,25(OH)_2D_3$. There was no conversion of ^{3}H-$25(OH)D_3$ in the cells that were transfected with the empty vector plasmid. These results provide proof of principle that if a cell can produce $1,25(OH)_2D_3$ then it has the capacity to downregulate cellular proliferation and induce maturation [44].

CLINICAL APPLICATIONS FOR THE ANTIPROLIFERATIVE ACTIVITY OF $1,25(OH)_2D_3$ AND ITS ANALOGS

With the recognition that skin cells have VDRs and that they respond to $1,25(OH)_2D_3$ by decreasing their proliferative activity and inducing their maturation, it was reasonable to consider using $1,25(OH)_2D_3$ and its analogs as a topical drug to treat the hyperproliferative skin disorder psoriasis. Topical $1,25(OH)_2D_3$ and its analogs calcipotriene, 22-oxo-1,25-dihydroxy-vitamin D_3 and 1,24-dihydroxyvitamin D_3 have all been demonstrated clinically to be effective in treating psoriasis [45–47]. It is a first-line treatment for psoriasis worldwide.

As early as 1980, the observation that $1,25(OH)_2D_3$ inhibited murine and human leukemic cell growth and induced them to mature suggested that $1,25(OH)_2D_3$ and its analogs could be developed for treating some leukemias and other cancers [13]. Unfortunately, $1,25(OH)_2D_3$ also causes hypercalcemia; patients with pre-leukemia who were treated with $1,25(OH)_2D_3$ initially responded to therapy but ultimately succumbed to their disease [48]. The likely explanations were that the patients developed severe hypercalcemia and that populations of cells either mutated and had defective or absent VDRs, thereby permitting the cells to grow rapidly in a blastic state, resulting in the death of the patient.

A huge effort is underway to develop analogs of $1,25(OH)_2D_3$ that have little calcemic activity but potent antiproliferative and maturation activity.

These analogs hold great promise as either adjunctive or primary therapy for solid tumors that have VDRs [13,49].

PREVENTION AND TREATMENT OF VITAMIN D DEFICIENCY

Humans evolved and have been bathed in sunlight. The skin has a huge capacity to produce vitamin D_3. Adults wearing bathing suits and exposed to 1 minimal erythemal dose (1 MED) resulted in an increase in circulating concentrations of vitamin D_3 in the circulation that was comparable to taking an oral dose of between 10,000 and 25,000 IU of vitamin D_2 (Fig. 6) [2,13]. The campaign by the American Academy of Dermatology and the sunscreen industry to encourage total sun protection increases the risk of vitamin D deficiency in infants, children, young, middle-aged, and older adults. A sensible approach for satisfying the body's vitamin D requirement is to encourage people of all skin types to have limited exposure to sunlight that is equivalent to about 25% of their MED. For example, consider a Caucasian living in Boston (latitude 42°N) who is exposed to 30 minutes of sunlight between the hours of 11 and 2 p.m. Eastern Daylight Savings time and

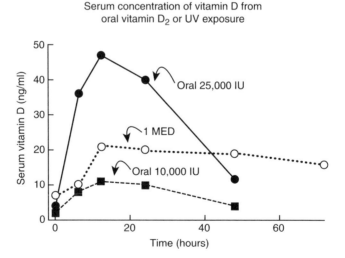

FIGURE 6 Comparison of serum vitamin D levels after a whole-body exposure to 1 MED (minimal erythemal dose) of simulated sunlight compared with a single oral dose of either 10,000 or 25,000 IU of vitamin D_2. (From Holick, M.F., Am. J. Clin. Nutr., 60, 619–630, 1994. With permission.)

ends up with a slight pinkness to the skin (1 MED); 25% of that time (*i.e.*, approximately 5- to 10-minute exposure of hands, face, and arms or arms and legs, two to three times a week) will satisfy that person's vitamin D requirement. If this exposure is maintained through the spring, summer, and fall, the excess vitamin D that is produced is stored in the body fat and slowly released into the circulation during the winter when vitamin D cannot be produced in the skin.

In the absence of adequate exposure to sunlight, most experts agree that the recommendation in 1997 by the Institute of Medicine of 200, 400, and 600 IU of vitamin D a day for those ages 0–50 years, 51–70 years, and 71 + years, respectively, is inadequate. A minimum of 1000 IU of vitamin D a day is necessary to maintain a healthy level of 25(OH)D, which is considered by many experts to be between 30 and 50 ng/mL [50–54].

Heaney *et al.* [54] have suggested that in the absence of sunlight the body requires 3000 to 5000 IU of vitamin D a day to fully satisfy its needs. We observed that healthy young and middle-aged adults who ingested 1000 IU of vitamin D a day from the end of the winter throughout the spring were able to maintain their 25(OH)D in the range of 30 to 40 ng/mL [50] (Fig. 7). Thus, exposure to sunlight or ingesting 1000 IU of vitamin D a day should satisfy the body's vitamin D requirement.

Because very few foods (*e.g.*, cod liver oil and oily fish) naturally contain vitamin D the only other sources of vitamin D come from fortified foods. Milk has been fortified with vitamin D since the 1930s and has helped eradicate rickets as a health problem in children in the United States, Canada, and a few European countries that permit fortification of milk with vitamin D. Unfortunately, because of an outbreak of vitamin D intoxication in the 1950s that was associated with over-fortification of milk with vitamin D, many European countries now forbid the fortification of dairy products with vitamin D. Margarine and some cereals are fortified with vitamin D.

A new approach for increasing vitamin D intake across the entire population has recently been introduced by the Minute Maid Corporation. They were the first to fortify orange juice with vitamin D_3, similar to milk (*i.e.*, 100 IU of vitamin D_3 per 8 oz.). The vitamin D_3 in orange juice is highly bioavailable (Fig. 7). It should be recognized, however, that milk, orange juice, and other fortified foods only contain a relatively small amount of vitamin D, and unless 6 to 10 glasses of milk or vitamin-D-fortified orange juice are drunk each day, it is difficult to obtain adequate vitamin D solely from the diet.

A simple way of correcting vitamin D deficiency is to give pharmacologic doses of vitamin D over a short period of time. For example, giving 50,000 IU of vitamin D which comes as a pill or capsule once a week for 8 weeks often

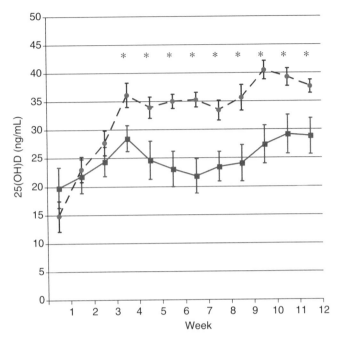

FIGURE 7   Weekly 25-hydroxyvitamin D [25(OH)D] levels in healthy adults ingesting vitamin D (1000 IU/8 oz./day) fortified (—■—) and unfortified orange juice (—●—). Error bars represent standard error of the means ($P < 0.05$, *$P \leq 0.01$). (From Tangpricha, V. et al., Am. J. Clin. Nutr., 77, 1478–1483, 2003. With permission.)

fills up the empty vitamin D tank [16]. A 25(OH)D level of at least 20 ng/mL should be achieved. Some patients who are severely vitamin D deficient may need an additional 8-week course. For patients who do not have very much exposure to sunlight, it is reasonable to give them 50,000 IU of vitamin D once every 2 to 4 weeks. Monitoring of serum 25(OH)D should be done once or twice a year. It should be noted that, although the upper limit of normal for 25(OH)D reported by many laboratories is 55 ng/mL, vitamin D intoxication usually does not occur until the 25(OH)D levels are above 150 ng/mL [42]. Alternative approaches are to give 500,000 IU of vitamin D intramuscularly twice a year or 400,000 IU of vitamin D once a month [55,56]. The problem with giving vitamin D intramuscularly is that it is often not bioavailable and it can be very uncomfortable. A multivitamin containing 400 IU of vitamin D will help the vitamin D status but usually will not maintain normal circulating concentrations of 25(OH)D above a healthy level of 30 ng/mL. A few companies are now marketing a vitamin D pill that contains 1000 IU of vitamin D.

Although vitamin D_2 is about 50–80% as effective as vitamin D_3, it is an excellent source of vitamin D. As long as 25(OH)D levels are maintained at at least 20 and preferably above 30 ng/mL, the use of either vitamin D_2 or vitamin D_3 is perfectly acceptable.

CONCLUSION

Vitamin D deficiency is insidious and has enormous health implications (Fig. 8). If, indeed, vitamin D evolved early in human evolution for controlling a wide variety of metabolic processes, including calcium and bone metabolism, immune function, cellular growth, and blood pressure regulation, then a program is needed to educate healthcare professionals and the population at large about their risk of vitamin D deficiency and its consequences. This is of particular concern for infants and young children for whom a vitamin D deficiency could impact the rest of their lives by increasing their risk of many chronic diseases, including type 1 diabetes, cardiovascular heart disease, and cancer.

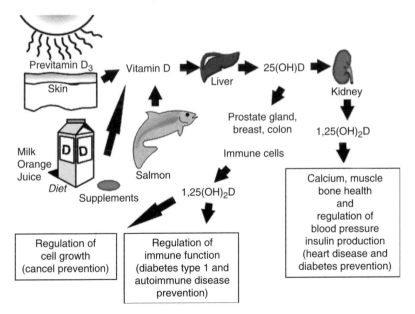

FIGURE 8 Schematic representation of the multitude of other potential physiologic actions of vitamin D for cardiovascular health, cancer prevention, regulation of immune function, and decreased risk of autoimmune diseases. (© Michael F. Holick, 2003. Used with permission.)

The promotion of the message to avoid all direct sun exposure on the skin needs to be tempered. Charles Schulz, who had great insights into life, promoted sensible sun exposure in one of his Peanuts® comic strips. Linus received in his school bag lunch several notes from his mother. She urged him to get good grades and to make friends, and then she said, "I hope that you are sitting in the sun, for a little sun is good as long as you don't overdo it; perhaps ten minutes a day this time of the year is about right." I could not have said it better myself. This simple recommendation could have an enormous impact on the overall health and well-being for all humans and could help decrease risk of many chronic diseases that plague them throughout their lives.

ACKNOWLEDGMENT

This work was supported in part by NIH grants MO1RR00533 and AR36963.

REFERENCES

1. Holick, M.F. (1989). Phylogenetic and evolutionary aspects of vitamin D from phytoplankton to humans, in *Vertebrate Endocrinology: Fundamentals and Biomedical Implications*, Vol. 3, Pang, P.K.T. and Schreibman, M.P., Eds., Academic Press, Orlando, FL, pp. 7–43.
2. Holick, M.F. (1994). McCollum Award Lecture, 1994: vitamin D—new horizons for the 21st century. *Am. J. Clin. Nutr.* 60: 619–630.
3. Holick, M.F. (2003). Vitamin D: a millennium perspective. *J. Cell. Biochem.* 88: 296–307.
4. MacLaughlin, J.A., Anderson, R.R., and Holick, M.F. (1982). Spectral character of sunlight modulates the photosynthesis of previtamin D_3 and its photo isomers in human skin. *Science* 1001–1003.
5. Holick, M.F., Tian, X.Q., and Allen, M. (1995). Evolutionary importance for the membrane enhancement of the production of vitamin D_3 in the skin of poikilothermic animals. *Proc. Natl. Acad. Sci. USA* 92: 3124–3126.
6. Webb, A.R., Kline, L., and Holick, M.F. (1988). Influence of season and latitude on the cutaneous synthesis of vitamin D_3: exposure to winter sunlight in Boston and Edmonton will not promote vitamin D_3 synthesis in human skin. *J. Clin. Endocrinol. Metab.* 67: 373–378.
7. Lu, Z., Chen, T.C., and Holick, M.F. (1992). Influence of season and time of day on the synthesis of vitamin D_3, in *Proceedings, Symposium on the Biological Effects of Light*, Holick, M.F. and Kligman, A., Eds., Walter De Gruyter & Co., Berlin, pp. 53–56.
8. Clemens, T.L., Henderson, S.L., Adams, J.S., and Holick, M.F. (1982). Increased skin pigment reduces the capacity of skin to synthesize vitamin D_3. *Lancet* 74–76.
9. Matsuoka, L.Y., Wortsman, J., Dannenberg, M.J., Hollis, B.W., Lu, Z., and Holick, M.F. (1992). Clothing prevents ultraviolet-B radiation-dependent photosynthesis of vitamin D_3. *J. Clin. Endocrinol. Metab.* 75: 1099–1103.
10. Matsuoka, L.Y., Ide, L., Wortsman, J., MacLaughlin, J., and Holick, M.F. (1987). Sunscreens suppress cutaneous vitamin D_3 synthesis. *J. Clin. Endocrinol. Metab.* 64: 1165–1168.

11. Holick, E.A., Lu, Z., Holick, M.T., Chen, T.C., Sheperd, J., and Holick, M.F. (2002). Production of previtamin D_3 by a mercury arc lamp and a hybrid incandescent/mercury arc lamp, in *Biologic Effects of Light 2001: Proceedings of a Symposium, Boston, Massachusetts*, Holick, M.F., Ed., Kluwer Academic, Boston, pp. 205–212.

12. Heaney, R.P., Dowell, M.S., Hale, C.A., and Bendich, A. (2003). Calcium absorption varies within the reference range for serum 25-hydroxyvitamin D. *J. Am. Coll. Nutr.* 22: 142–146.

13. Holick, M.F. (2002). Vitamin D: the underappreciated D-lightful hormone that is important for skeletal and cellular health. *Curr. Opin. Endocrinol. Diabetes* 9: 87–98.

14. McCary, L.C. and DeLuca, H.F. (1999). Functional metabolism and molecular biology of vitamin D action, in *Vitamin D: Physiology, Molecular Biology, and Clinical Applications*, Holick, M.F., Ed., Humana Press, Totowa, NJ, pp. 39–56.

15. Bouillon, R. (2001). Vitamin D: from photosynthesis, metabolism, and action to clinical applications, in *Endocrinology*, DeGroot, L.J. and Jameson, J.L., Eds., Saunders, Philadelphia, PA, pp. 1009–1028.

16. Malabanan, A., Veronikis, I.E., and Holick, M.F. (1998). Redefining vitamin D insufficiency. *Lancet* 351: 805–806.

17. Gloth, F.M., Gundberg, C.M., Hollis, B.W., Haddad, H.G., and Tobin, J.D. (1995). Vitamin D deficiency in homebound elderly persons. *JAMA* 274: 1683–1686.

18. Dawson-Hughes, B., Harris, S.S., Krall, E.A., and Dallal, G.E. (1997). Effect of calcium and vitamin D supplementation on bone density in men and women 65 years of age or older. *New Engl. J. Med.* 337: 670–676.

19. Lips, P. (2001). Vitamin D deficiency and secondary hyperparathyroidism in the elderly: consequences for bone loss and fractures and therapeutic implications. *Endocr. Rev.* 22: 477–501.

20. Chapuy, M.C., Preziosi, P., Maaner, M., Arnaud, S., Galan, P., and Hercberg, S. (1997). Prevalence of vitamin D insufficiency in an adult normal population. *Osteopor. Int.* 17: 439–443.

21. Kreiter, S.R., Schwartz, R.P., Kirkman, H.N., Charlton, P.A., Calikoglu, A.S., and Davenport, M. (2000). Nutritional rickets in African American breast-fed infants. *J. Pediatr.* 137: 02–06.

22. Tangpricha, V., Pearce, E.N., Chen, T.C., and Holick, M.F. (2002). Vitamin D insufficiency among free-living healthy young adults. *Am. J. Med.* 112: 659–662.

23. Nesby-O'Dell, S., Scanlon, K.S., Cogswell, M.E., Gillespie, C., Hollis, B.W., and Looker, A.C. (2002). Hypovitaminosis D prevalence and determinants among African American and white women of reproductive age: third national health and nutrition examination survey, 1988–1994. *Am. J. Clin. Nutr.* 76: 187–192.

24. Glerup, H., Mikkelsen, K., Poulsen, L., Hass, E., Overbeck, S., and Andersen, H. (2000). Hypovitaminosis D myopathy without osteomalacic bone involvement. *Calcif. Tissue Int.* 66: 419–424.

25. Holick, M.F. (2001). Sunlight "D"ilemma: risk of skin cancer or bone disease and muscle weakness. *Lancet* 357: 4–6.

26. Bischoff, H.A., Stähelin, H.B., Dick, W., Akos, R., Knecht, M., and Salis, C. (2003). Effect of vitamin D and calcium supplementation on falls: a randomized controlled study. *J. Bone Mineral Res.* 18: 343–351.

27. Apperly, F.L. (1941). The relation of solar radiation to cancer mortality in North America. *Cancer Res.* 1: 191–195.

28. Hernan, M.A., Olek, M.J., and Ascherio, A. (1999). Geographic variation of MS incidence in two prospective studies of U.S. women. *Neurology* 51: 1711–1718.

29. Rostand, S.G. (1979). Ultraviolet light may contribute to geographic and racial blood pressure differences. *Hypertension* 30: 150–156.

30. Scragg, R., Jackson, R., Holdaway, I.M., Lim, T., and Beaglehole, R. (1990). Myocardial infarction is inversely associated with plasma 25-hydroxyvitamin D_3 levels: a community-based study. *Int. J. Epidemiol.* 19: 559–563.

31. Mathieu, C., Waer, M., Laureys, J., Rutgeerts, O., and Bouillon, R. (1994). Prevention of autoimmune diabetes in NOD mice by 1:25 dihydroxyvitamin D_3. *Diabetologia* 37: 552–558.

32. Hypponen, E., Laara, E., Jarvelin, M.-R., and Virtanen, S.M. (2001). Intake of vitamin D and risk of type 1 diabetes: a birth-cohort study. *Lancet* 358: 1500–1503.

33. DeLuca, H.F. and Cantorna, M.T. (2001). Vitamin D: its role and uses in immunology. *FASEB J.* 15: 2579–2585.

34. Krause, R., Buhring, M., Hopfenmuller, W., Holick, M.F., and Sharma, A.M. (1998). Ultraviolet B and blood pressure. *Lancet* 352: 709–710.

35. Li, Y.C., Kong, J., Wei, M., Chen, Z.F., Liu, S.Q., and Cao, L.P. (2002). 1:25-dihydroxy-vitamin D_3 is a negative endocrine regulator of the renin-angiotensin system. *J. Clin. Invest.* 110: 229–238.

36. Garland, C., Shekelle, R.B., Barrett-Connor, E., Criqui, M.H., Rossof, A.H., and Oglesby, P. (1985). Dietary vitamin D and calcium and risk of colorectal cancer: a 19-year prospective study in men. *Lancet* 307–309.

37. Garland, C.F., Garland, F.C., Gorham, E.D., and Raffa, J. (1992). Sunlight, vitamin D, and mortality from breast and colorectal cancer in Italy, in *Biologic Effects of Light*, Holick, M.F., Ed., Walter de Gruyter & Co., New York, pp. 39–43.

38. Hanchette, C.L. and Schwartz, G.G. (1992). Geographic patterns of prostate cancer mortality. *Cancer* 70: 2861–2869.

39. Grant, W.B. (2002). An ecologic study of dietary and solar ultraviolet-B links to breast carcinoma mortality rates. *Am. Cancer Soc.* 94: 272–281.

40. Grant, W.B. (2002). An estimate of premature cancer mortality in the U.S. due to inadequate doses of solar ultraviolet-B radiation. *Cancer* 94: 1867–1875.

41. Garland, C.F., Garland, F.C., Shaw, E.K., Comstock, G.W., Helsing, K.J., and Gorham, E.D. (1989). Serum 25-hydroxyvitamin D and colon cancer: eight-year prospective study. *Lancet* 18: 1176–1178.

42. Koutkia, P., Chen, T.C., and Holick, M.F. (2001). Vitamin D intoxication associated with an over-the-counter supplement. *New Engl. J. Med.* 345: 66–67.

43. Schwartz, G.G., Whitlatch, L.W., Chen, T.C., Lokeshwar, B.L., and Holick, M.F. (1998). Human prostate cells synthesize 1:25-dihydroxyvitamin D_3 from 25-hydroxyvitamin D_3. *Cancer Epidemiol. Biomarkers Prev.* 7: 391–395.

44. Whitlatch, L.W., Young, M.V., and Schwartz, G.G. (2002). 25-Hydroxyvitamin D-1α-hydroxylase activity is diminished in human prostate cancer cells and is enhanced by gene transfer. *J. Steroid Biochem. Mol. Biol.* 81: 135–140.

45. Holick, M.F. (1998). Clinical efficacy of 1,25-dihydroxyvitamin D_3 and its analogues in the treatment of psoriasis. *Retinoids* 14: 12–17.

46. Kragballe, K., Beck, H.I., and Sogaard, H. (1988). Improvement of psoriasis by a topical vitamin D_3 analogue (MC903) in a double-blind study. *Br. J. Dermatol.* 119: 223–230.

47. Kato, T., Rokugo, M., Terui, T., and Tagami, H. (1986). Successful treatment of psoriasis with topical application of active vitamin D_3 analogue, α,24-dihydroxycholecalciferol. *Br. J. Dermatol.* 115: 431–433.

48. Koeffler, H.P., Hirjik, J., Iti, L., and The Southern California Leukemia Group. (1985). 1,25-Dihydroxyvitamin D_3: *in vivo* and *in vitro* effects on human preleukemic and leukemic cells. *Cancer Treat. Rep.* 69: 1399–1407.

49. Chen, T.C. and Holick, M.F. (2003). Vitamin D and prostate cancer prevention and treatment. *Trends Endocrinol. Metab.* 14: 423–430.

50. Tangpricha, V., Koutkia, P., Rieke, S.M., Chen, T.C., Perez, A.A., and Holick, M.F. (2003). Fortification of orange juice with vitamin D: a novel approach to enhance vitamin D nutritional health. *Am. J. Clin. Nutr.* 77: 1478–1483.
51. Holick, M.F. (1999). Calcium, in *Dietary Reference Intakes for Calcium, Phosphorus, Magnesium, Vitamin D, and Fluoride*, Institute of Medicine, National Academy Press, Washington, D.C., pp. 71–145.
52. Vieth, R., Chan, P.C., and MacFarlane, G.D. (2001). Efficacy and safety of vitamin D₃ intake exceeding the lowest observed adverse effect level. *Am. J. Clin. Nutr.* 73: 288–294.
53. Barger-Lux, M.J., Heaney, R.P., Dowell, S., Chen, T.C., and Holick, M.F. (1998). Vitamin D and its major metabolites: serum levels after graded oral dosing in healthy men. *Osteoporosis Int.* 8: 222–230.
54. Heaney, R.P., Davies, K.M., Chen, T.C., Holick, M.F., and Barger-Lux, M.J. (2003). Human serum 25-hydroxycholecalciferol response to extended oral dosing with cholecalciferol. *Am. J. Clin. Nutr.* 77: 204–210.
55. Heikinheimo, R.J., Ubjivaaram, J.A., Jantti, P.O., Maki-Jokela, P.L., Rajala, S.A., and Sievanen, H. (1994). Intermittant parenteral vitamin D supplementation in the elderly in nutritional aspects of osteoporosis, in *Challenges of Modern Science*, Burckhardt, P. and Heaney, R.P., Eds., Ares-Serono Symposia, Rome, pp. 335–340.
56. Trivedi, D.P., Doll, R., and Khaw, K.T. (2003). Effect of four monthly oral vitamin D₃ (cholecalciferol) supplementation on fractures and mortality in men and women living in the community: randomised double blind controlled trial. *Br. Med. J.* 326: 469–474.

CHAPTER 15

Evidence for the Breakpoint of Normal Serum 25-Hydroxyvitamin D: Which Level Is Required in the Elderly?

PAUL LIPS

Department of Endocrinology, Vrije Universiteit Medical Center, Amsterdam, The Netherlands

INTRODUCTION

Severe vitamin D deficiency may cause osteomalacia in the elderly. Moderate vitamin D deficiency causes secondary hyperparathyroidism and high bone turnover, which lead to bone loss, osteoporosis, and fractures [1]. More than 30 years ago, the high incidence of hip fractures in the elderly was found to be associated with vitamin D deficiency [2]. Randomized placebo-controlled trials studying the effects of vitamin D supplementation on fracture risk have led to discordant results. The different outcomes of the studies and the varying results of epidemiological studies have also resulted in controversy regarding the required serum concentration of 25-hydroxyvitamin D in the elderly population. This chapter deals with the available evidence on the required serum level of 25-hydroxyvitamin D in the elderly. In addition, the required dose of vitamin D in the elderly is

Nutritional Aspects of Osteoporosis, Second Edition

discussed, as well as which subgroups of the elderly might need vitamin D supplementation.

ASSESSING THE REQUIRED SERUM 25(OH)D CONCENTRATION

After production in the skin or intake with food, vitamin D_3 is hydroxylated in the liver to 25-hydroxyvitamin D [25(OH)D], which is subsequently hydroxylated in the kidney into 1,25-dihydroxyvitamin D [$1,25(OH)_2D$]; 25(OH)D is the main circulating metabolite, and $1,25(OH)_2D$ is the active metabolite stimulating the absorption of calcium from the gut. It has been found that $1,25(OH)_2D$ is subject to homeostatic regulation, including negative feedback [1]. Several methods to assess the required level of 25(OH)D are based on these homeostatic mechanisms. In case of vitamin D deficiency, the synthesis of $1,25(OH)_2D$ is substrate dependent; that is, it is dependent on available serum 25(OH)D [3]. A correlation between 25(OH)D and $1,25(OH)_2D$ only exists in cases of vitamin D deficiency. Above threshold serum 25(OH)D, this relationship no longer exists, and this level is probably the borderline required level. Of course, this finding could be assessed in a dynamic way by studying above which threshold level vitamin D supplementation does not lead to an increase of serum $1,25(OH)_2D$ [4].

The most commonly used method to assess the required serum 25(OH)D is based on the negative relationship between serum 25(OH)D and the serum parathyroid hormone (PTH) concentration. It has been known for a long time that serum PTH and serum 25(OH)D show an inverse seasonal relationship [5]. Whereas serum 25(OH)D reaches its maximum at the end of summer, serum PTH is maximal at the end of winter. When serum 25(OH)D is low, the serum $1,25(OH)_2D$ level drops and calcium absorption might decrease somewhat. This leads to an increase of serum PTH, which stimulates the production of $1,25(OH)_2D$. This mechanism maintains the serum $1,25(OH)_2D$ concentration at a very constant level between narrow limits, but in cases of vitamin D deficiency doing so is at the expense of an increase of serum PTH [1]. Most epidemiological studies show a negative relationship between serum 25(OH)D and serum PTH. In these relationships, there might be a breakpoint at the minimally required serum 25(OH)D level. This relationship can also be used in a dynamic study by showing at which baseline serum 25(OH)D levels vitamin D supplementation will cause a decrease of serum PTH. Another way to assess the required serum 25(OH)D level might be the relationship between serum 25(OH)D and bone mineral density (BMD).

EVIDENCE FROM EPIDEMIOLOGICAL AND INTERVENTION STUDIES

A vitamin D supplementation study in institutionalized elderly in the Netherlands compared the effects of vitamin D_3 doses of 400 IU/day and 800 IU/day with a control group. In that study, an increase of serum $1,25(OH)_2D$ was seen after vitamin D_3 supplementation but only when serum 25(OH)D at baseline was lower than 30 nmol/L [4]. It was concluded from this study that the minimally required serum 25(OH)D was 30 nmol/L. Evidence has also come from the Amsterdam Vitamin D Study, a double-blind, placebo-controlled study on the effect of vitamin D_3 (400 IU/day) or placebo on the incidence of hip fractures and other peripheral fractures [6]. In this study, a substudy was done on the relation of vitamin D supplementation with serum 25(OH)D, serum PTH, and bone mineral density. At baseline, a positive relationship was observed between serum 25(OH)D and the BMD of the femoral neck [7]. This relationship was significant only when serum 25(OH)D was lower than 30 nmol/L. At baseline, a negative correlation was observed between serum PTH and serum 25(OH)D. This relationship existed only when serum 25(OH)D was lower than 25 nmol/L. These data suggest that the breakpoint of serum 25(OH)D might be around 30 nmol/L. Vitamin D supplementation increased serum 25(OH)D in this study to 55 nmol/L in a sample of independently living elderly and to more than 60 nmol/L in institutionalized elderly [6,8]. After 2 years of vitamin D supplementation, the BMD in the femoral neck increased 2.2% compared with the placebo group [8]; however, vitamin D supplementation did not decrease the incidence of hip fractures or other peripheral fractures [6].

The Decalyos study, performed in Lyon, involved more than 3000 healthy nursing home residents who received vitamin D_3 (800 IU/day) and calcium (1200 mg/day) or double placebo. The vitamin D and calcium supplement did lead to a decrease of hip fractures and other non-vertebral fractures of more than 20% after 18 months [9]. Vitamin D supplementation caused a decrease of serum PTH of 50% and an increase of BMD in the femoral neck of 6% in this study. Some conclude that 800 IU/day is an adequate dose, and one may argue that the larger calcium supplement in the Lyon study is responsible for the different results found in the studies performed in Amsterdam and Lyon [1].

Another important point that emerged from these studies was the comparability of assays for serum 25(OH)D. The assays of Lyon and Amsterdam were cross-calibrated and it turned out that the correction factor was 0.45 to convert the Lyon serum levels to those measured in Amsterdam [10]. It appeared after correction that the patients in Lyon were more vitamin D deficient than those in Amsterdam. This cross-calibration is very important for the discussion on the breakpoint of serum 25(OH)D. Based on the assay differences, the breakpoint in Lyon would be 80% higher than that in Amsterdam.

The Suvimax study in postmenopausal women also showed a negative correlation between serum PTH and serum 25(OH)D. The breakpoint according to this study was at a serum 25(OH)D level of 78 nmol/L [11]. This is very similar to a study in medical inpatients done in the United States, where serum PTH increased when serum 25(OH)D was lower than 30 ng/mL or 75 nmol/L [12]. The baseline data of the MORE study, a global study on the effects of raloxifene on postmenopausal osteoporosis, showed higher serum PTH levels when serum 25(OH)D was lower than 50 nmol/L [13]. Finally, studies in Boston showed that the seasonal variation of serum PTH disappeared when serum 25(OH)D was higher than 95 nmol/L [14]. Of course, one might argue that a small increase of serum PTH when serum 25(OH)D is on the low side is an entirely appropriate physiological homeostatic mechanism. According to that view, only larger increases of serum PTH should be considered pathological. Levels of serum thyroid-stimulating hormone (TSH) and serum T4 are related. In patients with primary hypothyroidism one should not aim at completely suppressed serum TSH levels. Similarly, whether serum PTH should be completely suppressed or not should be discussed.

THE INFLUENCE OF CALCIUM INTAKE ON SERUM PTH AND VITAMIN D METABOLISM

An oral calcium dose of 1000 mg decreases the serum PTH level within 1 hour [15]. A considerable reduction in serum PTH over 24 hours can be obtained with oral calcium supplementation [16]. When serum PTH is low, the turnover of vitamin D metabolites is lower. On the other hand, when calcium intake is low, the half life of 25(OH)D is shorter. This is caused by the increased serum PTH (secondary hyperparathyroidism), which increases the turnover of vitamin D metabolites [17]. The importance of calcium supplementation has been clearly demonstrated by the Lyon vitamin D supplementation study (Decalyos study), where supplementation with vitamin D_3 (800 IU/day) and calcium (1200 mg/day) was very effective in decreasing the incidence of hip fractures and other non-vertebral fractures [9]. Another supplementation study was done in the United States with vitamin D_2 (15,000 IU/week) and calcium (1000–1500 mg/day). It appeared from this study that serum PTH decreased about 40% when serum

25(OH)D was lower than 40 nmol/L, it decreased about 20% when serum 25(OH)D was between 40 and 50 nmol/L, and it did not decrease when serum 25(OH)D was higher than 50 nmol/L [18]. So, this study also suggests that the breakpoint of serum 25(OH)D is at 50 nmol/L because above this level no decrease of serum PTH was observed after supplementation with vitamin D and calcium.

STAGING OF VITAMIN D DEFICIENCY

The following stages of vitamin D deficiency have been proposed [1]:

- Mild vitamin D deficiency when serum 25(OH)D is between 25 and 50 nmol/L
- Moderate vitamin D deficiency when serum 25(OH)D is between 12.5 and 25 nmol/L
- Severe vitamin D deficiency when serum 25(OH)D is lower than 12.5 nmol/L

The corresponding increases of serum PTH are 15% with mild vitamin D deficiency, between 15 and 30% for a moderate deficiency, and an increase greater than 30% with severe vitamin D deficiency. Limitations of assessing the breakpoint of normal serum 25(OH)D are the moderate comparability of assays for 25(OH)D and different dietary intakes of calcium; also, other determinants of serum PTH levels include renal function, estrogen status, and diuretics.

CONCLUSION

The assays for 25(OH)D vary widely which precludes an accurate assessment of the required level. Because of this variation, the breakpoint in one country might be 75 nmol/L and in another 50 nmol/L, but these breakpoints may actually be similar due to differences in the assays for serum 25(OH)D. The breakpoint between minor vitamin D deficiency and a vitamin D replete state also depends on calcium intake. A global average estimate is 50 nmol/L. A decrease of serum PTH or an increase of BMD after vitamin D supplementation does not prove anti-fracture efficacy. Vitamin D supplementation of 400 to 600 IU/day should be recommended for the house-bound elderly and nursing home residents and in any person with low serum 25(OH)D when sunshine exposure is not feasible. It is unlikely that more generous vitamin D supplementation should have measurable effects on bone health in the elderly population.

REFERENCES

1. Lips, P. (2001). Vitamin D deficiency and secondary hyperparathyroidism in the elderly: consequences for bone loss and fractures and therapeutic implications. *Endocr. Rev.* 22: 477–501.
2. Chalmers, J., Barclay, A., Davison, A.M., Macleod, D.A.D., and Williams, D.A. (1969). Quantitative measurements of osteoid in health and disease. *Clin. Orthop.* 63: 196–209.
3. Bouillon, R.A., Auwerx, J.H., Lissens, W.D., and Pelemans, W.K. (1987). Vitamin D status in the elderly: seasonal substrate deficiency causes 1,25-dihydroxycholecalciferol deficiency. *Am. J. Clin. Nutr.* 45: 755–763.
4. Lips, P., Wiersinga, A., van Ginkel, F.C., Jongen, M.J.M., Netelenbos, J.C., Hackeng, W.H.L., Delmas, P.D., and van der Vijgh, W.J.F. (1988). The effect of vitamin D supplementation on vitamin D status and parathyroid function in elderly subjects. *J. Clin. Endocrinol. Metab.* 67: 644–650.
5. Lips, P., Hackeng, W.H.L., Jongen, M.J.M., van Ginkel, F.C., and Netelenbos, J.C. (1983). Seasonal variation in serum concentrations of parathyroid hormone in elderly people. *J. Clin. Endocrinol. Metab.* 57: 204–206.
6. Lips, P., Graafmans, W.C., Ooms, M.E., Bezemer, P.D., and Bouter, L.M. (1996). Vitamin D supplementation and fracture incidence in elderly persons: a randomized, placebo-controlled clinical trial. *Ann. Intern. Med.* 124: 400–406.
7. Ooms, M.E., Lips, P., Roos, J.C., van der Vijgh, W.J.F., Popp-Snijders, C., Bezemer, P.D., and Bouter, L.M. (1995). Vitamin D status and sex hormone binding globulin: determinants of bone turnover and bone mineral density in elderly women. *J. Bone Mineral Res.* 10: 1177–1184.
8. Ooms, M.E., Roos, J.C., Bezemer, P.D., van der Vijgh, W.J.F., Bouter, L.M., and Lips, P. (1995). Prevention of bone loss by vitamin D supplementation in elderly women: a randomized double-blind trial. *J. Clin. Endocrinol. Metab.* 80: 1052–1058.
9. Chapuy, M.C., Arlot, M.E., Duboeuf, F., Brun, J., Crouzet, B., Arnaud, S., Delmas, P.D., and Meunier, P.J. (1992). Vitamin D3 and calcium to prevent hip fractures in elderly women. *New Engl. J. Med.* 327: 1637–1642.
10. Lips, P., Chapuy, M.C., Dawson-Hughes, B., Pols, H.A.P., and Holick, M.F. (1999). An international comparison of serum 25-hydroxyvitamin D measurements. *Osteoporosis Int.* 9: 394–397.
11. Chapuy, M.C., Preziosi, P., Maamer, M., Arnaud, S., Galan, P., Hercberg, S., and Meunier, P.J. (1997). Prevalence of vitamin D insufficiency in an adult normal population. *Osteoporosis Int.* 7: 439–443.
12. Thomas, M.K., Lloyd-Jones, D.M., Thadhani, R.I., Shaw, A.C., Deraska, D.J., Kitch, B.T., Vamvakas, E.C., Dick, I.M., Prince, R.L., and Finkelstein, J.S. (1998). Hypovitaminosis D in medical inpatients. *New Engl. J. Med.* 338: 777–783.
13. Lips, P., Duong, T., Oleksik, A.M., Black, D., Cummings, S., Cox, D., and Nickelsen, T. for the MORE Study Group. (2001). A global study of vitamin D status and parathyroid function in postmenopausal women with osteoporosis: baseline data from the multiple outcomes of raloxifene evaluation clinical trial. *J. Clin. Endocrinol. Metab.* 86: 1212–1221.
14. Krall, E.A., Sahyoun, N., Tannenbaum, S., Dallal, G.E., and Dawson-Hughes, B. (1989). Effect of vitamin D intake on seasonal variations in parathyroid secretion in postmenopausal women. *New Engl. J. Med.* 321: 1777–1783.
15. Lips, P., Netelenbos, J.C., van Doozn, L., Hackeng, W.H.L., and Lips, C.J.M. (1991). Stimulation and suppression of intact parathyroid hormone PTH (1–84) in normal subjects and hyperparathyroid patients. *Clin. Endocrinol. (Oxford)* 35: 35–40.

16. McKane, R., Khosla, S., Egan, K.S., Robins, S.P., Burritt, M.F., and Riggs, B.L. (1996). Role of calcium intake in modulating age-related increases in parathyroid function and bone resorption. *J. Clin. Endocrinol. Metab.* 81: 1699–1703.

17. Davies, M., Heys, S.E., Selby, P.L., Berry, J.L., and Mawer, E.B. (1997). Increased catabolism of 25-hydroxyvitamin D in patients with partial gastrectomy and elevated 1,25-dihydroxy-vitamin D levels: implications for metabolic bone disease. *J. Clin. Endocrinol. Metab.* 82: 209–212.

18. Malabanan, A.O., Veronikis, I.E., and Holick, M.F. (1998). Redefining vitamin D insufficiency. *Lancet* 351: 805–806.

CHAPTER 16

What is the Optimal Amount of Vitamin D for Osteoporosis?

REINHOLD VIETH

Department of Laboratory Medicine and Pathobiology, University of Toronto, and Pathology and Laboratory Medicine, Mount Sinai Hospital, Toronto, Canada

INTRODUCTION

For most nutrients, dietary intakes have offered a reasonable reference point for how much nutrient might be needed for health. When it comes to vitamin D, we have no comparable guide, so we need to look for other clues about our vitamin D requirements. Our biology was designed by evolution for life in equatorial Africa; therefore, consumption of those rare foods that do contain a meaningful amount of vitamin D, such as ocean fish, could not have played a role in determining human vitamin D requirements. All published 25-hydroxyvitamin D [25(OH)D] concentrations for healthy, non-human primates are, at the very least, near the top of what we currently regard as the normal range for humans. Current recommendations for vitamin D consumption by humans [1] produce 25(OH)D concentrations that are a better match for the levels in laboratory rats, nocturnal rodents [2], than the 25(OH)D concentrations published for all other primate species (Fig. 1). During evolution, requirements for vitamin D were satisfied by the life of the naked ape that became the species

Nutritional Aspects of Osteoporosis, Second Edition
211

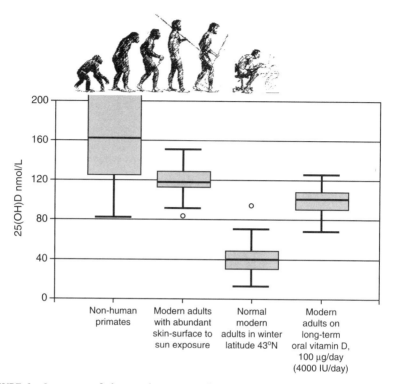

FIGURE 1   Summary of historical aspects of circulating 25(OH)D concentrations in non-human primates and in modern adults. Each character illustrated across the top of the figure represents the evolutionary stage of the data presented below it. Because modern humans evolved in tropical regions and without clothing, early vitamin D nutrition would have been similar to that of modern humans living under similar conditions. Results are published mean values for non-human primates [49–52] and for sun-rich adults—those given artificial tanning sessions as cited previously [29] (note that actual ranges extend even higher than the mean values shown). Data for modern adults in winter and their responses to vitamin D are individual data from hospital workers in Toronto, Canada [48]. These plots include whiskers that show the lowest and highest values for the data summarized; the boxes show the range of the central 50% of the sample group, with a line indicating the median value of the group. (From Vieth, R., in *Bone Loss and Osteoporosis in Past Populations: An Anthropological Perspective*, Agarwal, S.C. and Stout, S.D., Eds., Kluwer Academic, Dordrecht, 2003. With permission.)

Homo sapiens. It is plausible that we modern humans might benefit if we could compensate for the biological consequences of modern life. Potential disease consequences include hypertension and greater risks of breast, colon, and prostate cancers [3–5]. For now, we address the issue of how much vitamin D is optimal to prevent osteoporosis.

VITAMIN D AND OSTEOPOROSIS

Figure 2 summarizes randomized control trials looking at whether vitamin D, with or without calcium, affects risk of non-vertebral fracture. There has been no evidence that intake of vitamin D less than 20 µg (800 IU)/day is effective in preventing osteoporotic fractures. Whether or not additional calcium is needed in concert with vitamin D is difficult to tell, because most studies have combined groups receiving calcium and vitamin D for comparison to placebo groups receiving neither. Two randomized, controlled studies show that vitamin D₃ given by itself in doses of 100,000 IU (2500 µg) every 4 months [6] or 750 µg annually [7] reduces the occurrence of fractures.

Bone density declines more quickly during winter than during summer. Vitamin D supplements (about 20 µg or 800 IU per day) combined with calcium eliminate the faster fall in bone density during winter [8,9]. Furthermore, three studies show that the combination of calcium and 20 µg

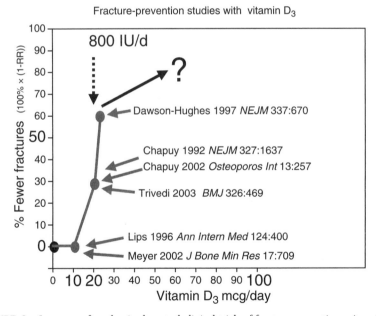

FIGURE 2   Summary of randomized-control clinical trials of fracture-prevention using vitamin D with or without calcium. None of the studies using doses of vitamin D₃ providing less than 20 µg/day was effective in reducing fracture risk [54]; however, all the studies in which there was a reduction in fracture risk used approximately 20 µg/day of vitamin D₃ [6,10–12]. This dose includes the known background intake; for the work by Dawson-Hughes, this background intake was 5 µg/day [11].

vitamin D together lower the fracture risk in adults older than 65 years [10–12].

Occurrence of fractures is reduced by about a third, even within the first year of these studies, when bone density is not increased by enough to account for the fewer fractures [11]. The explanation for this may be that vitamin D improves muscle strength and balance. This improvement reduces the occurrence of falls that bring about fractures as indicated by interventional studies with 20 μg/day of vitamin D [13,14]. Cross-sectional work shows similar benefits of vitamin D nutrition in elderly attending a falls clinic. Those with serum 25(OH)D levels of < 28 nmol/L had impaired balance, reflexes, and more falls than those with 25(OH)D levels over 44 nmol/L (>17.5 μg/L) [15].

In people less than 70 years old, risk of osteoporotic fracture is difficult to assess because nontraumatic fractures occur too rarely. Data from the Nurses Health Study, which involved more than 1 million person-years of follow-up, suggest a 37% lower risk of osteoporotic fracture in postmenopausal women younger than 65 who consume vitamin D in amounts of at least 12.5 μg/day, compared to women consuming less than 3.5 μg/day vitamin D [16]. The authors did not detect an effect of calcium intake on fractures but suggested a confounding effect because women at greater risk for fracture due to a family history of osteoporosis (thus at greater risk for fracture) would have been more likely to take calcium.

Other recent reports focusing on bone density preservation in the early postmenopausal period have failed to show any benefit of supplementing with vitamin D. Hunter et al. [17] randomized twins to take 20 μg/day of vitamin D_3 or placebo. Cooper et al. [18] randomized women to vitamin D_2 (250 μg/week) or placebo. In both these studies, mean 25(OH)D concentrations were already relatively high at baseline and in the control groups—25(OH)D = 70 to 83 nmol/L. The doses of vitamin D produced increases in 25(OH)D compared to the placebo of 35% [17] and 12% [18]. These effects on serum levels were so small it is not surprising that neither study produced a significant effect. The author is not aware of any other situation where such small increments of a drug or nutrient would be expected to produce meaningful effects. The study by Hunter et al. [17] suggests that when 25(OH)D concentrations approach 70 to 80 nmol/L the benefit of vitamin D for osteoporosis prevention may be reaching an asymptote.

25-Hydroxyvitamin D concentrations have modest effects on bone turnover markers. One small intervention study by Devine et al. [19] failed to detect changes in bone markers when 10 μg/day of vitamin D_3 was given to elderly women. A larger, cross-sectional study showed that higher 25(OH)D concentrations correlated with lower urinary excretions of hydroxyproline, pyridinoline, and deoxypyridinoline and lower plasma alkaline phosphatase and parathyroid hormone (PTH) concentrations [20]. Bischoff *et al.* [14] conducted a randomized controlled trial that showed that vitamin D supplementation of vitamin-D-insufficient elderly women suppresses bone turnover markers beyond the effect of calcium supplementation alone. The data available on bone markers indicate that 25(OH)D concentrations greater than 60 to 80 nmol/L may be approaching an asymptote in terms of bone *per se*, because there is no evidence of further suppression of bone turnover if initial 25(OH)D concentrations already exceed 60 nmol/L.

Several reports show that active absorption of calcium through the gut correlates better with 25(OH)D concentrations than it does with 1,25(OH)2D [14,19,21,22]. This relationship does not appear to reach a plateau, so that an "optimal" 25(OH)D concentration cannot be determined. What it does suggest is that the dietary requirements for calcium may decrease as 25(OH)D concentrations increase.

DOSAGE CONSIDERATIONS

The history of vitamin D intake reflects the arbitrary approaches used for dosage determinations in eras past. Cholecalciferol, or vitamin D_3, given in the form of cod liver oil has been a folk remedy in northern Europe since the 1700s. Empirically, a small teaspoonful daily was thought to help infants thrive. This arbitrary dose of cod liver oil has turned out to be a good guess, so far as infants are concerned. The 375 IU (9 μg) of vitamin D_3 contained in that teaspoon [23] was confirmed relatively recently as being appropriate for infants [24,25]. Compared to the adult, vitamin D nutrition in the infant and child has been well characterized. Until it became clear that vitamin D was important to the health of adults, there was very little thought directed at how much vitamin D adults might need to consume. The dose of 20 μg/day of vitamin D_3 (cholecalciferol) now recommended for prevention or treatment of osteoporosis [26] was originally selected because it represented a convenient doubling of the 10-μg/day dose present in formulations of vitamin D_2 (ergocalciferol). In the 1980s, Chapuy *et al.* [27] observed that 20 μg/day of ergocalciferol produced PTH suppression in the elderly. The group later changed the form of vitamin D that they used when carrying out their fracture-prevention studies. This was because of a report by Tjellesen *et al.* [28] that vitamin D_3 was more effective.

The fact that 20 μg of vitamin D_3 prevents fractures is not proof it is optimal for osteoporosis; it simply suggests that it is the lowest dose that shows a response along the dose–response curve for vitamin D and fracture prevention. No drug company would stop its development of a new drug at that point. Any owner of a proprietary pharmaceutical would continue to define the optimal dose for its product. The strategy to optimize dosage is very important for a proprietary drug, because if the dosage is not optimized it opens the market to another company with a more optimal dose of an alternative drug that will surely take over the market because of its greater efficacy. Unfortunately, because vitamin D is a nutrient and in the public domain, there is no comparable incentive to optimize the dose. There are no appropriate studies of osteoporosis prevention with vitamin D beyond the 20-μg/day dosage. It should be clear from Fig. 2 that our knowledge of the dose–response curve for vitamin D and osteoporosis is incomplete.

Figure 3 illustrates a dose–response curve reflecting the final average 25(OH)D concentrations attained in studies reported in the literature [5,29]. Table I summarizes incremental responses to different treatment strategies to raise 25(OH)D to steady-state concentrations. Responsiveness of vitamin D administration, as measured by the nmol/L increase per μg consumption per day, increases with: (1) lower vitamin D dosage, (2) lower initial 25(OH)D concentration, and (3) longer duration of supplementation. The latter suggests a long half-life and time to plateau.

The conventional way to improve vitamin D nutritional status has been to give vitamin D_3 or vitamin D_2 (ergocalciferol). Until recently, availability of 25(OH)D was another option (product discontinued by Organon, NJ). The company's discontinuation of 25(OH)D may have made sense, because the objective of increasing plasma 25(OH)D concentrations can be almost as easily achieved by providing enough vitamin D_3. Nonetheless, useful perspectives can be gained from previous experience with 25(OH)D. Barger-Lux and Heaney et al. [44] have shown that as 25(OH)D dosage increases, there is effectively a linear increase in the average 25(OH)D concentration achieved (Table I). However, when vitamin D_3 is used, the increment in 25(OH)D per μg per day of vitamin D_3 decreases as dose increases.

Because the increment in plasma 25(OH)D concentration per μg dose is at least 4 times higher for 25(OH)D administration than for vitamin D_3 administration, we can conclude that less than 25% of vitamin D molecules ever become 25(OH)D. Three quarters of the molecules of vitamin D that enter the body are removed by some other fate. The way this system is designed is wasteful in terms of vitamin D. This inefficiency is not surprising when we consider that our human biology evolved under conditions of abundant vitamin D supply, compared to what most of us acquire today (Fig. 1). We have poor capability to cope with a lack of vitamin D.

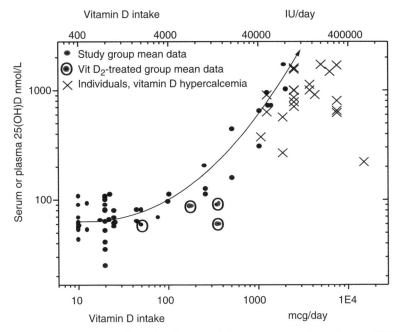

FIGURE 3   Dose–response relationship between daily vitamin D intake and mean 25(OH)D concentration based on data published in the literature. The solid points show mean results for groups of adults consuming the indicated doses of vitamin D. Results for groups of adults that unambiguously consumed vitamin D_2 are shown by the circled points. Vitamin D_3 is about 4 times as potent as vitamin D_2, based on tracing the circled points for subjects consuming vitamin D_2 back to the trend line based on vitamin D_3. Both axes are log scale. The results represented by the X's are for individuals showing the classic hypercalcemic response to toxic levels of prolonged vitamin D consumption. The data used to generate this graph were compiled and published previously [5,29].

HORMONAL 1,25(OH)$_2$D IS NOT AN ALTERNATIVE TO NUTRITIONAL VITAMIN D

For most of the 20th century, there was no debate, that vitamin D was a nutrient; it was known as the sunshine vitamin. Confusion arose when it was realized that the active form of the vitamin D molecule was 1,25-dihydroxyvitamin D [1,25(OH)$_2$D], or calcitriol, which is a hormone in the true sense of the word. A focus on the inadequacies of the term *vitamin* and a lack of consideration for the term *hormone* led to the misconception that vitamin D itself might be a hormone instead of a nutrient. Officially mandated nutritional committee reports in both North America [1] and

TABLE I   Strategies to Increase Circulating 25(OH)D Concentration in Adults: Effects of Compound, Dose, and Duration[a]

Compound	25(OH)D Increase per µg/day	Dose (µg/day)	Duration of Dose (weeks)	Absolute Increase in 25(OH)D (nmol/L)	Ref.
25(OH)D	4.1	50	4	206.4	[44]
25(OH)D	4.0	10	4	40	[44]
25(OH)D	3.8	20	4	76.1	[44]
Cholecalciferol	1.5	15	52	22	[45]
Cholecalciferol	1.4	20	8	27	[46]
Cholecalciferol	1.2	20	52	24.5	[17]
Cholecalciferol	1.1	25	8	28.6	[44]
Cholecalciferol	1.1	21	20	23.4	[47]
Cholecalciferol	0.8	100	52	81	[45]
Cholecalciferol	0.8	25	20	19	[48]
Cholecalciferol	0.7	138	20	102.7	[47]
Cholecalciferol	0.6	275	20	169.8	[47]
Cholecalciferol	0.6	250	8	146	[44]
Cholecalciferol	0.5	100	20	51.8	[48]
Cholecalciferol	0.5	1250	8	643	[44]
Ergocalciferol	0.3	36	104	—	[18]

[a]The results in this table represent recent work not included in Fig. 3. These data were assembled to permit comparison of efficacy doses of different strategies to increase 25(OH)D concentration. The results are sorted in order of decreasing response to the dose, based on the nmol/L increase in 25(OH)D per µg/day of oral dose used in these studies.

Europe [30] now state that nutritional vitamin D may be more suitably referred to as a hormone than a nutrient; however, vitamin D is no more a hormone than cholesterol is, because vitamin D is only the raw material needed for synthesis of $1,25(OH)_2D$.

Promotion of vitamin D nutrition is hindered by alarmist reactions justifiably associated with administration of any hormone. Use of a hormone implies that natural homeostatic control is circumvented, taken over by the physician; however, vitamin D does not generate an endocrine signal, $1,25(OH)_2D$ and its analogs do this. The purpose of supplementing with vitamin D is to optimize the natural functions of the endocrine/paracrine systems that require it.

Many studies have looked into the use of the hormone $1,25(OH)_2D$ and analogs of it in the prevention and treatment of osteoporosis [31]. I have a concern that $1,25(OH)_2D$ may be used too aggressively as an alternative to improved vitamin D nutrition for the prevention or treatment of osteoporosis. The point that 1,25(OH)2D almost certainly has a narrower therapeutic index (ratio of toxic versus therapeutic dose) than vitamin D has never been raised in analyses comparing them [31,32]. If osteoporosis occurs because the vitamin D system is somehow deficient or defective, it makes little sense to resort to the use of $1,25(OH)_2D$. Rickets and osteomalacia usually exist despite normal $1,25(OH)_2D$ concentrations. Increases in vitamin D supply will not increase $1,25(OH)_2D$ levels further [33,36]. As kidney function deteriorates, its endocrine capability also declines. Low serum $1,25(OH)_2D$ level reflects impaired renal function, not poor nutrition [36,37]. The effect that aging has on $1,25(OH)_2D$ levels can be overcome by increasing the $25(OH)D$ concentration [38,39]. Despite many studies looking into the use of $1,25(OH)_2D$ and its analogs to prevent or treat osteoporosis, the most complete meta-analysis of this topic by Papadimitropoulos [31] concludes that there is no evidence that $1,25(OH)_2D$ or its analogs offer any advantage over nutritional vitamin D at 20 μg/day.

SUMMARY

In 1997, when the Food and Nutrition Board last reviewed this nutrient, there was no evidence that intakes of vitamin D below 20 μg/day (800 IU/day) would have any measurable health effect in adults. Everything available at the time showed that to lower risk of fracture, adults needed to consume 20 μg/day [10,11,40]. The regrettable outcome is that final recommendations of the Food and Nutrition Board established values for vitamin D intakes of 15 μg/day for those over age 70 years and even lower for other adults [1]. By referring to the recommendations for vitamin D as adequate intakes (AIs), the Food and Nutrition Board openly admitted that there was no evidence that these intakes would do anything [41]. Since then, all of the new evidence that vitamin D does affect bone density, fractures, or muscle function confirms that adults need to consume at least 20 μg/day of vitamin D [6,12,14,42].

Returning to the question of what the "optimal" $25(OH)D$ concentration may be for the prevention of osteoporosis, current evidence points to 70 to 80 nmol/L as a $25(OH)D$ concentration above which an asymptote is approached, in terms of various features perceived as beneficial for prevention of osteoporosis and fractures. However, it should be clear from Fig. 2 that the dose–response curve for this nutrient has been explored only part way up the physiologic range that extends beyond 200 nmol/L (Fig. 1). The randomized controlled trials now published (Fig. 2) change the ethical background for future research in the field. It is unlikely that we can continue to use placebo doses of vitamin D in osteoporosis research. The ethics demand that we treat control groups according to the best knowledge to date [43]. To go beyond 20 μg/day will require

TABLE II   Two Versions of Opinions of the Author Regarding Optimal Doses of Vitamin D As They Relate to the Prevention and Treatment of Osteoporosis

	Current Public Recommendation	Research Target
What 25(OH)D level?	>70 nmol/L	100 nmol/L
How much vitamin D₃ to take?	2–25 μg/day (800–1000 IU/day)	100 μg/day (4000 IU/day)
Why?	Fracture prevention studies; realistic for use by general public because of products available	What we do not know yet; low PTH levels

dose-comparison studies, with 20 μg/day as the control compared to a higher dose. This will be a more demanding kind of research than what was done in the past, because the greatest increment in the response has almost certainly been achieved with 20 μg/day. Studies addressing the issue of an optimal dose of vitamin D will require greater numbers of participants than the studies published to date. Although doses of vitamin D higher than 20 μg/day are likely to offer additional benefits for osteoporosis, further research is faced with the need to deal with incrementally diminishing returns.

Table II summarizes the author's public and research perspectives of the topics discussed here and offers suggestions for 25(OH)D levels and vitamin D dosage as they relate to osteoporosis.

REFERENCES

1. Standing Committee on the Scientific Evaluation of Dietary Reference Intakes. (1997). *Dietary Reference Intakes: Calcium, Phosphorus, Magnesium, Vitamin D, and Fluoride*. National Academy Press, Washington, D.C.
2. Vieth, R., Milojevic, S., and Peltekova, V. (2000). Improved cholecalciferol nutrition in rats is noncalcemic, suppresses parathyroid hormone and increases responsiveness to 1,25-dihydroxycholecalciferol. *J. Nutr.* 130: 578–584.
3. Grant, W.B. and Garland, C.F. (2002). Evidence supporting the role of vitamin D in reducing the risk of cancer. *J. Intern. Med.* 252: 178–179.
4. Hanchette, C.L. and Schwartz, G.G. (1992). Geographic patterns of prostate cancer mortality. Evidence for a protective effect of ultraviolet radiation. *Cancer* 70: 2861–2869.
5. Vieth, R. (2001). Vitamin D nutrition and its potential health benefits for bone, cancer, and other conditions. *J. Nutr. Environ. Med.* 11: 275–291.
6. Trivedi, D.P., Doll, R., and Khaw, K.T. (2003). Effect of four monthly oral vitamin D₃ (cholecalciferol) supplementation on fractures and mortality in men and women living in the community: randomised double blind controlled trial. *Br. Med. J.* 326: 469–475.
7. Heikinheimo, R.J., Inkovaara, J.A., Harju, E.J. *et al.* (1992). Annual injection of vitamin D and fractures of aged bones. *Calcif. Tissue Int.* 51: 105–110.

8. Dawson-Hughes, B., Dallal, G.E., Krall, E.A., Harris, S., Sokoll, L.J., and Falconer, G. (1991). Effect of vitamin D supplementation on wintertime and overall bone loss in healthy postmenopausal women [see comments]. *Ann. Intern. Med.* 115: 505–512.

9. Rosen, C.J., Morrison, A., Zhou, H. *et al.* (1994). Elderly women in northern New England exhibit seasonal changes in bone mineral density and calciotropic hormones. *Bone Miner.* 25: 83–92.

10. Chapuy, M.C., Arlot, M.E., Duboeuf, F. *et al.* (1992). Vitamin D_3 and calcium to prevent hip fractures in the elderly women. *New Engl. J. Med.* 327: 1637–1642.

11. Dawson-Hughes, B., Harris, S.S., Krall, E.A., and Dallal, G.E. (1997). Effect of calcium and vitamin D supplementation on bone density in men and women 65 years of age or older [see comments]. *New Engl. J. Med.* 337: 670–676.

12. Chapuy, M.C., Pamphile, R., Paris, E. *et al.* (2002). Combined calcium and vitamin D_3 supplementation in elderly women: confirmation of reversal of secondary hyperparathyroidism and hip fracture risk: the Decalyos II study. *Osteoporosis Int.* 13: 257–264.

13. Pfeifer, M., Begerow, B., Minne, H.W., Abrams, C., Nachtigall, D., and Hansen, C. (2000). Effects of a short-term vitamin D and calcium supplementation on body sway and secondary hyperparathyroidism in elderly women. *J. Bone Mineral Res.* 15: 1113–1118.

14. Bischoff, H.A., Stahelin, H.B., Dick, W. *et al.* (2003). Effects of vitamin D and calcium supplementation on falls: a randomized controlled trial. *J. Bone Mineral Res.* 18: 343–351.

15. Dhesi, J.K., Bearne, L.M., Moniz, C. *et al.* (2002). Neuromuscular and psychomotor function in elderly subjects who fall and the relationship with vitamin D status. *J. Bone Mineral Res.* 17: 891–897.

16. Feskanich, D., Willett, W.C., and Colditz, G.A. (2003). Calcium, vitamin D., milk consumption, and hip fractures: a prospective study among postmenopausal women. *Am. J. Clin. Nutr.* 77: 504–511.

17. Hunter, D., Major, P., Arden, N. *et al.* (2000). A randomized controlled trial of vitamin D supplementation on preventing postmenopausal bone loss and modifying bone metabolism using identical twin pairs. *J. Bone Mineral Res.* 15: 2276–2283.

18. Cooper, L., Clifton-Bligh, P.B., Nery, M.L. *et al.* (2003). Vitamin D supplementation and bone mineral density in early postmenopausal women. *Am. J. Clin. Nutr.* 77: 1324–1329.

19. Devine, A., Wilson, S.G., Dick, I.M., and Prince, R.L. (2002). Effects of vitamin D metabolites on intestinal calcium absorption and bone turnover in elderly women. *Am. J. Clin. Nutr.* 75: 283–288.

20. Jesudason, D., Need, A.G., Horowitz, M., O'Loughlin, P.D., Morris, H.A., and Nordin, B.E. (2002). Relationship between serum 25-hydroxyvitamin D and bone resorption markers in vitamin D insufficiency. *Bone* 31: 626–630.

21. Heaney, R.P., Dowell, M.S., Hale, C.A., and Bendich, A. (2003). Calcium absorption varies within the reference range for serum 25-hydroxyvitamin D. *J. Am. Coll. Nutr.* 22: 142–146.

22. Heaney, R.P., Barger-Lux, M.J., Dowell, M.S., Chen, T.C., and Holick, M.F. (1997). Calcium absorptive effects of vitamin D and its major metabolites. *J. Clin. Endocrinol. Metab.* 82: 4111–4116.

23. Park, E.A. (1940). The therapy of rickets. *JAMA* 115: 370–379.

24. Cooke, R., Hollis, B., Conner, C., Watson, D., Werkman, S., and Chesney, R. (1990). Vitamin D and mineral metabolism in the very low birth weight infant receiving 400 IU of vitamin D. *J. Pediatr.* 116: 423–428.

25. Pittard, W.B., Geddes, K.M., Hulsey, T.C., and Hollis, B.W. (1991). How much vitamin D for neonates? *Am. J Dis. Child* 145: 1147–1149.

26. Brown, J.P. and Josse, R.G. (2002). 2002 clinical practice guidelines for the diagnosis and management of osteoporosis in Canada. *CMAJ* 167(suppl.): S1–S34.

27. Chapuy, M.C., Chapuy, P., and Meunier, P.J. (1987). Calcium and vitamin D supplements: effects on calcium metabolism in elderly people. *Am. J. Clin. Nutr.* 46: 324–328.
28. Tjellesen, L., Hummer, L., Christiansen, C., and Rodbro, P. (1986). Serum concentration of vitamin D metabolites during treatment with vitamin D_2 and D_3 in normal premenopausal women. *Bone Miner.* 1: 407–413.
29. Vieth, R. (1999). Vitamin D supplementation, 25-hydroxyvitamin D concentrations, and safety. *Am. J. Clin. Nutr.* 69: 842–856.
30. Health and Consumer Protection Directorate General. (2002). Opinion of the Scientific Committee on Food on the Tolerable Upper Intake Level of Vitamin D (http://europa.eu.int/comm/food/fs/sc/scf/out157_en.pdf).
31. Papadimitropoulos, E., Wells, G., Shea, B. *et al.* (2002). Meta-analyses of therapies for postmenopausal osteoporosis. VIII. Meta-analysis of the efficacy of vitamin D treatment in preventing osteoporosis in postmenopausal women. *Endocr. Rev.* 23: 560–569.
32. Lau, K.W. and Baylink, D.J. (1999). Vitamin D therapy of osteoporosis: plain vitamin D therapy versus active vitamin D analog (D-hormone) therapy. *Calcif. Tissue Int.* 65: 295–306.
33. Bouillon, R.A., Auwerx, J.H., Lissens, W.D., Pelemans, W.K. (1987). Vitamin D status in the elderly: seasonal disparate deficiency causes 1,25-dihydroxycholecalciferol deficiency. *Am. J. Clin. Nutr.* 45: 755–763.
34. Himmelstein, S., Clemens, T.L., Rubin, A., and Lindsay, R. (1990). Vitamin D supplementation in elderly nursing home residents increases 25(OH)D but not 1,25(OH)2D. *Am. J. Clin. Nutr.* 52: 701–706.
35. Landin-Wilhelmsen, K., Wilhelmsen, L., Wilske, J. *et al.* (1995). Sunlight increases serum 25(OH) vitamin D concentration whereas $1,25(OH)_2D_3$ is unaffected. Results from a general population study in Goteborg, Sweden (the WHO MONICA Project). *Eur. J Clin. Nutr.* 49: 400–407.
36. Vieth, R., Ladak, Y., and Walfish, P.G. (2003). Age-related changes in the 25-hydroxyvitamin D versus parathyroid hormone relationship suggest a different reason why older adults require more vitamin D. *J. Clin. Endocrinol. Metab.* 88: 185–191.
37. Ishimura, E., Nishizawa, Y., Inaba, M. *et al.* (1999). Serum levels of 1,25-dihydroxyvitamin D, 24,25-dihydroxyvitamin D, and 25-hydroxyvitamin D in nondialyzed patients with chronic renal failure. *Kidney Int.* 55(10): 19–27.
38. Kinyamu, H.K., Gallagher, J.C., Rafferty, K.A., and Balhorn, K.E. (1998). Dietary calcium and vitamin D intake in elderly women: effect on serum parathyroid hormone and vitamin D metabolites. *Am. J Clin. Nutr.* 67: 342–348.
39. Vieth, R., Dogan, M., Cole, D.E.C., Rubin, A., Bromberg, I.L., Josse, R., and Walfish, P.G. (2003). Vitamin D_3 at 90 or 700 μg weekly for 1 year: Responses of 25-(OH)D, PTH, urine, and plasma calcium. *Calcif. Tissue Int.* 72: 377–378 (abstr.).
40. Dawson-Hughes, B., Harris, S.S., Krall, E.A., Dallal, G.E., Falconer, G., and Green, C.L. (1995). Rates of bone loss in postmenopausal women randomly assigned to one of two dosages of vitamin D. *Am. J. Clin. Nutr.* 61: 1140–1145.
41. Vieth, R. and Fraser, D. (2002). Vitamin D insufficiency: no recommended dietary allowance exists for this nutrient. *CMAJ* 166: 1541–1542.
42. Pfeifer, M., Begerow, B., Minne, H.W. *et al.* (2001). Vitamin D status, trunk muscle strength, body sway, falls, and fractures among 237 postmenopausal women with osteoporosis. *Exp. Clin. Endocrinol. Diabetes* 109: 87–92.
43. Brody, B.A., Dickey, N., Ellenberg, S.S. *et al.* (2003). Is the use of placebo controls ethically permissible in clinical trials of agents intended to reduce fractures in osteoporosis? *J. Bone Mineral Res.* 18: 1105–1109.

44. Barger-Lux, M.J., Heaney, R.P., Dowell, S., Chen, T.C., Holick, M.F. (1998). Vitamin D and its major metabolites: serum levels after graded oral dosing in healthy men. *Osteoporos. Int.* 8: 222–230.
46. Harris S. (2002). Can vitamin D supplementation in infancy prevent type 1 diabetes? *Nutr. Rev.* 60: 118–121.
47. Heaney, R.P., Davies, K.M., Chen, T.C., Holick, M.F., and Barger-Lux, M.J. (2003). Human serum 25-hydroxycholecalciferol response to extended oral dosing with cholecalciferol. *Am. J. Clin. Nutr.* 77: 204–210.
48. Vieth, R., Chan, P.C., and MacFarlane, G.D. (2001). Efficacy and safety of vitamin D(3) intake exceeding the lowest observed adverse effect level. *Am. J. Clin. Nutr.* 73: 288–294.
49. Marx, S.J., Jones, G., Weinstein, R.S., Chrousos, G.P., and Renquist, D.M. (1989). Differences in mineral metabolism among nonhuman primates receiving diets with only vitamin D_3 or only vitamin D_2. *J. Clin. Endocrinol. Metab.* 69: 1282–1289.
50. Vieth, R., Fraser, D., and Kooh, S.W. (1987). Low dietary calcium reduces 25-hydroxycholecalciferol in plasma of rats. *J. Nutr.* 117: 914–918.
51. Adams, J.E., Gacad, M.A., Baker, A.J., and Rude, R.K. (1985). Serum concentrations of 1,25-dihydroxyvitamin D_3 in Platyrrhini and Cathrrhini: a phylogenetic appraisal. *Am. J. Primatol.* 9: 219–224.
52. Gacad, M.A. and Adams, J.S. (1992). Specificity of steroid binding in New World primate B95–8 cells with a vitamin D-resistant phenotype. *Endocrinology* 131: 2581–2587.
53. Lips, P., Graafmans, W.C., Ooms, M.E., Bezemer, P.D., and Bouter, L.M. (1996). Vitamin D supplementation and fracture incidence in elderly persons: a randomized, placebo-controlled clinical trial. *Ann. Intern. Med.* 124: 400–406.
54. Meyer, H.E., Smedshaug, G.B., Kvaavik, E., Falch, J.A., Tverdal, A., and Pedersen, J.I. (2002). Can vitamin D supplementation reduce the risk of fracture in the elderly? A randomized controlled trial. *J. Bone Miner. Res.* 17: 709–715.
55. Guo, Y.D., Strugnell, S., Back, D.W., and Jones, G. (1993). Transfected human liver cytochrome P-450 hydroxylates vitamin D analogs at different side-chain positions. *Proc. Natl. Acad. Sci. USA* 90: 8668–8672.

PART VI

Vitamin D—Second Part

CHAPTER 17

Serum 25-Hydroxyvitamin D and the Health of the Calcium Economy

ROBERT P. HEANEY

University Chair, Creighton University, Omaha, Nebraska

INTRODUCTION

Serum 25-hydroxyvitamin D [25(OH)D] is widely recognized as the functional indicator of vitamin D status. At the time this delineation was first formally made [1], it was not possible to assign numerical values that related serum levels to health status. Lacking such standards, clinicians and nutritionists have had to rely upon laboratory reference ranges in order to assess the ostensible normality of vitamin D status, either in groups under investigation or in patients being evaluated and treated. This is unsatisfactory on its face, as the reference ranges are not, *a priori*, "normal" but instead represent the levels prevailing in given populations of individuals who do not have evident rickets or osteomalacia. Thus, this approach begs the question of whether there are health consequences at 25(OH)D levels above those associated with evident rickets and osteomalacia. Additionally, reference ranges vary substantially from population to population, usually reflecting true differences in vitamin D status in groups with different

Nutritional Aspects of Osteoporosis, Second Edition

genetic makeup or living in different geographic situations or consuming different diets.

Despite this difficulty, there is a growing consensus among scientists that there may be health consequences associated with 25(OH)D values that are nevertheless well within various reference ranges. Establishing that fact has important consequences both for the diagnosis and treatment of individual patients and for the development of appropriate nutritional policy recommendations. The principal basis for this emerging consensus is the fact that there is an inverse relationship between serum parathyroid hormone (PTH) levels and serum 25(OH)D levels. Most of the papers reporting such a relationship have shown it to be curvilinear, with PTH values rising more steeply at lower values of 25(OH)D and becoming essentially flat at higher values. The point at which the curve flattens out can be estimated by various curve-fitting methods and will depend somewhat on the character of the equation selected to fit the data. The overwhelming majority of the reports to date find that the point at which the curve becomes flat is somewhere in the range of 75 to 120 nmol/L [2,3]. A few, principally Dutch, investigators [4,5], however, report lower values (e.g., 30–50 nmol/L); the reason for this discordance is unclear.

Often, the PTH values at the lower end of the 25(OH)D range are not themselves outside of the range of normal for that analyte, and it has been argued that such an elevation is a normal physiological adaptation and hence an appropriate response rather than an indicator of inadequacy; however, PTH is a principal determinant of bone remodeling, and increased remodeling is itself now recognized to be an independent risk factor for osteoporotic fracture [6]. Hence, elevated PTH values have to be presumed to be productive of morbidity until shown to be innocuous.

For all of these reasons, it has become important to find independent indicators of the functional status of systems dependent upon vitamin D at varying levels of vitamin D repletion, as reflected in different values for serum 25(OH)D. It is the purpose of this brief review to integrate four recent reports that measured vitamin-D-related health status outcomes and at the same time provided serum 25(OH)D concentration data. Three of them related to calcium absorption, and one was concerned with fractures in the elderly.

STUDIES OF CALCIUM ABSORPTION

The first study [7] compared calcium absorption efficiency from standard calcium supplement sources in 24 healthy postmenopausal women, studied twice in the spring of consecutive years (when serum vitamin D in the northern hemisphere is at its annual nadir). One year the participants were treated with vitamin D and in the other no vitamin D supplementation was used. Mean serum 25(OH)D without vitamin D supplementation averaged 50.2 nmol/L and with supplementation, 86.5 nmol/L. Both values were well within the applicable reference range. Calcium absorption was measured by pharmacokinetic methods, calculating the area under the curve for the calcemia induced following ingestion of a calcium source. Under otherwise identical conditions, calcium absorption averaged 22.5% without supplemental vitamin D and 35.3% with supplemental vitamin D ($P < 0.01$). Figure 1 shows the results for 14 of the 24 women who were common to both studies, for whom there were paired data. As can be seen, absorption rose with vitamin D in 12 of the 14 women; the mean change was $+42\%$ ($\pm 13\%$ SEM; $P < 0.02$). Fasting serum PTH fell as well, and fasting serum calcium was higher with vitamin D supplementation ($P < 0.01$ for both). While both sets of values for PTH and calcium were within their respective reference ranges, these changes would generally be recognized as consistent with the absorptive effect and indicative of improvement in the calcium economy generally. The 42% absorptive increase is of obvious importance for the maintenance of bone mass and the suppression of excess bone remodeling.

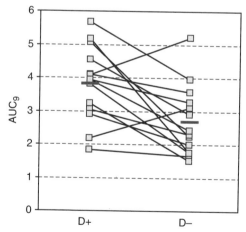

FIGURE 1   Paired values for area under the curve to 9 hours (AUC_9) for the absorptive rise in serum Ca from baseline in 14 postmenopausal women studied twice, once with vitamin D supplementation (D+) and once without (D–). These data are for the subset of women common to both studies [7]. The solid, horizontal bar symbols represent the means for these 14 women under the two vitamin D status conditions ($P < 0.02$). (© Robert P. Heaney, 2003. Used with permission.)

230

Study two [8] consisted of calcium absorption measurements in 26 healthy male outdoor summer workers, first at the end of summer, when their median serum 25(OH)D level was 127 nmol/L, and then at the end of winter, when median 25(OH)D was 74 nmol/L. While absorption efficiency was very slightly higher at the higher level of 25(OH)D, the difference was objectively small and not statistically significant. Figure 2 integrates this study with the prior one, plotting calcium absorption efficiency as a function of 25(OH)D status and showing that efficiency rises with serum 25(OH)D concentration to values in the range of 80 nmol/L and then apparently flattens out at higher levels. Thus, the curve is the approximate inverse of the PTH relationship which, as indicated above, also tends to flatten out in most studies in the region of 80 nmol/L.

In study three [9] Bischoff and colleagues reported results of a vitamin D intervention trial using falls as the primary investigative outcome. The investigators also reported data for serum 25(OH)D, serum PTH, and urine resorption biomarkers under conditions of calcium supplementation, with or without supplemental vitamin D. While true fractional absorption data, such as those in the two studies just cited, are not available for this study, it is nevertheless striking that in the group unsupplemented

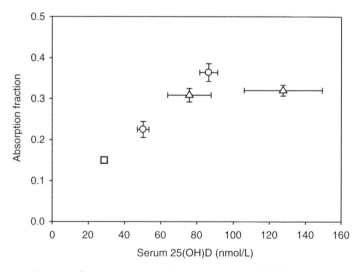

FIGURE 2   Absorption fraction plotted as a function of serum 25(OH)D concentration in three studies (see text). The paired ○ symbols represent the data of study one [7]; the paired △ symbols represent study two [8]; and the □ symbol is the estimated absorption for the subjects not treated with vitamin D in the study of Bischoff et al. [9]. (© Robert P. Heaney, 2003. Used with permission.)

with vitamin D, having a mean 25(OH)D level of 29 nmol/L, there was no change in PTH or in resorption biomarker excretion in response to a supplemental calcium intake of 1200 mg/day, indicating no net calcium absorption. By contrast, at a mean 25(OH)D level of 66 nmol/L and the same calcium load, PTH fell by 32% and bone resorption biomarkers by 26 to 30%. These differences indicate substantially greater calcium absorption in the presence of supplemental vitamin D. Because zero *net* absorption is equivalent to an absorption *fraction* of 10 to 15% [10], it is possible to add the untreated data from this study to Fig. 2 (the □ symbol). Note how closely this value approximates a downward extension of the data from study one.

In brief, studies one and three indicate clearly that absorption efficiency is impaired at circulating levels of 25(OH)D below 80 nmol/L, and they are consistent with previous reports indicating an important predictive relationship between circulating 25(OH)D levels and absorption across the range of 25(OH)D values usually encountered in healthy volunteers [11,12].

OSTEOPOROTIC FRACTURES

Differences in calcium absorptive performance would mean little if they did not have consequences for bone health. Evidence that they do have consequences comes from a recent double-blind, placebo-controlled vitamin D intervention trial. Trivedi *et al.* [13], using an intermittent vitamin D dosing regimen (100,000 units of vitamin D_3 by mouth every 4 months, averaging 820 IU per day), showed at the end of 5 years of supplementation that the vitamin-D-treated individuals had sustained 22% fewer clinically evident fractures than the unsupplemented group and 33% fewer fractures of the typical osteoporotic sort. In analysis of a subset of the nearly 2700 individuals in the study, they reported that the placebo-treated individuals had a mean 25(OH)D concentration of 53 nmol/L, whereas the supplemented individuals had a mean 25(OH)D level of 74 nmol/L. The close similarity of the serum 25(OH)D values in the fracture study of Trivedi *et al.* [13] and those of absorption study one from our group [7], just described, when taken together, mean that 25(OH)D values from the bottom half of the nominal reference range (up to about 80 nmol/L) are associated not only with impaired physiological functioning (malabsorption of calcium) but also explicit skeletal morbidity. Furthermore, the morbidity is precisely of the sort that would be predicted for the malabsorption we [7] and Bischoff [9] have reported.

COMMENT

The fact that absorptive impairment should occur at low serum 25(OH)D levels is not, in itself, particularly surprising, inasmuch as promotion of calcium absorption is perhaps the principal canonical function of vitamin D. Parfitt, for example, in his useful reconceptualization of the spectrum of vitamin D deficiency [14], cited calcium malabsorption and osteoporosis as the principal expressions of the degree of vitamin D deficiency commonly occurring in the industrialized nations. Hence, these studies help to define the "normal" range, as contrasted with the "reference" range. Given the abundant PTH data and the absorption experiments just cited, the evidence is now conclusive that 25(OH)D values below 80 nmol/L may well place an individual at risk for calcium malabsorption and hence for related bone loss and fragility fractures, just as Parfitt had conceptualized the issue.

In current practice, the term *deficiency* has been reserved for 25(OH)D levels in the range associated with rickets and osteomalacia. This implicitly reflects an assumption in the nutrition community that each nutrient has a single index disease, produced by a single mechanism: If one does not have rickets or osteomalacia, one could not be vitamin D deficient. Once articulated clearly in this manner, the presumption is readily seen to be untenable. As Parfitt defined the situation several years ago [14], severe vitamin D deficiency does produce rickets and osteomalacia, but less severe (and more common) degrees of deficiency produce osteoporosis. The current practice of the field to designate as "insufficient" 25(OH)D values that are subnormal but not yet so low as to be "deficient" must be seen to be a reflection of the one-nutrient/one-disease presumption. "Insufficiency" is an unhelpful term. I believe the evidence indicates that it should be abandoned, and that 25(OH)D values below 80 nmol/L should be recognized for what they are—*deficient*. Nutritional policy recommendations should be pointed toward achieving, at a population level, serum 25(OH)D values above 80 nmol/L for everyone.

REFERENCES

1. Food and Nutrition Board, Institute of Medicine. (1997). *Dietary Reference Intakes for Calcium, Magnesium, Phosphorus, Vitamin D, and Fluoride.* National Academy Press, Washington, D.C.
2. Thomas, M.K., Lloyd-Jones, D.M., Thadhani, R.I., Shaw, A.C., Deraska, D.J., Kitch, B.T., Vamvakas, E.C., Dick, I.M., Prince, R.L., and Finkelstein, J.S. (1998). Hypovitaminosis D in medical inpatients. *New Engl. J. Med.* 338: 777–783.

3. Chapuy, M.-C., Preziosi, P., Maamer, M., Arnaud, S., Galan, P., Hercberg, S., and Meunier, P.J. (1997). Prevalence of vitamin D insufficiency in an adult normal population. *Osteoporos. Int.* 7: 439–443.

4. Lips, P. (2001). Vitamin D deficiency and secondary hyperparathyroidism in the elderly: consequences for bone loss and fractures and therapeutic implications. *Endocr. Rev.* 22: 477–501.

5. Lips, P., Duong, T., Oleksik, A., Black, D., Cummings, S., Cox, D., and Nickelsen, T. (2001). A global study of vitamin D status and parathyroid function in postmenopausal women with osteoporosis: baseline data from the multiple outcomes of raloxifene evaluation clinical trial. *J. Clin. Endocrinol. Metab.* 86: 1212–1221.

6. Riggs, B.L., Melton III, L.J. (2002). Bone turnover matters: the raloxifene treatment paradox of dramatic decreases in vertebral fractures without commensurate increases in bone density. *J. Bone Mineral Res.* 17: 11–14.

7. Heaney, R.P., Dowell, M.S., Hale, C.A., and Bendich, A. (2003). Calcium absorption varies within the reference range for serum 25-hydroxyvitamin D. *J. Am. Coll. Nutr.* 22(2): 142–146.

8. Barger-Lux, M.J. and Heaney, R.P. (2002). Effects of above average summer sun exposure on serum 25-hydroxyvitamin D and calcium absorption. *J. Clin. Endocrinol. Metab.* 87(11): 4952–4956.

9. Bischoff, H.A., Stähelin, H.B., Dick, W., Akos, R., Knecht, M., Salis, C., Nebiker, M., Theiler, R., Pfeifer, M., Begerow, B., Lew, R.A., and Conzelmann, M. (2003). Effects of vitamin D and calcium supplementation on falls: a randomized controlled trial. *J. Bone Mineral Res.* 18(2): 3243–3351.

10. Heaney, R.P. (1991). Human calcium absorptive performance: a review, in *Nutritional Aspects of Osteoporosis*, Vol. 85, Burckhardt, P. and Heaney, R.P., Eds., Raven Press, New York, pp. 115–123.

11. Devine, A., Wilson, S.G., Dick, I.M., and Prince, R.L. (2002). Effects of vitamin D metabolites on intestinal calcium absorption and bone turnover in elderly women. *Am. J. Clin. Nutr.* 75: 283–288, 2002.

12. Barger-Lux, M.J., Heaney, R.P., Lanspa, S.J., Healy, J.C., and DeLuca, H.F. (1995). An investigation of sources of variation in calcium absorption efficiency. *J. Clin. Endocrinol. Metab.* 80: 406–411.

13. Trivedi, D.P., Doll, R., and Khaw, K.T. (2003). Effect of four monthly oral vitamin D_3 (cholecalciferol) supplementation on fractures and mortality in men and women living in the community: randomised double blind controlled trial. *Br. Med. J.* 326: 469–474.

14. Parfitt, A.M. (1990). Osteomalacia and related disorders, in *Metabolic Bone Disease and Clinically Related Disorders*, 2nd ed., Avioli, L.V. and Krane, S.M., Eds., Saunders, Philadelphia, PA, pp. 329–396.

CHAPTER 18

Defining Optimal 25-Hydroxyvitamin D Levels in Younger and Older Adults Based on Hip Bone Mineral Density

HEIKE A. BISCHOFF-FERRARI[1] and BESS DAWSON-HUGHES[2]

[1]Division of Aging and Robert B. Brigham Arthritis and Musculoskeletal Diseases Clinical Research Center, Brigham and Women's Hospital, Boston, Massachusetts; [2]Bone Metabolism Laboratory, Jean Mayer U.S.D.A. Human Nutrition Research Center on Aging, Tufts University, Boston, Massachusetts

ABSTRACT

Current efforts to assess optimal levels of 25-hydroxyvitamin D (25-OHD) for bone health have been largely targeted to Caucasian elderly, and the common means to defining optimal 25-OHD has been a surrogate marker, serum parathyroid hormone (PTH). This approach has led to a large range of suggested optimal 25-OHD levels (20 to 110 nmol/L), and a consensus has not been reached. The rationale for defining optimal 25-OHD status in the older population is to prevent fractures; equally important is its role in optimizing peak bone mass in the younger part of the population. Therefore, bone mineral density (BMD) may be a better endpoint than PTH for the estimation of optimal 25-OHD levels in a large part of the population. Open questions include: Is there a threshold for optimal 25-OHD status in regard BMD? If so, does this threshold differ by age and ethnicity?

In this chapter, we explored the association between 25-OHD levels and hip bone mineral density (BMD) as a way to define optimal 25-OHD status

Nutritional Aspects of Osteoporosis, Second Edition

in different age groups and ethnicities using a representative sample of U.S. ambulatory adults (the third National Health and Nutrition Examination Survey, or NHANES III). We found a significant positive association between 25-OHD levels and total hip BMD in both younger and older adults of Caucasian, Mexican-American, and African-American ethnicity. BMD increased continuously with higher 25-OHD levels throughout the reference range (22.5–94 nmol/L) in all subgroups, suggesting that it is advantageous to be at the upper end of the reference range (90–100 nmol/L) for men and women of younger and older age and different ethnical background.

PTH VERSUS BMD IN THRESHOLD ASSESSMENT FOR OPTIMAL 25-OHD LEVELS

Several investigators have defined optimal vitamin D status as the 25-OHD level that maximally decreases parathyroid hormone (PTH) [1,2]. This is desirable because PTH promotes bone resorption and bone loss. Concerns related to this approach are several. PTH levels fluctuate in relation to diet [3,4], time of day [5], and renal function [3] and may be falsely low in elderly persons with immobility-induced bone loss and hypercalcemia [6]. Estimates of optimal 25-OHD status using PTH vary widely from 20 to 110 nmol/L (9 to 38 ng/mL) [7–12], basically covering most of the reference range of 25-OHD (22.5–94 nmol/L). Also, threshold definitions based on PTH were typically assessed in the elderly Caucasian population and generalizability to younger adults or other ethnicities have not been evaluated. Indeed, PTH levels are less suitable to assess bone health in the younger population, where PTH levels are expected to be low. However, as vitamin D is essential for bone growth [13,14] and preservation [15], establishing optimal 25-OHD levels in younger age groups is important, and benefits may extend beyond maximal suppression of PTH.

Bone mineral density, on the other hand, may be a better endpoint for the estimation of optimal 25-OHD levels in regard to bone health in a large part of the population. BMD is an established index of skeletal development and definition of peak bone mass in young adults. In the elderly, BMD is a strong predictor of fracture risk [16]. Furthermore, BMD measurement integrates the lifetime impact of many influences on the skeleton, including PTH, and is a more stable measure of bone health than PTH.

RATIONALE FOR ASSESSMENT OF OPTIMAL 25-OHD IN THE NON-WHITE POPULATION

Optimal 25-OHD status has not been addressed in any age group of the non-white population, despite the fact that several investigators described an increased risk for decreased vitamin D levels in African-Americans compared to Caucasians [17,18]. The clinical importance of this finding might be questioned because African-Americans have higher BMD than do Caucasians throughout adulthood [19,20]. However, hip fractures in African-American individuals, similar to Caucasians, increase exponentially after age 70, with vitamin D deficiency being a risk factor [21]. In addition, recent reports indicate a rising prevalence of rickets in babies of African-American mothers [22]. Therefore, the exploration of a possible threshold for 25-OHD and BMD in different ethnicities may be of considerable clinical importance, despite the differences in BMD among these groups.

METHODS APPLIED TO STUDY THE ASSOCIATION BETWEEN 25-OHD AND BMD IN A POPULATION-BASED SAMPLE

In this study, we used data from the NHANES III, which was conducted between 1988 and 1994 to study the health and nutritional status of the non-institutionalized U.S. population. The study analyzed data for 13,432 individuals, including data on 25-OHD serum levels and hip BMD. Racial/ethnic composition of the study population was as follows: 45% were non-Hispanic Caucasians (whites), 28% were non-Hispanic African-Americans (blacks), and 27% were Mexican-Americans. The age range of subjects was 20 to 90 + years (younger adults: 20–49 years; older adults: ≥ 50 years).

Dual-energy x-ray absorptiometry (Lunar DPX; GE Medical Systems, Waukesha, WI) was used to measure areal bone density (bone mass per unit of area scanned) at the hip [23,24]. Serum 25-hydroxyvitamin D concentrations were assayed with radioimmunoassay kits (DiaSorin, Stillwater MN) [25]. The reference range for the assay is 22.5 to 94 nmol/L (9–37.6 ng/mL). Information on cigarette smoking was obtained in the household interview. Calcium intake in milligrams per day was calculated from a 24-hour dietary recall. The poverty income ratio (PIR) was computed as the ratio of family income versus the poverty threshold as produced annually by the Census Bureau, adjusted for changes caused by inflation, and is a marker for socioeconomic status. Body mass index (BMI; weight in kilograms divided by height in meters squared) was measured at the time of the household interview. The variable "any estrogen use" (never, former, current) was created from the response on the use and duration of use of "birth control pills" and "estrogen or female hormone pills."

STATISTICAL ANALYSES

Linear regression models were used to model the association between serum 25-hydroxyvitamin D levels and bone mineral density. Four covariates—gender, age-category, estrogen use, and race/ethnicity [24,26]— were considered as potential effect modifiers. Our regression analyses showed that the two age groups (20–49 years; ≥ 50 years) and the three race/ethnicity groups significantly modified the association, whereas gender and estrogen use did not. Therefore, results are presented in six subgroups stratified by age and ethnicity. Serum levels of 25-OHD were divided into quintiles within each age group and race/ethnic group. The following potential confounders were included in the linear regression models: gender, age, BMI, smoking, PIR, daily calcium intake, and estrogen use among women. In addition, the model controlled for month of measurement to adjust for seasonal changes in vitamin D levels [11]. All effect estimates reported were calculated accounting for NHANES III sample weights, stratification, and clustering [27]. Thus, the point estimates are generalizable to the non-institutionalized, civilian U.S. population at the time of NHANES III. To evaluate the dose–response relationship more closely and to assess possible thresholds, we conducted a locally weighted regression smoothing (Lowess) of bone mineral density on serum 25-hydroxyvitamin D levels, after adjustment for the same covariates as the linear regression models.

RESULTS

Mean unadjusted 25-OHD levels were highest in whites (young adults $= 82.8$ nmol/L ± 30.6 SD; older adults $= 72.1$ nmol/L ± 26.0 SD), intermediate in Mexican-Americans (younger adults $= 61.5$ nmol/L ± 22.9 SD; older adults $= 59.3$ nmol/L ± 23.5 SD), and lowest in blacks (younger adults $= 46.8$ 46.8 nmol/L ± 19.9 SD; older adults $= 52.4$ nmol/L ± 24.4 SD) in both age groups. Among the younger age group, 21% of whites, 48% of Mexican-Americans, and 76% of blacks had 25-OHD levels below the midpoint of the reference range (< 58.25 nmol/L). Among the older adults, 32% of whites, 55% of Mexican-Americans, and 67% of blacks had 25-OHD levels below the midpoint of the reference range (Fig. 1).

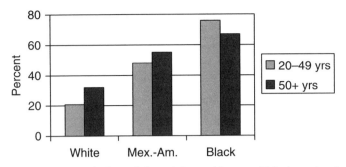

FIGURE 1   Percent of subjects below 58.25 nmol/L serum 25-hydroxyvitamin D.

Blacks had the highest BMD, highest BMI, lowest daily calcium intake, lowest current estrogen use, and lowest income as measured by the PIR. Whites were on the other end of the spectrum for these measures. The percentage of current or past smokers was highest among the whites, and the percentage of never-smokers was highest among Mexican-Americans. In the younger age group, former estrogen use was highest among the blacks, while among the older age group former estrogen use was highest in the whites.

A significant positive association (trend test) between BMD and quintiles of 25-hydroxyvitamin D was present in younger ($P < 0.001$) and older ($P < 0.001$) whites, younger ($P = 0.004$) and older ($P = 0.01$) Mexican-Americans, and older blacks ($P = 0.03$). A similar trend was found in younger blacks ($P = 0.08$). The strongest association between 25-hydroxyvitamin D level and bone mineral density was observed in younger and older whites, for whom, in addition to the significant trend test, each quintile of 25-hydroxyvitamin D was significantly different from the reference category. Compared to the lowest quintile of 25-hydroxyvitamin D, the highest quintile showed a 4.1% improvement in BMD in young whites, 4.8% in older whites; 1.8% in young Mexican-Americans, 3.6% in older Mexican-Americans; and 1.2% in young blacks, 2.5% in older blacks. Race-specific lowest and highest quintiles of 25-hydroxyvitamin D were lowest in whites (≤ 52.9 nmol/L), highest in whites (≥ 98.1 nmol/L); lowest in Mexican-Americans (≤ 41.2 nmol/L), highest in Mexican-Americans (>79.6 nmol/L); and lowest in blacks (≤ 31.4 nmol/L), highest in blacks (≥ 64.6 nmol/L).

In the regression plots, BMD continued to rise throughout and beyond the reference range in younger whites (up to 180 nmol/L). Similarly, but less pronounced, BMD increased within and beyond the reference range in younger Mexican-Americans (up to 120 nmol/L). In blacks, BMD rose throughout most of the reference range (up to 90–100 nmol/l), but there were very few observations at levels above the reference range.

In older whites, the association between BMD and 25-OHD level had a steep positive slope throughout the reference range and appeared to plateau in the range of 90 to 100 nmol/L. In older Mexican-Americans and older blacks, higher 25-OHD was associated with higher BMD throughout the reference range.

Among whites, other significant determinants of higher BMD were, in order of importance, higher BMI, male gender, younger age within age category, former estrogen use, current estrogen use, not smoking more than 11 cigarettes per day, higher PIR, and higher calcium intake. Among Mexican-Americans, the significant factors were higher BMI, male gender, and lower age. Among blacks, higher BMI, male gender, lower age, and former estrogen use were significant determinants of higher BMD.

DISCUSSION

Hip BMD increased continuously with higher 25-OHD levels throughout the reference range in all subgroups of this representative sample of the U.S. population. This suggests that it may be advantageous in younger and older adults to have 25-OHD levels between 90 and 100 nmol/L (36–40 ng/mL), the upper end of the reference range. The association did not differ between men and women and was present in Caucasian, Mexican-American, and African-American individuals. Several other cross-sectional studies have identified a positive association between 25-OHD levels and BMD at the spine [28,29] and femoral neck [28–30] in postmenopausal women and BMD at the forearm in adolescent females [31] and males [32]; however, a threshold of such an association was not studied before. In younger whites, we found no identifiable threshold where higher 25-OHD levels were not associated with additional increases in BMD, even beyond the reference range (up to 180 nmol/L). Because BMD is generally stable in men and women ages 20 to 40 years, this is consistent with the concept that higher levels of 25-OHD may contribute to the development of higher peak bone mass. Within the reference range, younger Mexican-American and younger African-American individuals had a similar but less pronounced pattern than did Caucasian subjects. BMD rose to about 90 to 100 nmol/L in all three racial/ethnic groups.

There is some support in the literature for the observation that 25-OHD levels at the upper end of the reference range may be preferable to levels as high as the midpoint of the reference range (57 nmol/L) in older adults. In a recent randomized controlled trial (RCT), vitamin D supplementation that increased mean 25-OHD levels from 53 to 74 nmol/L significantly reduced total fracture risk by 22% in 2686 elderly subjects treated for 5 years [33].

In a trial that tested vitamin D together with calcium, increases in 25-OHD from 71 to 112 nmol/L were associated with lower fracture rates [34]. Other fracture trials have involved supplementing subjects with lower starting 25-OHD levels; in these studies, vitamin D supplementation has had positive [35,36] and neutral [37,38] effects on fracture rates. Among trials examining the impact of supplemental vitamin D on changes in BMD, supplementation that increased 25-OHD from 60.6 to 92.1 nmol/L increased BMD at the spine and total body [39]; increases from 66.3 to 100.1 nmol/L improved BMD at the spine, total body, and femoral neck [40]. Increases from 27 to 62 nmol/L were also beneficial at the femoral neck [41].

As indicated earlier, the use of PTH suppression as a determinant of optimal 25-OHD levels has resulted in a wide range of 25-OHD estimates, from 20 to 110 nmol/L [7–12]; however, most of these estimates are clustered between 75 and 110 nmol/L [9–12]. Differences in 25-OHD assays certainly account for some but probably not a large proportion of the variability in many of these threshold estimates [42]. Collectively, these studies are compatible with our finding that it is possible to improve the bone status of older subjects who have 25-OHD levels as high as the midpoint of the reference range (50 to 65 nmol/L) by supplementing them to levels near the upper end of the reference range (80–100 nmol/L).

This study confirms the high prevalence of low 25-OHD levels in the general population and the higher prevalence among African-Americans [17,18]. The clinical importance of this finding might be questioned because African-American subjects have higher BMD than do Caucasian subjects [19,20]; however, vitamin D deficiency has been found to be a risk factor for hip fractures among African-Americans [21].

The vitamin D intakes needed to increase 25-OHD to desirable levels of 90 to 100 nmol/L exceed the currently recommended intakes of 200 IU/day for young adults, 400 IU/day of those ages 51 to 70, and 600 IU/day for those over age 70 [43]. Supplementation of vitamin D with 700 to 1000 IU/day brings mean 25-hydroxyvitamin D levels to 90 to 100 nmol/L [2,44,45]. The intake required to bring a large majority of adults into this 25-OHD range, however, has not been defined.

The strength of the study is its population-based design. The large sample size provided enough power to perform stratification by ethnicity and age group. The consistency of the association between 25-OHD and BMD across race/ethnicity and age groups lends credibility to the main findings. The endpoint BMD is important in regard to bone health in younger and older adults. In addition, serum 25-OHD was assessed with a widely used and well-validated assay, so levels in this study can be compared with those in the other studies [42]. We were able to adjust the analyses for a number of important

242   Nutritional Aspects of Osteoporosis

determinants of BMD: BMI, calcium intake, age, gender, smoking, estrogen use, and poverty income ratio.

There are also limitations to our study. One limitation is the cross-sectional design of the analyses, which cannot be used to establish a causal relationship between vitamin D levels and BMD; however, a causal relationship between these factors has been demonstrated in several randomized controlled trials [34,35].

In conclusion, a significant positive association between 25-OHD levels and total hip BMD in young and older Caucasian, Mexican-American, and African-American adults was observed throughout the reference range. In young Caucasian and Mexican-American individuals, the association between 25-OHD levels and BMD remained positive above the reference range of 25-OHD. This study adds support to the concept that 25-OHD levels at the upper end of the reference range are preferable to lower 25-OHD levels for better BMD. Given the high prevalence of low 25-OHD levels in this national survey and the positive association between 25-OHD and hip BMD, higher doses of vitamin D than are customary will be needed to achieve optimal 25-OHD levels. Public health efforts to promote higher vitamin D intake for optimal bone health may be warranted with regard to recommending that supplementation begin no later than early adulthood and continue throughout life, for Caucasian as well as Mexican-American and African-American individuals.

REFERENCES

1. Lips, P. (2001). Vitamin D deficiency and secondary hyperparathyroidism in the elderly: consequences for bone loss and fractures and therapeutic implications. *Endocr. Rev.* 22: 477–501.
2. Tangpricha, V., Pearce, E.N., Chen, T.C., and Holick, M.F. (2002). Vitamin D insufficiency among free-living healthy young adults. *Am. J. Med.* 112: 659–62.
3. Freaney, R., McBrinn, Y., and McKenna, M.J. (1993). Secondary hyperparathyroidism in elderly people: combined effect of renal insufficiency and vitamin D deficiency. *Am. J. Clin. Nutr.* 58: 187–191.
4. Dawson-Hughes, B., Stern, D.T., Shipp, C.C., and Rasmussen, H.M. (1988). Effect of lowering dietary calcium intake on fractional whole body calcium retention. *J. Clin. Endocrinol. Metab.* 67: 62–68.
5. Kitamura, N., Shigeno, C., Shiomi, K. *et al.* (1990). Episodic fluctuation in serum intact parathyroid hormone concentration in men. *J. Clin. Endocrinol. Metab.* 70: 252–263.
6. Bischoff, H., Stahelin, H.B., Vogt, P. *et al.* (1999). Immobility as a major cause of bone remodeling in residents of a long-stay geriatric ward. *Calcif. Tissue. Int.* 64: 485–489.
7. Lips, P., Wiersinga, A., van Ginkel, F.C. *et al.* (1988). The effect of vitamin D supplementation on vitamin D status and parathyroid function in elderly subjects. *J. Clin. Endocrinol. Metab.* 67: 644–650.
8. Malabanan, A., Veronikis, I.E., and Holick, M.F. (1998). Redefining vitamin D insufficiency. *Lancet* 351: 805–806.

9. Peacock, M. (1998). Effects of calcium and vitamin D insufficiency on the skeleton. *Osteoporos Int.* 8: S45–S51.
10. Chapuy, M.C., Preziosi, P., Maamer, M. *et al.* (1997). Prevalence of vitamin D insufficiency in an adult normal population. *Osteoporos Int.* 7: 439–443.
11. Dawson-Hughes, B., Harris, S.S., and Dallal, G.E. (1997). Plasma calcidiol, season, and serum parathyroid hormone concentrations in healthy elderly men and women. *Am. J. Clin. Nutr.* 65: 67–71.
12. Krall, E.A., Sahyoun, N., Tannenbaum, S., Dallal, G.E., and Dawson-Hughes, B. (1989). Effect of vitamin D intake on seasonal variations in parathyroid hormone secretion in postmenopausal women. *New Engl. J. Med.* 321: 1777–1783.
13. Specker, B.L., Ho, M.L., Oestreich, A. *et al.* (1992). Prospective study of vitamin D supplementation and rickets in China. *J. Pediatr.* 120: 733–739.
14. Aksnes, L. and Aarskog, D. (1982). Plasma concentrations of vitamin D metabolites in puberty: effect of sexual maturation and implications for growth. *J. Clin. Endocrinol. Metab.* 55: 94–101.
15. Smith, R. and Dent, C.E. (1969). Vitamin D requirements in adults: clinical and metabolic studies on seven patients with nutritional osteomalacia. *Bibl. Nutr. Dieta* 13: 44–45.
16. Cummings, S.R., Nevitt, M.C., Browner, W.S. *et al.* (1995). Risk factors for hip fracture in white women: Study of Osteoporotic Fractures Research Group. *New Engl. J. Med.* 332: 767–773.
17. Nesby-O'Dell, S., Scanlon, K.S., Cogswell, M.E. *et al.* (2002). Hypovitaminosis D prevalence and determinants among African American and white women of reproductive age: third National Health and Nutrition Examination Survey, 1988–1994. *Am. J. Clin. Nutr.* 76: 187–192.
18. Harris, S.S., Soteriades, E., Coolidge, J.A., Mudgal, S., Dawson-Hughes, B. (2000). Vitamin D insufficiency and hyperparathyroidism in a low income, multiracial, elderly population. *J. Clin. Endocrinol. Metab.* 85: 4125–4130.
19. Bell, N.H., Gordon, L., Stevens, J., and Shary, J.R. (1995). Demonstration that bone mineral density of the lumbar spine, trochanter, and femoral neck is higher in black than in white young men. *Calcif. Tissue Int.* 56: 11–13.
20. Bachrach, L.K., Hastie, T., Wang, M.C., Narasimhan, B., and Marcus, R. (1999). Bone mineral acquisition in healthy Asian, Hispanic, black, and Caucasian youth: a longitudinal study. *J. Clin. Endocrinol. Metab.* 84: 4702–4712.
21. Bohannon, A.D., Hanlon, J.T., Landerman, R., and Gold, D.T. (1999). Association of race and other potential risk factors with nonvertebral fractures in community-dwelling elderly women. *Am. J. Epidemiol.* 149: 1002–1009.
22. Biser-Rohrbaugh, A. and Hadley-Miller, N. (2001). Vitamin D deficiency in breast-fed toddlers. *J. Pediatr. Orthop.* 21: 508–511.
23. Wahner, H.W., Looker, A., Dunn, W.L., Walters, L.C., Hauser, M.F., and Novak, C. (1994). Quality control of bone densitometry in a national health survey (NHANES III) using three mobile examination centers (PG-951-60). *J. Bone Mineral Res.* 9: 951–960.
24. Looker, A.C., Johnston, C.C., Jr., Wahner, H.W. *et al.* (1995). Prevalence of low femoral bone density in older U.S. women from NHANES III (PG-796-802). *J. Bone Mineral Res.* 10: 796–802.
25. Gunter, E.W., Lewis, B.L., and Konkikowski, S.M. (1996). *Laboratory Methods Used for the Third National Health and Nutrition Examination Survey (NHANES II), 1988–1994* [CD-ROM]. Centers for Disease Control, Hyattsville, MD (available from National Information Service, Springfield, VA).
26. Looker, A.C., Dawson-Hughes, B., Calvo, M.S., Gunter, E.W., and Sahyoun, N.R. (2002). Serum 25-hydroxyvitamin D status of adolescents and adults in two seasonal subpopulations from NHANES III. *Bone* 30: 771–777.
27. Korn, E.L. and Graubard, B.I. (1991). Epidemiologic studies utilizing surveys: accounting for the sampling design (PG-1166-73). *Am. J. Public Health* 81: 1166–1173.

28. Mezquita-Raya, P., Munoz-Torres, M., Luna, J.D. *et al.* (2001). Relation between vitamin D insufficiency, bone density, and bone metabolism in healthy postmenopausal women. *J. Bone Mineral Res.* 16: 1408–1415.

29. Collins, D., Jasani, C., Fogelman, I., and Swaminathan, R. (1998). Vitamin D and bone mineral density. *Osteoporos Int.* 8: 110–114.

30. Fradinger, E.E. and Zanchetta, J.R. (2001). Vitamin D and bone mineral density in ambulatory women living in Buenos Aires, Argentina. *Osteoporos Int.* 12: 24–27.

31. Outila, T.A., Karkkainen, M.U., and Lamberg-Allardt, C.J. (2001). Vitamin D status affects serum parathyroid hormone concentrations during winter in female adolescents: associations with forearm bone mineral density. *Am. J. Clin. Nutr.* 74: 206–210.

32. Lamberg-Allardt, C.J., Outila, T.A., Karkkainen, M.U., Rita, H.J., Valsta, L.M. (2001). Vitamin D deficiency and bone health in healthy adults in Finland: could this be a concern in other parts of Europe? *J. Bone Mineral Res.* 16: 2066-73.

33. Trivedi, D.P., Doll, R., and Khaw, K.T. (2003). Effect of four monthly oral vitamin D3 (cholecalciferol) supplementation on fractures and mortality in men and women living in the community: randomised double blind controlled trial. *Br. Med. J.* 326: 469.

34. Dawson-Hughes, B., Harris, S.S., Krall, E.A., and Dallal, G.E. (1997). Effect of calcium and vitamin D supplementation on bone density in men and women 65 years of age or older. *New Engl. J. Med.* 337: 670–676.

35. Chapuy, M.C., Arlot, M.E., Duboeuf, F. *et al.* (1992). Vitamin D3 and calcium to prevent hip fractures in the elderly women. *New Engl. J. Med.* 327: 1637–1642.

36. Heikinheimo, R.J., Inkovaara, J.A., Harju, E.J. *et al.* (1992). Annual injection of vitamin D and fractures of aged bones. *Calcif. Tissue Int.* 51: 105–110.

37. Lips, P., Graafmans, W.C., Ooms, M.E., Bezemer, P.D., and Bouter, L.M. (1996). Vitamin D supplementation and fracture incidence in elderly persons: a randomized, placebo-controlled clinical trial. *Ann. Intern. Med.* 124: 400–406.

38. Meyer, H.E., Smedshaug, G.B., Kvaavik, E., Falch, J.A., Tverdal, A., and Pedersen, J.I. (2002). Can vitamin D supplementation reduce the risk of fracture in the elderly? A randomized controlled trial. *J. Bone Mineral Res.* 17: 709–715.

39. Dawson-Hughes, B., Dallal, G.E., Krall, E.A., Harris, S., Sokoll, L.J., and Falconer, G. (1991). Effect of vitamin D supplementation on wintertime and overall bone loss in healthy postmenopausal women. *Ann. Intern. Med.* 115: 505–512.

40. Dawson-Hughes, B., Harris, S.S., Krall, E.A., Dallal, G.E., Falconer, G., and Green, C.L. (1995). Rates of bone loss in postmenopausal women randomly assigned to one of two dosages of vitamin D. *Am. J. Clin. Nutr.* 61: 1140–1145.

41. Ooms, M.E., Roos, J.C., Bezemer, P.D., van der Vijgh, W.J., Bouter, L.M., and Lips, P. (1995). Prevention of bone loss by vitamin D supplementation in elderly women: a randomized double-blind trial. *J. Clin. Endocrinol. Metab.* 80: 1052–1058.

42. Lips, P., Chapuy, M.C., Dawson-Hughes, B., Pols, H.A., and Holick, M.F. (1999). An international comparison of serum 25-hydroxyvitamin D measurements. *Osteoporos Int.* 9: 394–397.

43. Intakes, Standing Committee on the Scientific Evaluation of Dietary Intakes. *Dietary Reference Intakes: Calcium, Phosphorus, Magnesium, Vitamin D, and Fluoride.* National Academy Press, Washington, D.C., 1997.

44. Barger-Lux, M.J., Heaney, R.P., Dowell, S., Chen, T.C., and Holick, M.F. (1998). Vitamin D and its major metabolites: serum levels after graded oral dosing in healthy men. *Osteoporos Int.* 8: 222–230.

45. Dawson-Hughes, B. (2002). Impact of vitamin D and calcium on bone and mineral metabolism in older adults, in *Biologic Effects of Light 2001*, Holick, M.F., Ed. Kluwer Academic, Boston, MA, pp. 175–183.

CHAPTER 19

Vitamin D Supplementation in Postmenopausal Black Women Improves Calcium Homeostasis and Bone Turnover in Three Months

JERI W. NIEVES, BARBARA AMBROSE, ELIZABETH VASQUEZ, MARSHA ZION, FELICIA COSMAN, and ROBERT LINDSAY

Clinical Research, Helen Hayes Hospital, West Haverstraw, New York

ABSTRACT

Black women often have low serum vitamin D levels with associated increases in serum parathyroid hormone (PTH). It is unclear, however, whether this relative insufficiency of vitamin D in comparison to a white population has any negative impact on bone turnover and loss in postmenopausal black women. We initiated a 2-year, placebo-controlled, randomized clinical trial in 91 black postmenopausal women to determine whether vitamin D supplementation (1000 IU/day) can improve calcium homeostasis and reduce bone turnover and subsequent bone loss. Results for the first 3 months are presented here. Women were eligible for the study if three of four grandparents were black and if screening serum 25-hydroxyvitamin D [25(OH)D] was less than 20 ng/mL. Three weeks before randomization to vitamin D or placebo, the calcium intake of all participants was increased to at least 1000 mg/day, with calcium supplements, if needed. At baseline and 3 months after randomization, the following biochemical parameters were evaluated in serum: 25(OH)D; PTH; 1,25-dihydroxyvitamin D [1,25(OH)$_2$D];

Nutritional Aspects of Osteoporosis, Second Edition
Copyright © 2004 by Elsevier Science (USA)

ionized calcium; osteocalcin (OC); propeptide of human type I procollagen (PICP); and, in urine, free deoxypyridinoline (fDPD), calcium, and creatinine. At baseline average serum 25(OH)D was 12 ng/mL; PTH was 48 pg/mL. There were no significant group differences in either baseline biochemical variable. Baseline 25(OH)D was correlated with baseline PTH ($R = -0.207$; $P = 0.05$) and with fDPD ($R = -0.187$; $P = 0.08$). At 3 months, in the vitamin-D-supplemented group, there was a 130% increase in 25(OH)D ($P < 0.001$), a 10% decrease in PTH ($P < 0.01$), a 25% increase in 1,25(OH)$_2$D ($P < 0.005$), and a small 2.2% ($P < 0.01$) increase in urine calcium compared to baseline. There were no significant changes in the placebo group. The marker of bone resorption, fDPD, was reduced by 7% in the vitamin D group ($P < 0.01$), whereas fDPD increased 12% in the placebo group (group difference $P < 0.006$). Both markers of bone formation, OC and PICP, increased by 6% ($P = 0.07$) and 8% ($p = 0.02$), respectively, in the vitamin D group, with no change in either marker in the placebo group. In conclusion, vitamin D supplementation in black women with insufficient levels of serum 25(OH)D improves calcium homeostasis and improves bone turnover toward higher formation and lower resorption rates. It remains to be seen whether these changes in calcium homeostasis and bone turnover result in a long-term impact of vitamin D supplementation on bone density in postmenopausal black women.

INTRODUCTION

Black women are believed to be at lower risk for fracture than white women, but the risk of fracture is still substantial and the consequences of fracture may be greater in black women who have been reported to have higher post hip-fracture morbidity and mortality [1,2]. Although the bone density of black women is reported to be 12% higher than age-matched white women throughout life [3], in the Study of Osteoporotic Fractures [4], the rate of bone loss in elderly black women (>65 years old) was reported to be twice that of elderly white women. In several previous studies, it has been found that the majority of black women had low levels of serum vitamin D and higher levels of PTH, yet lower rates of bone turnover than whites [3–7].

Low vitamin D intake and low serum 25(OH)D are linked to bone loss and fracture in white women. Serum levels of 25(OH)D have been used to define vitamin D status as normal (>20 ng/mL or 50 nmol/L), insufficient (10–20 ng/mL or 25–50nmol/L), or deficient (<10 ng/mL or 25 nmol/L). It has been shown that vitamin D supplementation of postmenopausal white women can reduce bone turnover, bone loss, and fracture rates in several studies of vitamin D supplementation, typically in combination with calcium (500 to 1200 mg/day). The difference in BMD between groups treated with vitamin D or placebo on average was 1.0, 1.2, and 0.2%, respectively, for the spine, femoral neck, and forearm [11–20]. Significant reductions (26 to 54% reduction in hip and non-spine fracture rates) in fracture have also been seen in those randomized clinical trials where calcium was given in conjunction with vitamin D [12,15,21–22]. In the one study where fractures were not reduced, the participants had higher baseline serum 25(OH)D levels, were not given additional calcium, and were given a lower dose of vitamin D (400 IU daily) [23].

Almost no data exist evaluating the effects of vitamin D in black women, although a small uncontrolled study reported that vitamin D supplementation (800 IU) for 3 months in 10 postmenopausal black women increased 25(OH)D, decreased PTH, and reduced bone turnover [24]. We began a 2-year randomized controlled study to determine if vitamin D supplementation (1000 IU) can improve mineral metabolism and reduce bone turnover and bone loss in black postmenopausal women with insufficient serum levels of 25(OH) D at baseline. The changes in calcium metabolism and bone turnover during the first 3 months of vitamin D supplementation are presented here.

METHODS

We telephone screened 201 women, and 131 women came in for a screening visit. Black race was assessed by a self-report of three of four grandparents being black. All women were over 45 years of age with natural spontaneous menopause or surgical ovariectomy at least 1 year prior to recruitment and reported no diseases or medication use known to influence bone or calcium metabolism. Three weeks before randomization, serum 25(OH)D was measured, and the calcium intake of all participants was maintained at or increased to 1000 mg per day with calcium supplements, if needed. A total of 107 black women enrolled who met the entry criteria of serum 25(OH) D less than 20 ng/mL. These women were randomized to vitamin D (1000 IU/day) or placebo capsules for 2 years. Calcium homeostasis and bone turnover were measured at baseline and 3 months in 79 women.

Calcium homeostasis variables and bone turnover markers included serum 25(OH)D, parathyroid hormone (PTH), $1,25(OH)_2D$; osteocalcin (OC), and C-terminal propeptide of human type I procollagen (PICP), as well as free deoxypyridinoline (fDPD), calcium, and creatinine in urine. Diasorin radioimunnoassays were used for 25(OH)D and $1,25(OH)_2D$, as well as PICP. PTH was analyzed by Nichols immunoradiometric assay (IRMA) and osteocalcin by Immunotopics IRMA. Free urinary deoxypyridinoline was measured using a Quidel enzyme-linked immunosorbent assay (ELISA). Inter-assay and intra-assay coefficient of variations for all above assays were less than 10 and 12%, respectively.

RESULTS

STUDY SUBJECTS

Baseline characteristics of the study groups are presented in Table I. Both groups were similar in terms of age and years since menopause. The females were above average weight with a mean BMI of over 30. The spine and hip BMD values were similar, with the corresponding z-scores approximately 0.5 standard deviations above the race-matched normal population, even though all these women had deficient levels of 25(OH)D.

BASELINE

Baseline mean serum 25(OH)D in this population was 12 ng/mL, with a range of 5 to 20 ng/mL, as expected, because of the study inclusion criterion that 25(OH)D be ≤20 ng/mL. In fact, half of these women (56%) had serum 25(OH)D in the frankly deficient range, below 10 ng/mL. Serum PTH was at the upper limit of normal, with a mean of 48 pg/mL (range 17–111 pg/mL). Fifteen women (19%), at baseline, had serum PTH above 65 pg/mL, likely indicating secondary hyperparathyroidism. Spot urinary calcium/creatinine was similar at baseline in both groups. There was a significant difference in $1,25(OH)D_2$ between the groups, with the placebo group having higher baseline levels. At baseline, 25(OH) D was modestly inversely correlated with

TABLE I Demographic Variables at Baseline

Variable	Placebo ($n = 38$) (mean ± SEM)	Vitamin D ($n = 41$) (mean ± SEM)
Age	61.0 ± 1.1	62.8 ± 1.2
Years from menopause	15.5 ± 1.9	15.5 ± 1.8
Weight (kg)	81.8 ± 2.2	84.0 ± 2.6
Body mass index (kg/m²)	31.5 ± 0.8	31.5 ± 0.9
Spine bone mineral density	1.22 ± 0.02	1.16 ± 0.02
Hip bone mineral density	1.05 ± 0.02	1.04 ± 0.02

TABLE II   Calcium Homeostasis Variables at Baseline and 3 Months

	Placebo (mean ± SEM)		Vitamin D (mean ± SEM)	
	Baseline	3 Months	Baseline	3 Months
25(OH)D	12.5 ± 0.98	13.8 ± 1.1	11.7 ± 0.83	24.9 ± 1.3[a]
Parathyroid hormone	45.8 ± 2.8	47.0 ± 3.1	48.4 ± 2.8	43.2 ± 2.6[a]
1,25(OH)$_2$ D	47.6 ± 2.3	42.4 ± 1.7	40.3 ± 2.1	48.3 ± 2.7[a]
Urine Ca/Cr	0.085 ± 0.00	0.087 ± 0.011	0.087 ± 0.009	0.119 ± 0.014[a]

[a]$P < 0.05$ paired t-test baseline to 3 months.

both baseline PTH ($R = -0.207$; $P = 0.05$) and bone resorption as measured by fDPD ($R = -0.187$; $p = 0.08$).

CALCIUM HOMEOSTASIS OVER 3 MONTHS

Table II provides the baseline and 3-month values for the calcium homeostasis variables in the placebo and vitamin-D-supplemented groups. There was no difference in the baseline values of 25(OH)D between the two treatment groups, nor was there a difference from baseline to 3 months in the placebo group. However, the vitamin-D-supplemented group had a 139% increase ($P < 0.001$) in 25(OH)D, indicating excellent compliance in the vitamin D group and adequacy of the 1000 IU daily dose in raising 25(OH)D levels to the sufficient range. In addition, only one individual in the vitamin-D-supplemented group had a 25(OH)D level that remained less than 10 ng/mL at 3 months, whereas 23 of these women had 25(OH)D less than 10 ng/mL at baseline. Serum PTH decreased 8.5% in the vitamin-D-supplemented group ($P < 0.05$) and increased 3% in the placebo group (not significant). At 3 months, there was a 25% increase in urinary calcium/creatinine in the vitamin D group ($P < 0.05$) and a non-significant increase of 2% in the placebo group. After 3 months, the placebo group had a non-significant 4% decrement in 1,25(OH)D$_2$, while the vitamin-D-supplemented group had a 27% increase ($P < 0.05$).

BONE TURNOVER CHANGES OVER 3 MONTHS

When the population of women deficient in 25(OH)D was supplemented with 1000 IU/day of vitamin D, deoxypyridinoline (a marker of bone resorption) decreased by 6.5% ($P < 0.05$), but it increased 14% in the placebo

TABLE III   Percent Change in Bone Turnover from Baseline to 3 Months

	Placebo (%) (mean ± SEM)	Vitamin D (%) (mean ± SEM)
Deoxypyridinoline	+14 ± 5.8	−6.5 ± 4.9[a]
Osteocalcin	+0.75 ± 2.5	+6.7 ± 3.8[a]
Propeptide type1 procollagen	+3.0 ± 3.1	+8.7 ± 4.2[a]

[a]$P < 0.05$ paired t-test baseline to 3 months.

group ($P < 0.05$; Table III). The markers of bone formation, osteocalcin and propeptide of type I procollagen, both increased significantly in the vitamin-D-supplemented group, with no significant change being observed in the placebo group (Table III).

DISCUSSION

Although there have been many reports that black women have higher BMD than white women, fractures in black women remain an important public health issue. Several studies have shown that vitamin D supplementation, often with calcium, can prevent bone loss and fractures in white women [11–22]. Vitamin D has the potential to provide a low-risk, low-cost treatment for women of all races but may be particularly useful in black women who are prone to have very low serum levels of 25(OH)D.

There were limitations in this study that should be mentioned. These are short-term (3 month) results, and the more long-term effects are not yet known. Although bone density will be assessed as part of the final outcome, fracture outcome will not be assessed in this small study; however, as bone turnover results may have an effect independent of BMD changes on any potential fracture reduction, both BMD and bone turnover have been assessed in this trial. The drop-out rate was fairly high (25%) in this population, and it is unknown how this might impact the results. The optimal 25(OH)D serum level for postmenopausal black women is not known, thus standard values for white women were applied to this population. In fact, there remains debate over the optimal level of serum 25(OH)D for all races [25]. However, at the time the study was initiated, serum 25(OH)D below 20 ng/mL (50 nmol/L) was routinely described as insufficient or even deficient.

In conclusion, vitamin D supplementation in black women with insufficient levels of 25(OH)D improves calcium homeostasis and improves bone turnover toward higher formation and lower resorption rates. These changes may result in improved bone quality, reduced bone loss, and possibly reduced fracture rates in postmenopausal black women.

ACKNOWLEDGMENT

This study was funded by the National Institute of Aging (A61406705).

REFERENCES

1. Furtenber, A.L. and Mezey, M.D. (1987). Differences in outcome between black and white elderly hip fracture patients. *J. Chronic Dis.* 40: 931–938.
2. Kellie, S.E. and Brody, J.A. (1990). Sex specific and race specific hip fracture rates. *Am. J. Public Health* 80: 326–328.
3. Looker, A.C., Johnston, C.C., Wahner, H.W., Dunn, W.L., Calvo, M.S., Harris, T.B. *et al.* (1994). Prevalence of low femoral bone density in older U.S. women from NHANES III. *J. Bone Mineral Res.* 10: 796–802.
4. Cauley, J.A., Ensrud, K.E., Kuller, L.H., and Cummings, S.R. (1996). Hip bone loss increases with age among elderly African American women: the Study of Osteoporotic Fractures. *J. Bone Mineral Res.* 11(suppl.): S1–S154.
5. Cosman, F., Morgan, D.C., Nieves, J.W., Shen, V., Luckey, M.M., Dempster, D.W., Lindsay, R., and Parisien, M. (1997). Resistance to bone resorbing effects of PTH in black women. *J. Bone Mineral Res.* 12: 958–966.
6. Bell, N.H., Green, A., Epstein, S., Oexmann, M.J., Shaw, S., and Shary, J. (1985). Evidence for alteration of vitamin D endocrine system in blacks. *J. Clin. Invest.* 76(2): 470–473.
7. M'Buyamba-Kabangu, J.R., Fagard, R., Lijnen, P., Boullon, R., Lissens, W., and Amery, A. (1987). Calcium, vitamin D-endocrine system and parathyroid hormone in black and white males. *Calcif. Tissue Int.* 41: 70–74.
8. Fuleihan, G.E., Gunberg, C., Gleason, R., Brown, E.M., Stromski, M.E., Grant, F.D. *et al.* (1994). Racial differences in parathyroid hormone. *J. Bone Mineral Res.* 79: 1642–1647.
9. Harris, S.S., Soteriades, E., and Dawson-Hughes, B. (2001). Secondary hyperparathyroidism and bone turnover in elderly blacks and whites. *J. Clin. Endocrinol. Metab.* 86(8): 3801–3804.
10. Harris, S.S., Soteriades, E., Coolidge, J.A., Mudgal, S., and Dawson-Hughes, B. (2000). Vitamin D insufficiency and hyperparathyroidism in a low income, multiracial, elderly population. *J. Clin. Endocrinol. Metab.* 85: 4125–4130.
11. Baeksgaard, L., Andersen, K.P., and Hyldstrup, L. (1998). Calcium and vitamin D supplementation increases spinal BMD in healthy postmenopausal women. *Osteoporosis Int.* 8: 255–260.
12. Dawson-Hughes, B., Harris, S.S., Krall, E.A., and Dallal, G.E. (1997). Effect of calcium and vitamin D supplementation on bone density in men and women 65 years of age or older. *New Engl. J. Med.* 337: 670–676.
13. Ooms, M.E., Roos, J.C., Bezemer, P.D., van der Vigh, W.J.F., Bouter, L.M., and Lips, P. (1995). Prevention of bone loss by vitamin D supplementation in elderly women: a randomized double-blind trial. *J. Clin. Endocrinol. Metab.* 80: 1052–1058.

14. Ushiroyama, T., Okamura, S., Ikeda, A., and Ueki, M. (1995). Efficacy of ipriflavone and 1 alpha vitamin D therapy for the cessation of vertebral bone loss. *Int. J. Gynaecol. Obstet.* 48(3): 283–288.

15. Chapuy, M.C., Arlot, M.E., Duboeuf, F., Brun, J., Crouzet, B., Arnaud, S., Delmas, P.D., Meunier, P.J. (1992). Vitamin D and calcium to prevent hip fractures in elderly women. *New Engl. J. Med.* 327: 1637–1642.

16. Dawson-Hughes, B., Harris, S.S., Krall, E.A., Dallal, G.E., Falconer, G., and Green, C.L. (1995). Rates of bone loss in postmenopausal women randomly assigned to one of two dosages of vitamin D. *Am. J. Clin. Nutr.* 61: 1140–1145.

17. Orwoll, E.S., Oviatt, S.K., McClung, M.R., Defios, L.J., and Sexton, G. (1990). The rate of bone mineral loss in normal men and the effects of calcium and cholecalciferol supplementation. *Ann. Intern. Med.* 112: 29–34.

18. Lau, E.M.C., Woo, J., Lam, V., and Hong, A. (2001). Milk supplementation of the diet of postmenopausal Chinese women on a low calcium intake retards bone loss. *J. Bone Mineral Res.* 16(9): 1704–1709.

19. Adams, J.S., Kantorovich, V., Wu, C., Javanbakht, M., and Hollis, B.W. (1999). Resolution of vitamin D insufficiency in osteopenic patients results in rapid recovery of bone mineral density. *J. Clin. Endocrinol. Metab.* 86: 1212–1221.

20. Peacock, M., Liu, G., Carey, M. *et al.* (2000). Effect of calcium or 25-OH vitamin D_3 dietary supplementation on bone loss at the hip in men and women over the age of 60. *J. Clin. Endocrinol. Metab.* 85: 3011–3019.

21. Komulainen, M.H., Kroger, H., Tuppurainen, M.T. *et al.* (1998). HRT and vitamin D in prevention of non-vertebral fractures in postmenopausal women: a 5 year randomized trial. *Maturitas* 31: 45–54.

22. Chevalley, T., Rizzoli, R., Nydegger, V. *et al.* (1994). Effects of calcium supplements on femoral bone mineral density and vertebral fracture rate in vitamin D replete elderly patients. *Osteoporosis Int.* 4: 245–252.

23. Lips, P., Graafmans, W.C., Ooms, M.E., Bezemer, P.D., and Bouter, L.M. (1996). Vitamin D supplementation and fracture incidence in elderly persons: a randomized, placebo-controlled clinical trial. *Ann. Intern. Med.* 124: 400–406.

24. Kyriakidou-Himonas, M., Aloia, J.F., and Yeh, J.K. (1999). Vitamin D supplementation in postmenopausal black women. *J. Clin. Endocrinol. Metab.* 84: 3988–3990.

25. Holick, M.F. (1998). Vitamin D requirements for humans of all ages: new increased requirements for women and men 50 years and older. *Osteoporosis Int.* 8(suppl.): S24–S29.

CHAPTER 20

Adherence to Vitamin D Supplementation in Elderly Patients After Hip Fracture*

Elena Segal,[1] H. Zinnman,[2] B. Raz,[3] A. Tamir,[4,5] and S. Ish-Shalom[1,4]

[1]Metabolic Bone Diseases Unit, Rambam Medical Center, Haifa, Israel; [2]Orthopedic Surgery Department, Rambam Medical Center, Haifa, Israel; [3]Endocrine Laboratory, Rambam Medical Center, Haifa, Israel; [4]The Bruce Rappaport Faculty of Medicine, Technion–Israel Institute of Technology, Haifa, Israel; [5]Department of Community Medicine and Epidemiology, Carmel Medical Center, Haifa, Israel

ABSTRACT

Objectives: To evaluate adherence to calcium and vitamin D supplements in hip fracture patients after hospital discharge in the frame of postsurgical follow-up program; to assess factors that influenced adherence. Design: Longitudinal observational study. Setting: Academic medical center. Participants: Ninety-six hip fracture patients, mean age 72.7 ± 8.8. Measurements: Serum levels of $25(OH)D_3$ and PTH, adherence to treatment. Intervention: Treatment with 1200 mg of calcium carbonate and 800 IU of vitamin D was started during the hospital stay. Three months after hospital discharge, adherence to the prescribed supplements was checked and the levels of $25(OH)D_3$ and PTH were re-evaluated. Results: Fifty-eight (60.4%) patients had a low initial $25(OH)D_3$ level; 73 (75.8%) patients did not adhere to the treatment. Adherence was significantly higher in women than in men (29% versus 5.3%; $P < 0.039$) and in patients provided with written treatment recommendation in the hospital discharge letters: 45.8% of patients having the recommendation (11 patients) versus 16.6% not having one (12 patients)

---

*An edited version of this chapter has previously been published as a Letter to the Editor in The Journal of the American Geriatrics Society in April 2004.

($P = 0.002$). Three months later, compliance increased to 70.8% for the whole group, while, in previously non-compliant patients, the compliance reached 66.9%. The mean serum $25(OH)D_3$ level was significantly higher at that visit (15.63 ± 5.45 ng/L versus 12.81 ± 5.52 ng/L, $P < 0.001$). The mean serum PTH level in the vitamin D deficient patients decreased from 45.5 ± 26.5 to 38.5 ± 20.34 ng/mL ($P = 0.048$). *Conclusion:* Adherence of elderly hip fracture patients to calcium and vitamin D supplements is low and could be significantly influenced by written recommendations in the hospital discharge letter and by participation in a follow-up program.

INTRODUCTION

Normal vitamin D status is crucial to bone health, especially in aging patients. The decrease in the 25-hydroxyvitamin D_3 [$25(OH)D_3$] level in elderly people is well known. Vitamin D and calcium supplements have been shown to reduce incidence of non-vertebral and hip fractures [1–3]. It is also well known that hip fractures account about 10% of all fractures [4] and the rate of hip fractures increases by 1 to 3% per year [5]. About 10% of these patients sustain repeat hip fractures [6], and, according to Dolk [7], the frequency of two hip fractures in the course of an individual's life could reach 20%. Treatment with vitamin D and calcium supplements and improvement of vitamin D status play an important role in the osteoporosis therapeutic strategy and in the prevention of hip fractures in the elderly, decreasing by 30% the hip fracture rate in treated versus untreated patients [3]. Adherence to chronic treatment, which does not have an immediately perceivable effect on pain relief or on general performance, may be low in this group. These patients are candidates for anti-resorptive therapy with bisphosphonates that were effective in vitamin D replenished patients; therefore it is important to keep the normal serum level of $25(OH)D_3$. The aim of our study was to evaluate compliance with vitamin D supplements in elderly hip fracture patients after discharge from the Orthopedic Department.

PATIENTS AND METHODS

SUBJECTS

The study included 96 consecutive patients, 77 women and 19 men, ages 50 to 90 years (mean age, 72.7 ± 8.8), who underwent surgical repair of hip fracture in the Department of Orthopedic Surgery.

Methods

Follow-Up Program

The patients were enrolled in a post-surgical follow-up program that was created to perform continuous follow-up for hip fracture patients; the program was started during the hospital stay and continued later in the Metabolic Bone Diseases Unit. Patients currently receiving any antiosteoporotic treatment and patients with severe cognitive impairment were not included in this program. Three months after hospital discharge, the patients were examined in the Metabolic Bone Diseases Unit. At that first visit, 25(OH)D$_3$ and parathyroid hormone (PTH) serum levels were re-evaluated and the adherence to treatment was checked; the patients were required to bring to the office visit all the medications that they were currently using and were questioned about the regularity of the use of these medications. An additional similar evaluation was performed 3 months later.

Laboratory Evaluation

Calcium and inorganic phosphate concentration in serum and serum levels of creatinine, albumin, and liver enzymes were determined using standard laboratory techniques (Hitachi 747, Roche, Basel, Switzerland). 25(OH)D$_3$ was assessed by ^{125}I-radioimmunoassay (DiaSorin, Stillwater, MN), and intact PTH by Nichols immunoradiometric assay (IRMA; Nichols Institute Diagnostics, San Juan Capistrano, CA). Laboratory evaluation was performed in all patients during the initial hospital stay and at two consecutive follow-up visits (3 and 6 months after hospital discharge).

Calcium and Vitamin D Supplementation.

Supplementation with 1200 mg of calcium carbonate daily and 800 units of vitamin D daily was initiated during the hospital stay.

Hospital Charts Review

Recommendations for calcium and vitamin D supplements were retrieved from the charts.

Statistical analysis

Student's paired t-test was used to compare variables between two visits. The chi-square test was performed to evaluate association between categorical variables.

TABLE I   25(OH)D₃ Level in Hospitalized Hip Fracture Patients

25(OH)D$_3$ level (ng/mL)	No.	%
<10	35	36.5
10–15	23	23.9
15–25	36	37.5
>25	2	2.1
Total	96	100

RESULTS

We found that 58 (60.4%) hip fracture patients had 25(OH)D$_3$ serum levels
< 15 ng/mL at the time of hospitalization (Table I). Four (4.2%) patients
had secondary hyperparathyroidism. Three months after hospital discharge,
only 23 (24.2%) patients had adhered to the recommended supplements,
while 73 (75.8%) patients stopped the treatment. The compliance rate was
significantly higher in women compared to men: 28.9% (22 women) versus
5.3% (1 man) ($P < 0.039$). Hospital discharge letter analysis revealed that
written recommendations about vitamin D and calcium supplements was
included in one of four of the letters. Patients having the recommendations—
11 patients 45.8%—were more compliant with supplementation compared to
12 (16.6%) who did not have the written recommendations ($P = 0.002$).
Three months later, at the second visit to the Metabolic Bone Diseases Unit,
68 patients (70.8% of the entire group) were compliant with the treatment,
while 49 of 73 previously non-compliant patients (66.9%) adhered to the
treatment. The mean 25(OH)D$_3$ level was significantly higher at that visit
(15.63 ± 5.44 ng/L versus 12.47 ± 5.4 ng/mL; $P < 0.001$). The mean PTH level
decreased from 45.5 ± 26.5 ng/L to 38.5 ± 20.34 ng/L in the vitamin-D-
deficient patients ($P = 0.048$).

DISCUSSION

Vitamin D$_3$ synthesis, which takes place in the skin under the influence
of ultraviolet light, decreases with aging due to insufficient sunlight
exposure and decreased functional capacity of the skin [8]. According to
recommendations of the Food and Nutrition Board of the Institute
of Medicine, adequate intake of vitamin D is 400 IU daily for people
51 to 70 years old and 600 IU for 71 years and older [9]. Vitamin D
deficiency appears to be a widespread, but under-recognized, condition.

Thirty-seven percent of those whose daily vitamin D intake was above the recommended daily amount and 66% of those who consumed less than the recommended daily amount of vitamin D were found to be vitamin D deficient [8,10,11]. Low vitamin D intake (less than 100 IU/day) was associated with an increased risk for hip fracture (RR = 3.9, CI = 1.7–9.3) [8,12]. Frequency of vitamin D deficiency is about 60% in the healthy elderly [13]. Increased hypovitaminosis D rate after hip fracture was reported by Sahota et al. [14] in 68% of patients and by Ryan [15] in 88% of patients. Sato et al. [16] reported a hazard ratio of 6.5 for hip fracture in vitamin D deficient patients after stroke [25(OH)D$_3$ serum level ≤ 10 ng/mL] versus vitamin D insufficient patients [25(OH)D$_3$ serum level 10 to 20 ng/mL].

Subclinical vitamin D deficiency is characterized by mild secondary hyperparathyroidism and enhanced risk of osteoporotic fractures due to an increase in bone turnover. Secondary hyperparathyroidism was observed in half of the Sahota et al. [14] patients; this group attempted to maintain calcium homeostasis at the expense of increased bone turnover, leading to amplified hip bone loss. Bone turnover markers are reported to be increased in vitamin D deficient patients [18].

Vitamin D and PTH status are important parts of metabolic evaluation, but these parameters are not routinely evaluated even after an event of osteoporotic fracture. Davidson et al. [19] assessed the management of hip fracture patients 12 months after the event. Only 15% of this group had had a vitamin D level measured, and in 69% it was found to be low. Another study [20] reported that diagnosis of osteoporosis was made in 15.4% of patients discharged after hip fracture; osteoporosis treatment including calcium and vitamin D therapy was started in about 20% of these patients. How many of them continued with the prescribed treatments is unknown. In the recent study of Bahl et al. [21], no difference in calcium and vitamin D supplementation was shown between hospitalized hip fractures and pneumonia patients. Supplementation with 800 IU of vitamin D and 1 g of elemental calcium in vitamin D deficient patients increased the 25(OH)D$_3$ level and decreased the PTH level by 50%, as well as the level of bone turnover markers [22]. A decrease in hip fracture risk with calcium and vitamin D supplements was observed in the Decalyos studies [22] in elderly patients with secondary hyperparathyroidism (RR = 1.7; PTH was reduced to normal in 6 months). The decrease in PTH on vitamin D supplementation is followed by a decrease in bone turnover [8,23]. Mean PTH decreased significantly in the vitamin D deficient patients in our study group, but not in the entire cohort, probably due to lack of compliance of patients with the highest serum PTH level at inclusion.

Supplementation with calcium and vitamin D was observed to reduce bone loss in the femoral neck and in the spine and total body as well as the incidence of non-vertebral fractures by 25 to 50% [1,8,24–26]. Vitamin D repletion was also associated with a decrease in PTH and a 4 to 5% increase in BMD both at the lumbar spine and the femoral neck [27]. A positive relationship was observed between 25(OH)D$_3$ level and BMD [8,28,29]. Fracture rate reduction in vitamin D therapy can also be partially explained by a reduction in body sway and the risk of falling [30,31].

There is strong evidence that patients who sustain hip fracture are at greater risk of developing another fracture [6]; therefore, osteoporosis treatment in these patients is crucial, but it is not widely implemented right now [32]. Compliance with taking these supplements in elderly patients is problematic and under-evaluated. Chevalley et al. [33] assessed compliance with osteoporotic treatments in a group of patients with low-trauma fractures after entering the special "osteoporosis clinical pathway" and found it to be 67%. We have demonstrated that low compliance with calcium and vitamin D supplements could be significantly modified by clear written recommendations in hospital discharge letters and could be markedly increased by participation in a post-surgical follow-up program, reaching as high as 70% at the second visit.

Treatment with calcium and vitamin D must be part of a fracture-preventing strategy in the treatment of osteoporosis. According to Bendich et al. [34], 134,764 hip fractures and $2.6 billion of direct medical costs could have been avoided (data for 1995) if individuals ≥50 years had been taking 1200 mg of a calcium supplement for the prevention of primary osteoporotic hip fractures.

The less expensive the therapeutic regimen is, the more cost effective it is [35]. The secondary prevention of osteoporosis using a "fracture liaison service" [36] or "osteoporotic pathway" [33] represents a real clinical option; educational programs [37] and specialty follow-up have significantly raised patients' compliance with osteoporotic medications: from 24.2 to 70.8% in our group and from 45 to 71% as reported by Paccione et al. [37]. "It is never too early to pay attention to the risk of osteoporosis, and never too late to prevent hip fractures" [2].

CONCLUSION

About two-thirds of elderly patients hospitalized with hip fracture presented with hypovitaminosis D. The minority of the patients were compliant with vitamin D and calcium supplements after hospital discharge; the compliance was higher in women. A quarter of the discharge letters from the Department of Orthopaedic Surgery included a recommendation to continue with vitamin D and calcium supplements; the compliance rate was higher in those patients who had been given this written recommendation. Compliance rose dramatically after the first visit in the Metabolic Bone Diseases Unit. Participation in a post-surgical follow-up program can significantly influence patients' compliance and could be part of a therapeutic strategy to reduce the incidence of hip fractures.

REFERENCES

1. Dawson-Hughes, B., Harris, S.S., Krall, E.A., Dallal, G.E. (1997). Effect of calcium and vitamin D supplementation on bone density in men and women 65 years of age or older. *New Engl. J. Med.* 337: 670–676.
2. Chapuy, M.C. and Meunier, P.J. (1995). Physiopathology and prevention of fractures of the proximal end of the femur. *Rev. Pract.* 45: 1120–1123.
3. Chapuy, M.C. and Meunier, P.J. (1996). Prevention of secondary hyperparathyroidism and hip fracture in elderly women with calcium and vitamin D3 supplements. *Osteoporosis Int.* 6(suppl. 3): 60–63.
4. Eastell, R., Reid, D.M., Compston, J., Cooper, C., Fogelman, I., Francis, R.M., Hay, S.M., Hosking, D.J., Puride, D.W., Ralston, S.H., Reeve, J., Russel, R.G., and Stevenson, J.C. (2001). Secondary prevention of osteoporosis: when should a non-vertebral fracture be a trigger for action? *Q. J. Med.* 94: 575–597.
5. Cummings, S.R. and Melton, L.J. (2002). Epidemiology and outcomes of osteoporotic fractures. *Lancet* 359: 1761–1767.
6. Bischoff, H.A., Solomon, D.H., Dawson-Hughes, B. *et al.* (2001). Repeat hip fractures in a population-based sample of Medicare recipients in the U.S.: rates, timing and gender differences. *J. Bone Mineral Res.* 16(suppl. 1): 291.
7. Dolk, T. (1989). Influence of treatment factors on the outcome after hip fractures. *Upsala J. Med. Sci.* 94: 209–221.
8. Lips, P. (2001). Vitamin D deficiency and secondary hyperparathyroidism in the elderly: consequences for bone loss and fractures and therapeutic implications. *Endocrinol. Rev.* 22: 477–501.
9. Standing Committee on the Scientific Evaluation of Dietary Reference Intakes, Institute of Medicine. (1997). *Dietary Reference Intakes: Calcium, Phosphorus, Magnesium, Vitamin D and Fluoride.* National Academy Press, Washington, D.C.
10. Thomas, M.K., Lloyd-Jones, D.M., Thadhani, R.I. et al. (1998). Hypovitaminosis D in medical inpatients. *New Engl. J. Med.* 338: 777–783.
11. Meunier, P.J. (1993). Prevention of hip fractures. *Am. J. Med.* 95: S75–S78.
12. Meyer, H.E., Henriksen, C., Falch, J.A. *et al.* (1995). Risk factors for hip fracture in a high incidence area: a case-control study from Oslo, Norway. *Osteoporosis Int.* 5: 239–246.
13. Sourberbielle, J.C., Cormier, C., Kindermans, C. *et al.* (2001). Vitamin D status and redefining serum parathyroid hormone reference range in the elderly. *J. Clin. Endocrinol. Metab.* 86: 3086–3090.
14. Sahota, O., Gaynor, K., Harwood, R.H. *et al.* (2001). Hypovitaminosis D and "functional hypoparathyroidism": the NoNoF (Nottingham Neck of Femur) study. *Age Aging* 30: 467–472.

15. Ryan, P.J. (2002). Hypovitaminosis D in clinical practice. *J. Bone Mineral Res.* 17(suppl. 1): 316.
16. Sato, Y., Asoh, T., Kondo, I. *et al.* (2001). Vitamin D deficiency and risk of hip fractures among disabled elderly stroke patients. *Stroke* 32: 1673–1677.
17. Cummings, S.R., Browner, W.S., Bauer, D. *et al.* (1998). Endogenous hormones and the risk of hip and vertebral fractures among older women. *New Engl. J. Med.* 339: 733–738.
18. Brazier, M., Kamel, S., Maamer, M. *et al.* (1995). Markers of bone remodeling in the elderly subject: effects of vitamin D insufficiency and its correction. *J. Bone Mineral Res.* 10: 1753–1761.
19. Davidson, C.W., Merrilees, M.J., Wilkinson, T.J. *et al.* (2000). Hip fracture mortality and morbidity: can we do better? *New Zealand Med. J.* 114: 329–332.
20. Jubi, A.G. and De Geus-Wenceslau, C.M. (2002). Evaluation of osteoporosis treatment in seniors after hip fracture. *Osteoporosis Int.* 13: 205–210.
21. Bahl, S., Coates, P.S., and Greenspan, S.L. (2002). The management of osteoporosis after hip fracture: have we improved our care? *J. Bone Mineral Res.* 17(suppl. 1): 358.
22. Chapuy, M.C., Pamphile, R., Paris, E. *et al.* (2002). Combined calcium and vitamin D_3 supplementation in elderly women: confirmation of reversal of secondary hyperparathyroidism and hip fracture risk—the Decalyos 11 study. *Osteoporosis Int.* 13: 257–264.
23. Ooms, M.E., Roos, J.C., Bezemer, P.D. *et al.* (1995). Prevention of bone loss by vitamin D supplementation in elderly women: a randomized double-blind trial. *J. Clin. Endocrinol. Metab.* 80: 1052–1058.
24. Meunier, P.J., Chapuy, M.C., Arlot, M.E. *et al.* (1994). Can we stop bone loss and prevent hip fractures in the elderly? *Osteoporosis Int.* 4(suppl. 1): 71–76.
25. Gillespie, W.J., Avenell, A., Henry, D.A. *et al.* (2001). Vitamin D and vitamin D analogues for preventing fractures associated with involutional and post-menopausal osteoporosis [Cochrane Review]. *Cochrane Database Syst. Rev.* 1: CD000227.
26. Chapuy, M.C., Arlot, M.E., Dudoeuf, F. *et al.* (1992). Vitamin D_3 and calcium to prevent hip fractures in elderly women. *New Engl. J. Med.* 327: 1637–1642.
27. Adams, J.S., Kantorovich, V., Wu, C. *et al.* (1999). Resolution of vitamin D deficiency in osteopenic patients results in rapid recovery of bone mineral density. *J. Clin. Endocrinol. Metab.* 84: 2799–2830.
28. Khaw, K.T., Sneyd, M.J., and Compston, J. (1998). Bone density, parathyroid hormone and 25-hydroxyvitamin D concentrations in middle-aged women. *Br. Med. J.* 305: 273–277.
29. Egmosse, C., Lund, B., McNair, P. *et al.* (1987). Low serum levels of 25-hydroxyvitamin D in institutionalized old people: influence of solar exposure and vitamin D supplementation. *Age Aging* 16: 35–40.
30. Pfeifer, M., Begerov, B., and Minne, H.W. (2002). Vitamin D and muscle function. *Osteoporosis Int.* 13: 187–194.
31. Pfeifer, M., Begerov, B., Minne, H.W. *et al.* (2000). Effects of short-term vitamin D and calcium supplementation on body sway and secondary hyperparathyroidism in elderly women. *J. Bone Mineral Res.* 15: 1113–1118.
32. Kamel, H.K. and Duyhie, E.H. (2002). The underuse of therapy in the secondary prevention of hip fractures. *Drugs Aging* 19: 1–10.
33. Chevalley, T., Hoffmeyer, P., Bonjour, J.P. *et al.* (2002). An osteoporosis clinical pathway for the medical management of patients with low-trauma fracture. *Osteoporosis Int.* 13: 450–455.
34. Bendich, A., Leader, S., and Muhuri, P. (1999). Supplemental calcium for the prevention of hip fracture: potential health-economic benefits. *Clin. Ther.* 21: 1058–1072.
35. Vestergaard, P., Rejnmark, L., and Mosekilde, L. (2001). Hip fracture prevention: cost-effective strategies. *Pharmacoeconomics* 19(5, pt. 1): 449–468.

36. McLellan, A.R. and Fraser, M. (2002). A 28-month audit of the efficacy of the fracture liaison service in offering secondary prevention for patients with osteoporotic fractures. *J. Bone Mineral Res.* 17(suppl.1): 358.
37. Paccione, P., Powell, R., O'Neill, J. *et al.* (2002). Impact of an educational intervention for the prevention and treatment of osteoporosis: a health plan's perspective. *J. Bone Mineral Res.* 17(suppl. 1): 477.

CHAPTER 21

Vitamin D Round Table*

BESS DAWSON-HUGHES,[1] ROBERT P. HEANEY,[2] MICHAEL HOLICK,[3]
PAUL LIPS,[4] PIERRE J. MEUNIER,[5] and REINHOLD VIETH[6]

[1]Bone Metabolism Laboratory, Jean Mayer U.S.D.A. Human Nutrition Research Center on Aging at Tufts University, Boston, Massachusetts, USA; [2]University Chair, Creighton University, Omaha, Nebraska; [3]Department of Endocrinology, Boston University School of Medicine, Boston, Massachusetts, USA; [4]Department of Endocrinology, Vrije Universiteit Medical Center, Amsterdam, The Netherlands; [5]Rheumatology and Bone Disease, Edouard Herriot Hopital, Lyon, France; [6]Department of Laboratory Medicine and Pathobiology, University of Toronto, and Pathology and Laboratory Medicine, Mt. Sinai Hospital, Toronto, Canada

INTRODUCTION

This round table discussion addressed the following two questions:

- What is the optimal level of 25-hydroxyvitamin D [25(OH)D] for the skeleton and why?
- How much vitamin D_3 (cholecalciferol) is needed to reach the optimal level of 25(OH)D?

The participants in the roundtable were Paul Lips, M.D., Ph.D.; Michael Holick, M.D., Ph.D.; Robert P. Heaney, M.D.; Pierre Meunier, M.D.; Reinhold Vieth, Ph.D.; and Bess Dawson-Hughes, M.D. Each of the participants spent 5 minutes presenting his or her answers to these questions along with supporting evidence. The presentations were followed by a 45-minute general

*This material is based on work supported by the U.S. Department of Agriculture, under agreement No. 58-1950-9001. Any opinions, findings, conclusions, or recommendations expressed in this publication are those of the authors and do not necessarily reflect the view of the U.S. Department of Agriculture.

263

discussion with audience participation. This paper summarizes the views expressed during the round table.

WHAT IS THE OPTIMAL LEVEL OF 25(OH)D FOR THE SKELETON AND WHY?

The participants considered several criteria by which the optimal 25-hydroxyvitamin D [25(OH)D] level might be defined. These included the level needed to maximally suppress the circulating parathyroid hormone (PTH) concentration and the 25(OH)D level associated with the highest bone mineral density (BMD), with greatest calcium absorption, with reduced rates of bone loss, and with reduced fracture rates. The issue of vitamin D status and risk of falling was addressed in the discussion.

Dr. Lips pointed out that the 25(OH)D level associated with maximal suppression of PTH in his study was 30 nmol/L [1]. Several participants cited other estimates. Dr. Meunier noted that studies have placed the estimate at 75 to 80 nmol/L [2], 70 to 75 nmol/L [3], 65 to 75 nmol/L [4], and 50 nmol/L [5]. Dr. Dawson-Hughes standardized 25(OH)D levels from several studies to DiaSorin equivalent values using the cross-calibration study of Lips [6]. This resulted in threshold 25(OH)D values of 55 nmol/L [2], 75 nmol/L [7], 82 nmol/L [8], and 99 nmol/L [9]. Thus, the estimates of 25(OH)D required for maximal PTH suppression vary widely from 30 to 99 nmol/L, and there is a cluster of estimates in the 75 to 80 nmol range. Dr. Holick noted that the inverse association in 25(OH)D and PTH is also present in healthy young adults, in whom he identified a threshold 25(OH)D level of 75 nmol/L [10]. Dr. Vieth pointed out that the relationship between PTH and 25(OH)D changes with age; for example, if you are older than 70 years and desire a PTH equivalent to that of a young adult, your 25(OH)D level needs to exceed 100 nmol/L [11].

With regard to 25(OH)D levels and calcium absorption, Dr. Heaney cited his recent observation that calcium absorption increases with increasing 25(OH)D levels and that calcium absorption was 65% greater at serum 25(OH)D levels averaging 86.5 nmol/L than at levels averaging 50 nmol/L [12]. Increased absorption of calcium results in an increase in the circulating level of ionized calcium and a reduction in the circulating PTH level. Thus, Dr. Heaney's finding describes the metabolic basis for the observation that increasing the 25(OH)D level to 75 to 80 nmol/L lowers the circulating level of PTH.

Dr. Lips noted that 25(OH)D and BMD of the hip are positively associated at 25(OH)D levels below 30 nmol/L, but not at higher 25(OH)D levels [13].

In contrast, hip BMD increased with increasing 25(OH)D levels up to 90 to 100 nmol/L, according to an earlier presentation at the meeting by Dr. Bischoff. The latter analysis included men and women age 51 and older who participated in the third National Health and Examination Survey (NHANES III).

With regard to the effect of vitamin D on change in BMD, Dr. Dawson-Hughes noted that bone loss during the wintertime was reduced with vitamin D supplementation that increased serum 25(OH)D levels from about 60 to 90 nmol/L [14,15]. These studies in healthy older women also demonstrated that vitamin D supplements reduced bone loss from the hip [14] and spine [15] year-round.

Concerning the most important endpoint—fractures—Heaney highlighted the randomized controlled trial recently published in Great Britain in which elevating mean serum 25(OH)D from 53.4 to 74.3 nmol/L produced a 33% reduction in typical osteoporotic fractures over a 5-year treatment period [16]. The available randomized, controlled supplement studies were summarized by Dr. Meunier, who noted that studies in which supplementation brought mean serum 25(OH)D levels up to the range of 74 to 112 nmol/L significantly lowered fracture rates, whereas the study in which 25(OH)D increased to only 54 nmol/L per day did not significantly change fracture rates [16,17–21] (Table I). Published serum 25(OH)D values and values that have been standardized to DiaSorin equivalent values are also shown in Table I. Dr. Meunier noted that the higher supplement doses were associated with bigger decrements in serum PTH.

TABLE I   Serum 25(OH)D, PTH, and Non-Vertebral Fracture Responses to Supplementation with Vitamin D₃

Study	Gender	Dose Vitamin D₃ (IU/day)	Published Serum 25(OH)D Values (nmol/L)	Standardized Serum 25(OH)D Values[a] (nmol/L)	Effect on Serum PTH (%)	Preventative Effect on Non-Vertebral Effects (Hip and Others)
Chapuy et al. [17,21]	F	800	100	71	−47	+ +
Chapuy et al. [18]	F	800	100	71	−33	+
Dawson-Hughes et al. [19]	M, F	700	112	99	F, −33M, −23	+
Trivedi et al. [16]	M, F	820	74	—	—	+
Lips et al. [20]	M, F	400	54	54	−6	Not significant

[a]Serum 25(OH)D values standardized to DiaSorin equivalent values (i.e., HPLC followed by a competitive protein binding assay), based on a cross-calibration study [24].

An audience participant raised the issue that part of the reduction in fracture rates seen with vitamin D supplementation may be related to the effect of vitamin D on lowering the risk of falling. Indeed, supplementation that increased 25(OH)D levels from 30 to 65 nmol/L has been shown to lower the number of falls occurring in very elderly institutionalized women [22]. This mechanism may have been a factor in the vitamin D intervention trials conducted in very elderly and vitamin-D-deficient subjects, such as the trials reported by Chapuy et al. [17,18]; however, there is no evidence that it was a significant factor in a younger cohort of men and women, mean age 71 years [19]. In that study, the fall rate was found to be similar in the supplemented and placebo groups [19].

HOW MUCH VITAMIN D₃ IS NEEDED TO REACH THE OPTIMAL LEVEL OF 25(OH)D?

Dr. Vieth pointed out that at low daily doses of supplemental vitamin D_3, the increase in 25(OH)D per microgram is 1.2 nmol/L. According to the findings of Drs. Vieth and Heaney, at higher doses, this figure drops to 0.7 nmol/L for every microgram of vitamin D_3 given as a daily oral dose [12,23]. Dr. Lips noted that the increase in serum 25(OH)D following supplementation with 400 to 600 IU/day is very much dependent upon the baseline serum 25(OH)D level. He observed a large increase when baseline serum 25(OH)D was low and a small increase when it was high [24]. Vitamin D_2 gives a smaller increment of only 0.3 nmol/L for every microgram [25]. Dr. Holick finds that for patients with starting 25(OH)D levels over 50 nmol/L, 50,000 IU of vitamin D_2 twice per month will maintain their levels between 75 and 100 nmol/L. Patients with lower starting levels will need loading doses of vitamin D. Dr. Dawson-Hughes noted that, of the 389 participants in her study who took 700 IU/day of vitamin D_3 (together with 500 mg of supplemental calcium), 90% of the men and 87% of the women had 25(OH)D levels of 80 nmol/L or higher (measured year-round), whereas only 57% of the men and 28% of the women in the placebo group had levels as high as 80 nmol/L [26]. These subjects consumed an average of 200 IU of vitamin D per day in their diets. Dr. Vieth summarized the relationship between vitamin D_3 dose and outcomes in fracture prevention trials (Fig. 1). Fracture risk was reduced at vitamin D_3 dosages of 700 and 800 IU/day, but not at lower doses.

In closing, the participants' answers to the two questions are summarized in Table II. There is some convergence of opinion that the optimal 25(OH)D level for bone health is around 75 nmol/L and that an intake of

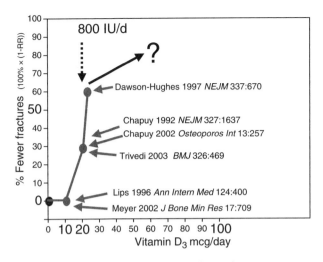

FIGURE 1   Fracture prevention studies with Vitamin D_3.

TABLE II   Round Table Participants' Views of the Optimal 25(OH)D Levels and the Doses of Vitamin D_3 Needed To Achieve Those Levels

Participant	Optimal 25(OH)D Level (nmol)	Oral Vitamin D_3 Dose Needed To Reach Average Optimal 25(OH)D Level μg/day	IU/day
Lips	50	10–15	400–600
Holick	75	25	1000[a]
Heaney	80	40[b]	1600[b]
Meunier	75	20	800
Vieth	70	25[c]	1000
Dawson-Hughes	80	25	1000

[a]Consistent with recent observation that 1000 IU of vitamin D_3 per day in orange juice maintained an average 25(OH)D level of 94 ± 20 nmol/L [27].
[b]Based on data in the Trivedi et al. paper [16].
[c]Estimated dose to deliver an *average* 25(OH)D level of 70 nmol/L is given in the table, but the dose needed to provide the level of 70 nmol/L for practically all healthy adults (criterion for an RDA) would be 100 μg/day.

800 to 1000 IU of vitamin D_3 is needed to attain the desired 25(OH)D level of 75 nmol/L. The group agreed with Dr. Meunier that this reappraisal of the lower limit of vitamin D sufficiency has two important clinical consequences: Vitamin D insufficiency is much more common than previously believed, and this is relevant to larger possibilities of vitamin D supplements for preventing fractures, particularly in elderly subjects; in

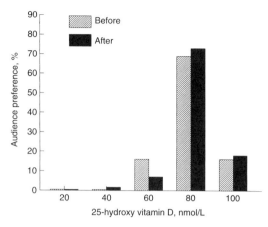

FIGURE 2   Scientific audience views of optimal 25(OH)D levels for bone health before and after the round table.

addition, it is important to ensure that the serum 25(OH)D level obtained after vitamin D supplementation reaches this new threshold. However, Dr. Lips expressed the view that at this time the criterion for broad-based supplementation is not fulfilled.

An audience opinion poll was taken at the beginning and again at the end of the round table. Participants were asked to vote for the 25(OH)D level that was closest to their view of optimal, given the choices of 0, 20, 40, 60, 80, and 100 nmol/L. The results of the poll are shown in Fig. 2. There is a clear preference among these scientists in the general nutrition community for a 25(OH)D level of 80 nmol/L; however, we all concede that the questions addressed in this workshop are not yet fully answered and will require ongoing evaluation of data from a variety of studies.

REFERENCES

1. Lips, P., Wiersinga, A., van Ginkel, F.C., Jongen, M.J., Netelenbos, J.C., Hackeng, W.H., Delmas, P.D., and van der Vijgh, W.J. (1988). The effect of vitamin D supplementation on vitamin D status and parathyroid function in elderly subjects. *J. Clin. Endocrinol. Metab.* 67: 644–650.
2. Chapuy, M.C., Preziosi, P., Maamer, M., Arnaud, S., Galan, P., Hercberg, S., and Meunier, P.J. (1997). Prevalence of vitamin D insufficiency in an adult normal population. *Osteoporosis Int.* 7: 439–443.
3. McKenna, M.J. (1992). Differences in vitamin D status between countries in young adults and the elderly. *Am. J. Med.* 93: 69–77.

4. Thomas, M.K., Lloyd-Jones, D.M., Thadhani, R.I., Shaw, A.C., Deraska, D.J., Kitch, B.T., Vamvakas, E.C., Dick, I.M., Prince, R.L., and Finkelstein, J.S. (1998). Hypovitaminosis D in medical inpatients. *New Engl. J. Med.* 338: 777–783.

5. Malabanan, A., Veronikis, I.E., and Holick, M.F. (1998). Redefining vitamin D insufficiency. *Lancet* 351: 805–806.

6. Lips, P., Chapuy, M.C., Dawson-Hughes, B., Pols, H.A., and Holick, M.F. (1999). An international comparison of serum 25-hydroxyvitamin D measurements. *Osteoporosis Int.* 9: 394–397.

7. Peacock, M. (1998). Effects of calcium and vitamin D insufficiency on the skeleton. *Osteoporosis Int.* 8: S45–S51.

8. Krall, E.A., Sahyoun, N., Tannenbaum, S., Dallal, G.E., and Dawson-Hughes, B. (1989). Effect of vitamin D intake on seasonal variations in parathyroid hormone secretion in postmenopausal women. *New Engl. J. Med.* 321: 1777–1783.

9. Dawson-Hughes, B., Harris, S.S., and Dallal, G.E. (1997). Plasma calcidiol, season, and serum parathyroid hormone concentrations in healthy elderly men and women. *Am. J. Clin. Nutr.* 65: 67–71.

10. Tangpricha, V., Pearce, E.N., Chen, T.C., and Holick, M.F. (2002). Vitamin D insufficiency among free-living healthy young adults. *Am. J. Med.* 112: 659–662.

11. Vieth, R., Ladak, Y., and Walfish, P.G. (2003). Age-related changes in the 25-hydroxyvitamin D versus parathyroid hormone relationship suggest a different reason why older adults require more vitamin D. *J. Clin. Endocrinol. Metab.* 88: 185–191.

12. Heaney, R.P., Dowell, M.S., Hale, C.A., and Bendich, A. (2003). Calcium absorption varies within the reference range for serum 25-hydroxyvitamin D. *J. Am. Coll. Nutr.* 22: 142.

13. Ooms, M.E., Lips, P., Roos, J.C., van der Vijgh, W.J., Popp-Snijders, C., Bezemer, P.D., and Bouter, L.M. (1995). Vitamin D status and sex hormone binding globulin: determinants of bone turnover and bone mineral density in elderly women. *J. Bone Mineral Res.* 10: 1177–1184.

14. Dawson-Hughes, B., Harris, S.S., Krall, E.A., Dallal, G.E., Falconer, G., and Green, C.L. (1995). Rates of bone loss in postmenopausal women randomly assigned to one of two dosages of vitamin D. *Am. J. Clin. Nutr.* 61: 1140–1145.

15. Dawson-Hughes, B., Dallal, G.E., Krall, E.A., Harris, S., Sokoll, L.J., and Falconer, G. (1991). Effect of vitamin D supplementation on wintertime and overall bone loss in healthy postmenopausal women. *Ann. Intern. Med.* 115: 505–512.

16. Trivedi, D.P., Doll, R., and Khaw, K.T. (2003). Effect of four monthly oral vitamin D3 (cholecalciferol) supplementation on fractures and mortality in men and women living in the community: randomised double blind controlled trial. *Br. Med. J.* 326: 469.

17. Chapuy, M.C., Arlot, M.E., Duboeuf, F., Brun, J., Crouzet, B., Arnaud, S., Delmas, P.D., and Meunier, P.J. (1992). Vitamin D_3 and calcium to prevent hip fractures in the elderly women. *New Engl. J. Med.* 327: 1637–1642.

18. Chapuy, M. C., Pamphile, R., Paris, E., Kempf, C., Schlichting, M., Arnaud, S., Garnero, P., and Meunier, P.J. (2002). Combined calcium and vitamin D_3 supplementation in elderly women: confirmation of reversal of secondary hyperparathyroidism and hip fracture risk—the Decalyos II study. *Osteoporosis Int.* 13: 257–264.

19. Dawson-Hughes, B., Harris, S.S., Krall, E.A., and Dallal, G.E. (1997). Effect of calcium and vitamin D supplementation on bone density in men and women 65 years of age or older. *New Engl. J. Med.* 337: 670–676.

20. Lips, P., Graafmans, W.C., Ooms, M.E., Bezemer, P.D., and Bouter, L.M. (1996). Vitamin D supplementation and fracture incidence in elderly persons: a randomized, placebo-controlled clinical trial. *Ann. Intern. Med.* 124: 400–406.

21. Chapuy, M.C., Arlot, M.E., Delmas, P.D., and Meunier, P.J. (1994). Effect of calcium and cholecalciferol treatment for three years on hip fractures in elderly women. *Br. Med. J.* 308: 1081–1082.

22. Bischoff, H.A., Stahelin, H.B., Dick, W., Akos, R., Knecht, M., Salis, C., Nebiker, M., Theiler, R., Pfeifer, M., Begerow, B., Lew, R.A., and Conzelmann, M. (2003). Effects of vitamin D and calcium supplementation on falls: a randomized controlled trial. *J. Bone Mineral Res.* 18: 343–351.

23. Vieth, R., Chan, P.C., and MacFarlane, G.D. (2001). Efficacy and safety of vitamin D₃ intake exceeding the lowest observed adverse effect level. *Am. J. Clin. Nutr.* 73: 288–294.

24. Lips, P., Duong, T., Oleksik, A., Black, D., Cummings, S., Cox, D., and Nickelsen, T. (2001). A global study of vitamin D status and parathyroid function in postmenopausal women with osteoporosis: baseline data from the multiple outcomes of raloxifene evaluation clinical trial. *J. Clin. Endocrinol. Metab.* 86: 1212–1221.

25. Cooper, L., Clifton-Bligh, P.B., Nery, M.L., Figtree, G., Twigg, S., Hibbert, E., and Robinson, B.G. (2003). Vitamin D supplementation and bone mineral density in early postmenopausal women. *Am. J. Clin. Nutr.* 77: 1324–1329.

26. Dawson-Hughes, B. and Harris, S.S. (2000). Definition of the optimal 25OHD status for bone. in Norman, A., Ed., *Vitamin D Endocrine System: Structural, Biological, Genetic and Clinical Aspects.* University of California, Riverside, pp. 909–915.

27. Tangpricha, V., Koutkia, P., Rieke, S.M., Chen, T.C., Perez, A.A., and Holick, M.F. (2003). Fortification of orange juice with vitamin D: a novel approach for enhancing vitamin D nutritional health. *Am. J. Clin. Nutr.* 77: 1478–1483.

28. Meyer, H.E., Smedshaug, G.B., Kvaavik, E., Falch, J.A., Tverdal, A., and Pedersen, J.I. (2002). Can vitamin D supplementation reduce the risk of fracture in the elderly? A randomized controlled trial. *J. Bone Mineral Res.* 17: 709–715.

PART VII

Acid Load From Food—First Part

Effects of Diet Acid Load on Bone Health

LYNDA A. FRASSETTO, R. CURTIS MORRIS, JR., and ANTHONY SEBASTIAN
Department of Medicine and General Clinical Research Center, University of California, San Francisco, California

ABSTRACT

Alveolar ventilation, renal acid–base regulatory activity, and the diet acid and base loads together determine the setpoint at which the concentrations of blood hydrogen ion and plasma bicarbonate are regulated. The diet acid load results from catabolism of the sulfur-containing amino acids cysteine and methionine and from incompletely oxidized dietary-supplied or metabolically produced organic acids. The combination of high acid load (from protein and cereal grain products) and a low base load (from non-grain plant foods) in diets in industrialized countries leads to a net endogenous production of acid (NEAP) that the body must dispose of either by renal excretion or by titration of internal base reservoirs. When NEAP exceeds about 40 mEq/day (0.55–0.65 mEq/kg body weight), renal net acid excretion (RNAE) falls below NEAP in about 50% of individuals, suggesting chronic titration of internal base reservoirs in those individuals.

In *in vitro* systems, adding metabolic acids to either living or dead bone causes three distinct effects: physicochemical exchange of bone minerals to

Nutritional Aspects of Osteoporosis, Second Edition

buffer the hydrogen ions, including sodium, potassium, and calcium; release of the bicarbonate-yielding anionic salts of bone (carbonates, phosphates, hydroxides); and activation of osteoclastic bone resorption and inhibition of osteoblastic bone production. Conversely, addition of base decreases bone mineral exchange and the release of bicarbonate and increases osteoblastic bone production while decreasing osteoclastic bone breakdown. At all pH levels, addition of parathyroid hormone (PTH) or vitamin D to the system increases bone breakdown, while inactivating or killing the bone cells (both the osteoblasts and osteoclasts) decreases bone breakdown. And, under all experimental conditions and in a linear fashion, as the hydrogen ion concentration falls from a pH of 7.1 to 7.6 so does release of bone mineral salts from bone.

The decline in bone breakdown observed with declining systemic acid content (or increased base content) in *in vitro* systems may parallel events in *in vivo* systems. If so, then the addition of diet net acid loads sufficient to exceed RNAE should lead to trade-offs that induce increases in the amount of bone mineral released and over many years should contribute to the low bone mineral densities typically found in older subjects in industrialized countries. Subjects with low net diet acid loads would be expected to have higher bone mineral densities than subjects with high net acid loads. Under research conditions at steady state, neutralization of dietary acid with basic salts of potassium to reduce RNAE to near zero decreases both blood hydrogen ion levels and urine calcium excretion, decreases release of biomarkers of bone breakdown, and may stabilize or improve bone mineral densities in subjects with calcium metabolic disorders, such as those with hypercalciuric nephrolithiasis. Whether chronic neutralization of NEAP or chronic diet net base loads would improve bone health is not yet known.

DETERMINANTS OF THE SETPOINT AT WHICH BLOOD ACIDITY AND PLASMA BICARBONATE CONCENTRATION ARE REGULATED IN NORMAL SUBJECTS

RESPIRATORY DETERMINANTS

In normal subjects ingesting self-selected diets, plasma hydrogen ion concentration ($[H^+]$) differs among individuals by as much as 10 nEq/L, which is 25% of the mean value (40 nEq/L) [1]. The homeostatic mechanisms that minimize deviations in plasma acidity within an individual during disturbances of acid–base balance are well defined [2–6]. The factors that account for differences among individuals under ordinary physiological conditions have only recently been extensively investigated.

Madias *et al.* [1] were the first to propose that the interindividual differences in plasma acidity in normal subjects can be partly accounted for by differences in the level at which plasma carbon dioxide (P_{CO2}) is regulated by the respiratory system, such as primary hypo- or hyperventilation. Madias carried out studies in 25 normal subjects demonstrating a positive correlation between plasma [H^+] and P_{CO2} among the subjects; that is, as P_{CO2} increased, so did hydrogen ion concentration. The possibility that plasma acidity rather than carbon dioxide tension was the independent variable was excluded because primary differences in plasma acidity would be expected to correlate negatively rather than positively with plasma P_{CO2}, inasmuch as acidemia is known to stimulate alveolar ventilation and alkalemia to suppress it. At the same time, plasma bicarbonate concentration ([HCO_3^-]) was also found to vary directly with P_{CO2} among subjects, as individuals with greater rates of alveolar ventilation (lower P_{CO2}) would be expected to have correspondingly lower plasma [HCO_3^-], and vice versa.

In the Madias study [1], the interindividual differences in steady state plasma P_{CO2} accounted for approximately 35% of the interindividual differences in plasma [H^+] and approximately 50% of those in plasma [HCO_3^-]. In subsequent studies, Kurtz *et al.* [7] confirmed the findings of Madias *et al.* in normal subjects.

METABOLIC DETERMINANTS

Diet

Kurtz *et al.* [7] were the first consider whether "metabolic" factors might also play a role in determining the interindividual differences in blood acidity and plasma [HCO_3^-] in normal subjects. Conceivably, differences in such factors as dietary sodium chloride intake or plasma aldosterone could alter steady-state blood acidity in normal subjects independent of carbon dioxide tension. Kurtz *et al.* focused their attention on the potential role of interindividual differences in the diet-dependent rate of endogenous acid production. Under normal physiological circumstances, endogenous acid production is partly due to intake of acids determined by the composition of the diet.

Net endogenous noncarbonic acid production (NEAP) in normal subjects eating self-selected diets may differ by nearly tenfold, with a range of approximately 20 to 120 mEq/24 hr [8,9]. Under ordinary physiological conditions, these differences reflect to a major extent differences in the composition of the diet. It is well known that plasma acidity is maintained at an increased level and plasma [HCO^{3-}] at a decreased level in clinical conditions that result in a sustained pathological increases in endogenous acid production [10–12], as well as in experimental conditions in which the net systemic acid load is maintained at an greatly increased level by exogenous acid loading [2,13,14]. It seemed reasonable to consider whether increases in endogenous acid production secondary to normal variations in diet composition might also appreciably increase plasma acidity and bicarbonate concentration in the steady state.

In their study, Kurtz et al. fed 19 normal subjects various diets producing net acid excretion rates varying from 14 to 154 mEq/day, similar to the normal range established by Lennon et al. [8]. In the steady state, there was a significant direct relationship between plasma acidity and RNAE and a significant inverse relationship between plasma [HCO^{3-}] and RNAE; that is, as RNAE increased, steady-state hydrogen ion concentration increased, and steady-state plasma bicarbonate concentration decreased. These findings indicate that normal subjects eating typical net acid-producing diets have a low-grade metabolic acidosis of a severity determined by the magnitude of the net acid load of their diet.

The Aging Kidney

Another potential influence on the net amount of acid in the system would be the interindividual differences in acid excretion. The kidney is ultimately responsible for excreting non-carbonic (or "metabolic") acids from the body, but, with increasing age, renal excretory capacity declines. To evaluate this, Frassetto et al. [15] carried out an analysis of measurements of blood hydrogen ion concentration and carbon dioxide tension, plasma bicarbonate concentration, renal net acid excretion, and glomerular filtration rate (GFR; estimated as 24-hour creatinine clearance) in 64 healthy adult men and women over a wide range of ages, each of whom was in a steady state on a controlled diet while residing in a clinical research center. Those studies identified age as an independent determinant of the blood acid–base composition in adult humans. From young adulthood to old age (17–74 years), otherwise healthy men and women develop a progressive increase in blood acidity and decrease in plasma bicarbonate concentration, indicative of an increasingly worsening low-grade metabolic acidosis (Fig. 1). At constant GFR, Frassetto et al. [15] also confirmed the findings of Kurtz et al. [7] in normal subjects.

Taken together, the studies of Kurtz et al. and Frassetto et al. established that over the normal ranges of variation of P$_{CO2}$ and RNAE, P$_{CO2}$ is about

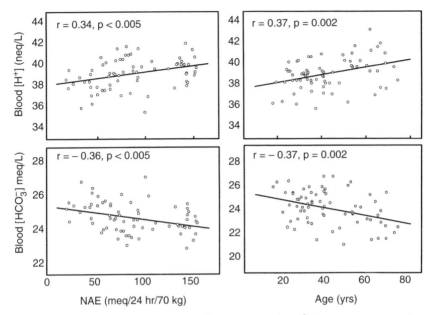

FIGURE 1   Relationship between blood $[H^+]$ and plasma $[HCO_3^-]$ concentrations, renal net acid excretion, and age in normal adult humans $(n = 64)$. Each data point represents the mean steady-state value in a subject eating a constant normal diet.

1.7 times more potent than RNAE in influencing plasma $[H^+]$ and about 3.0 times more potent than RNAE in influencing plasma $[HCO_3^-]$. In view of this strong effect of interindividual differences in respiratory setpoint, it is not surprising that the respiratory component would have been recognized earlier than the dietary metabolic component.

Estimating the Diet Net Acid Load

It is possible to quantify net endogenous noncarbonic acid production in normal subjects ingesting whole food diets by measurements of the quantity of the inorganic constituents of diet, urine, and stool and of the total organic anion content of the urine [8]; however, such studies are extremely time consuming and labor intensive. In their studies, Kurtz et al. utilized renal net acid excretion as a quantitative index of net endogenous non-carbonic acid production, because under steady-state conditions there is a predictable relation between these two variables [8,16] and because RNAE is more readily measured. In 16 normal subjects studied by Lennon et al. [8]

by independently measuring NEAP and RNAE, nearly 90% of the variance in RNAE among the subjects was accounted for by differences in NEAP.

Acid Balance

Computing external hydrogen ion balance as the steady-state difference between the net rate of endogenous noncarbonic acid production and the rate of renal net acid excretion, Lennon *et al.* [8] reported that, on the average, external hydrogen ion balance was not significantly different from zero in normal subjects ingesting diets yielding endogenous acid production rates ranging from 20 to 120 mEq/day. However, on closer inspection of the data reported by Lennon *et al.* [8], it is evident that external hydrogen ion balance was positive in many of the subjects studied by Kurtz' analysis; well over 50% of normal subjects who consumed diets that produced 40 mEq of net acid per day or more were in a state of continuing positive hydrogen ion balance (Fig. 2). Because the average net acid load of free-living Americans is in the range of 40 to 50 mEq/day [9,17], a substantial fraction of the American population is possibly in a state of continuing positive hydrogen ion balance, suggesting chronic titration of internal base reservoirs.

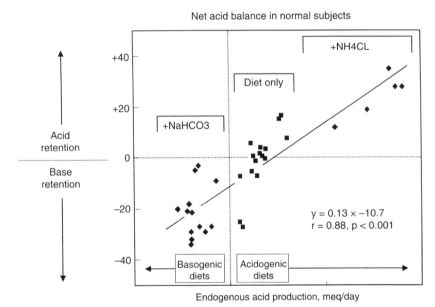

FIGURE 2   Relationship between renal net acid excretion and external acid balance at steady state in normal subjects under conditions of normal diet intake and external acid (NH_4Cl) or base ($NaHCO_3$) loading.

However, a diet net acid load of 40 mEq/day may be an overestimate of the daily net acid load required to initiate continuing hydrogen ion retention by the body in the steady state, as that figure was arrived at without a consideration of the potentially large amplifying effect of age-related declines in renal function. Lennon *et al.* did not report the age of the subjects they studied. Such studies of metabolic balance in normal subjects are often carried out in younger, not older, subjects. With increasing age, the amount of hydrogen ion retained per day might be greater for any given value of NEAP, with the result that the value of NEAP at which net acid balance is zero might be lower. That is, diet net acid loads even lower than 40 mEq/day might sustain continuing hydrogen ion retention by the body. Thus, it may be considered that middle-aged and older individuals with typical age-related declines of renal function will not only be chronically acidotic but persistently retaining hydrogen ions in the body despite relatively small daily net acid loads. The implications of such retention of hydrogen ions, or "diet and age-related low-grade metabolic acidosis" by the body persisting over decades must be considered. That consideration will be important in understanding the clinical impact of the constant background acidosis induced by eating typical net-acid-producing diets.

CHRONIC METABOLIC ACIDOSIS AND BONE WASTING

The effects of more profound degrees of systemic acid–base perturbations have been studied in many organ systems, including bone. In both acute and chronic states, metabolic acidosis reduces bone mass [18–20]. Bone serves as an ion exchange reservoir that exchanges potassium and sodium ions for hydrogen ions [19,21–25], the net result of which during acidosis is loss of bone potassium and sodium in exchange for buffering hydrogen ion. Bone is also a large reservoir of base in the form of alkaline salts of calcium (phosphates, carbonates), which are released into the systemic circulation in response to acid loads to the systemic circulation [2,19,26–37]. The liberated base mitigates the severity of the attendant systemic acidosis and thus contributes to systemic acid–base homeostasis. The liberated calcium and phosphorus are lost in the urine, without compensatory increase in gastrointestinal absorption, and thus bone mineral content declines [28,35,38,39]. That result may be viewed as an unavoidable disadvantage of the participation of bone in the body's normal acid–base homeostatic response to the acid load.

The response of bone to acute acidosis has been studied most extensively by Bushinsky and coworkers using a variety of in vitro models [18]. Those studies demonstrate the prompt initiation of a physicochemical process by acute metabolic acidosis that results in buffering of hydrogen by bone carbonate, with attendant release of sodium, potassium, and calcium [24,29,40,41].

When acid loading continues over days to weeks, bone continues to participate in systemic acid–base homeostasis, helping to stop the progressive acid-ward shift in systemic acid–base equilibrium, to its own detriment [2,28,35,42]. Net external acid balance remains positive without accompanying progressively worsening acidemia and hypobicarbonatemia, indicating continuing internal titration of the net acid load. Mobilization of bone base persists, and the bone minerals (calcium and phosphorus) accompanying that base continue to be wasted in the urine, without compensatory increases in intestinal absorption [42,43]. With chronicity of the acidosis, bone mineral content and bone mass progressively decline [27,44–48]. Morphologically, osteoporosis develops [20,44–51].

The biologic importance of the skeleton's homeostatic contribution in titrating chronic net acid loads is underscored by the fact that the process is not solely a passive physicochemical dissolution of bone mineral by an acidic extracellular fluid but also an active process involving cell-mediated bone resorption and cell-mediated bone formation signaled by increased extracellular fluid hydrogen ion concentration and decreased bicarbonate concentration [20,52–59]. Extracellular acidification (acidemia with hypobicarbonatemia) increases the activity of osteoclasts, the cells that mediate bone resorption [53–56,58], and suppresses the activity of osteoblasts, the cells that mediate bone formation [53,54]. The inhibition of bone formation [20,53,54] can be viewed as contributing to acid–base homeostasis, as the result would be lesser utilization of extracellular base for bone formation.

It is not only the mineral phase of bone that is lost during chronic acidosis but also the organic phase. Release of bone mineral by osteoclasts is accompanied by osteoclastic degradation of bone matrix [20,44–51,59,60]. Likewise, because inhibition of osteoblastic bone formation inhibits both matrix and mineral deposition, the acid–base homeostatic contribution of osteoblasts likewise affects both the mineral and organic phases of bone. In human studies, evidence that matrix resorption is increased and formation is decreased during chronic acid loading is the finding that urinary hydroxyproline excretion increases [28,60,61].

Bushinsky et al. [62–65] also demonstrated that addition of PTH or vitamin D to the bone environment increased bone calcium loss, while inhibiting or killing the bone cells decreased the amount of bone calcium decreased.

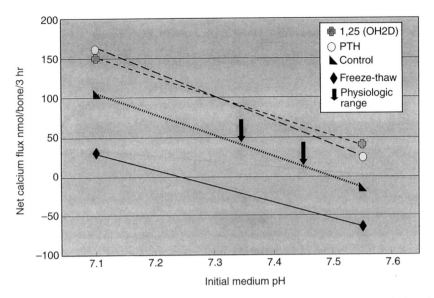

FIGURE 3   Calcium efflux in mouse calvariae cultured under different conditions. (Adapted from Bushinsky and Frick [93]. With permission.)

And, over the range of pH from 7.1 to 7.6, as hydrogen ion concentration increased (pH decreased), bone calcium loss increased (Fig. 3). That is, in these *in vitro* systems, going from a so-called normal human systemic pH of 7.35 to a pH of 7.45 caused a decline in bone calcium loss, which was evident whether or not mitigating influences such as PTH or vitamin D were present.

PLASMA ACID–BASE BALANCE AND DIET ACID LOAD IN HUMANS

THE TRADE-OFF HYPOTHESIS

In vitro studies such as those mentioned above are usually carried out in systems without the range of checks and balances that occur in *in vivo* systems. As Alpern [66], Alpern and Sakhaee [67], and Krapf *et al.* [68] have noted, in conditions causing metabolic acidosis, the severity of acidosis as reflected in plasma acid–base composition underestimates the severity of the pathophysiological injury attributable to the condition inducing the acidosis. During the acute or chronic acid loading discussed above, the skeletal contribution to the defense of systemic pH is in part a physicochemical response of the mineral phases of bone accessible directly or indirectly to extracellular fluid compositional changes and an active process involving acid–base-regulated cell-mediated resorption and formation of whole bone, both mineral and organic components.

With diet-dependent chronic metabolic acidosis, renal and extrarenal homeostatic adaptations are activated that serve to minimize disturbances in blood $[H^+]$ and plasma $[HCO_3^-]$ but which at the same time have trade-off detrimental effects. Those adaptations include decreased renal citrate excretion (renal base conservation) [69,70], dissolution of bone (skeletal base mobilization) [44], hypercalciuria and hyperphosphaturia (promotes skeletal base mobilization) [28,71], skeletal muscle protein catabolism (supply amino acid nitrogen for renal ammonia production and attendant acid excretion as ammonium) [72–76], and renal proliferative and hypertrophic growth (promoting renal acid–base regulatory function) [77]. The trade-offs are increased risks for renal calcification and stone formation (hypocitraturia, hypercalciuria), osteoporosis (dissolution of bone), muscle wasting (skeletal muscle protein catabolism), and progression of renal disease (renal cellular hypertrophy and proliferation) [78–81]. Thus, although the degree of diet-induced, age-amplified metabolic acidosis may be mild as judged by the degree of perturbation of blood acid–base equilibrium from currently accepted norms, its pathophysiologic significance cannot be judged exclusively from the degree of that perturbation. Adaptations of the skeleton, skeletal muscle, kidney, and endocrine systems that serve to mitigate the degree of that perturbation impose a cost in cumulative organ damage that the body pays out over decades of adult life.

EFFECT OF CHANGING THE DIET ACID LOAD ON PLASMA ACID–BASE COMPOSITION IN HEALTHY SUBJECTS: INTERVENTIONAL STUDIES

The cross-sectional observation that individuals eating higher net-acid-producing diets have greater blood acidity and lower plasma bicarbonate concentrations than individuals eating lower net-acid-producing diets does not establish a cause-and-effect relation between diet acid load and plasma acid–base composition. Because the question is whether, within individuals, differences in diet net acid load within the usual dietary range influence plasma acid–base composition, the simplest study would be to examine the effect of changing the body's net acid load *within that range* by administration of an acid or base supplement to the diet while otherwise maintaining constancy of the diet.

Sebastian *et al.* [61] carried out such a study in postmenopausal women eating a constant whole-foods diet that produced a net acid load within the normal range, wherein we supplemented the diet with potassium bicarbonate in amounts sufficient to reduce the body's net acid load on average to nearly zero. In the steady state, prior to starting the base supplement, blood pH was 7.39 ± 0.02, plasma bicarbonate concentration was 23.7 ± 1.3 mEq/L, and RNAE was 71 ± 9 mEq/day. When potassium bicarbonate (60–120 mmols/day) was added to the diet for 18 days, blood pH increased by 0.02 ± 0.01 units, plasma bicarbonate concentration increased by 1.8 ± 1.1 mEq/L, and RNAE decreased to 13 ± 22 mEq/day, while the absolute values of all variables remained within the so-called normal range [82]. When the potassium bicarbonate supplement was discontinued, all measures returned to their pre-$KHCO_3$ levels (Fig. 4). That is, systemic acid–base equilibrium adjusted its setpoint to differences in diet net acid load within the so-called normal range of diet net acid loads. Because blood acidity decreased significantly, and plasma bicarbonate increased significantly, when the diet-dependent net acid load was reduced to near zero, the pre-existing "normal" net acid load clearly had been significantly influencing the setpoint of systemic acid–base equilibrium, in effect causing a low-grade metabolic acidosis.

Taken together with the results of the cross-sectional studies of Kurtz *et al.* [7] and Frassetto *et al.* [15] discussed earlier, these results support the conclusion that under ordinary physiological conditions a low-grade metabolic acidosis is the norm for otherwise healthy individuals who are eating typical net-acid-producing diets and that the severity of the acidosis is proportional to the net acid load of the diet. By this formulation, the blood acidity and plasma bicarbonate concentration at which an otherwise healthy subject under ordinary physiological conditions would be expected not to have metabolic acidosis (or metabolic alkalosis) are those that prevail when the habitual diet net acid load is zero. In other words, if one habitually eats a net-acid-producing diet, one remains acidotic on average, if only a little bit (thanks to homeostatic mechanisms).

EVIDENCE THAT CHRONIC DIET-INDUCED LOW-GRADE METABOLIC ACIDOSIS CHRONICALLY MOBILIZES SKELETAL BASE

For any level of acid loading, if bone is contributing to acid–base homeostasis, it should be found that, even though blood acid–base equilibrium appears to be relatively stable over months to years, not all of the daily net acid load can

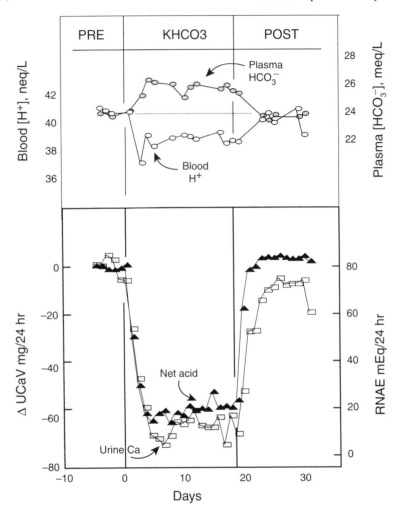

FIGURE 4   Improvement in steady-state blood acidity and urine calcium loss with sufficient dietary bicarbonate supplementation to reduce net acid excretion to near zero in 18 postmenopausal women.

be recovered in the urine [2,28]; that is, acid appears to be accumulating in the body on a daily basis. Existing data support the possibility that continued acid retention occurs in a substantial fraction of the otherwise healthy population consuming diet net acid loads within the normal range. By Kurtz's analysis [7], well over 50% of normal subjects who consumed diets that produced 40 mEq of net acid per day or more were in a state of continuing positive hydrogen ion balance (Fig. 2). Because the average net acid load of

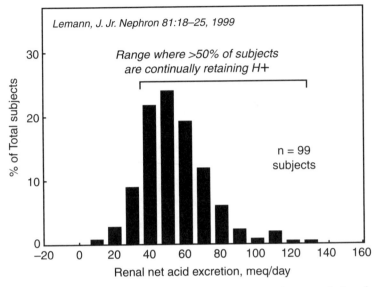

FIGURE 5 Renal net acid excretion in free-living Americans eating normal diets ($n = 99$). (Adapted from data provided by Lemann [9].)

free-living Americans is in the range of 40 to 50 mEq/day [9,17], that raises the possibility that a substantial fraction of the American population is in a state of continuing hydrogen ion balance (Figs. 2 and 5). In such subjects, stability of blood acid–base equilibrium would provide evidence of the existence of an internal reservoir of base that continually delivers base to the systemic circulation in an amount equal to the fraction of the net acid load that the kidneys fail to excrete. Bone is the major such internal reservoir of base known to exist.

With decades-long metabolic acidosis, it is not necessary to postulate that the amounts of base released per day to the extracellular fluid (ECF) be large relative to the ongoing rate of endogenous acid production in order to account for acidosis-induced bone wasting. With high rates of NEAP induced experimentally by oral administration of acid precursors, sustained until plasma bicarbonate concentration stabilizes, bone base contributes substantially to buffering of the acid load [2,42].

On theoretical grounds, Oh and colleagues [83,84] have argued that with chronicity of metabolic acidosis over years and decades, bone base cannot continue to contribute substantially (e.g., tens of milliequivalents per day) to the titration of endogenous acid, inasmuch as calculations reveal that the total buffer capacity of bone is too small to last more than a few years at those rates. Nevertheless, their considerations should not be construed as arguing against the role of decades-long metabolic acidosis in stimulating bone wasting, since even 1 or 2 meq/day of skeletal base mobilization per day, over decades, would result in substantial depletion of bone mineral. For example, using the reference data of Oh *et al.* [84], only 1 meq/day of base loss from bone as calcium hydroxyapatite over 40 years (*e.g.*, ages 30–70 years) would equal 14,600 meq of base, which is equivalent to nearly 32,000 meq of calcium, or somewhat over 50% of total bone calcium content. Yet, 1 meq/day per day of base is only about 2% of NEAP in free-living Americans eating their usual diets [9,17]. Thus, in relation to typical diet net acid loads, the daily net acid retention required to sustain skeletal demineralization in the long run need not be very large.

Unlike chemical buffers, which are internal to the system and serve as readily reversible temporary proton stores, bone and kidney may be regarded as external proton sinks by virtue of their ability to generate new base for input to the system. The two sinks operate in parallel. When net acid is produced endogenously, the bone does not wait to see whether the kidney will keep up by net acid excretion (new bicarbonate generation). Bone and kidney are simultaneously exposed to the acid-loaded systemic circulation and will respond concurrently with new base input to the systemic circulation, each according to its sensitivity and capacity. As blood recirculates systemically, to whatever extent bone supplies base in response to its encounter with the acid-loaded blood, to that extent the kidney sees less acid (as reflected by blood acidity and plasma bicarbonate concentration); therefore, in the steady state, it is not being signaled to generate new bicarbonate at the full rate of NEAP. It is not surprising, then, that the kidney does not keep up with NEAP. Or, to put it in other words, if bone can respond at all to the acid-loaded blood, however small a fraction of NEAP its base input to the systemic circulation may be, to that extent RNAE will lag behind NEAP, and the apparent balance of hydrogen ion will be positive. As we pointed out above, in free-living adults eating typical net-acid-producing diets, bone need contribute base at no more than 2% of NEAP to substantially demineralize itself over decades of adult life. The potential cumulative demineralizing effect, over decades, of small acidosis-mediated effluxes of bone mineral has long been recognized [37].

It might be argued that as long as the kidney generates any new bicarbonate (*viz.*, through net acid excretion), base will be redeposited into bone; therefore, the net daily external balance of hydrogen ion need not necessarily be positive nor bone base stores necessarily become progressively depleted. That might be true if the base lost from bone were readily redepositable. But, unlike the case with acute acid loading, where the initial response of bone is to buffer changes in hydrogen ion concentration by physicochemical exchange for sodium and potassium ions on the mineral surface of the bone, with chronic acid loading bone titrates hydrogen ion by means of cell-mediated dissolution of the alkaline salts of calcium in the bone matrix, with subsequent disposal of the dissolved calcium in the urine. Generation of new bicarbonate is not accompanied by generation of new calcium or even conservation of the skeletally mobilized calcium, the excretion rate of which varies directly in the urine among subjects with the net acid load of the diet (Fig. 5) [9], nor would it be expected to relieve the acidosis-induced activation of cell-mediated bone resorption, as acid excretion is always playing catch-up with the diet net acid load. Interdicting progressive loss of base from the skeletal reservoir requires relieving the chronic acidosis-induced inhibition of renal calcium reabsorption and activation of cell-mediated bone calcium resorption. Those can be achieved by neutralizing the diet net acid load.

Given that the calcium efflux from bone accompanying acidosis-mediated base efflux is disposed of in urine, it is not surprising that urinary calcium excretion correlates positively with NEAP (as reflected in RNAE) in free-living Americans eating typical net-acid-producing diets [9] (Fig. 5) and that Americans eating diets of average calcium intake (~800 mg/day) [85] are commonly in negative calcium balance [86,87]. Individuals eating diets containing substantially higher than average amounts of calcium are not in negative calcium balance [86], but the NEAP of such diets is not known. Conceivably the NEAP of such diets is much lower than average and too low to sustain net bone base efflux. High calcium diets may reduce NEAP by displacement of higher with lower net-acid producing foods (e.g., milk and/or calcium-rich plant foods for meat and cereal grains) and/or by increasing dietary base input (e.g., organic anions in calcium-rich plant foods). The most common forms of dietary calcium supplements (calcium citrate and calcium carbonate) also supply base. For example, as judged by the change in RNAE, 1000 mg of calcium as calcium carbonate yields about 15 mEq of absorbed base, for a minimal yield of about 30% of ingested base absorbed [88]. The yield from calcium citrate is similar [89]. Barzel [19] suggested that this base supply is a critical component of the beneficial skeletal effect of dietary calcium supplementation.

Another way to test whether persisting bone loss occurs in response to chronic low-level, diet-induced metabolic acidosis is to examine the effect of sustained neutralization of the diet net acid load by addition of exogenous base. Such studies have been carried out in postmenopausal women [61]. Potassium bicarbonate, when administered in doses that nearly completely neutralize the diet net acid load, reduces urinary wasting of calcium and phosphorus, improves preexisting negative balances of calcium and phosphorus, and, as indicated by biochemical markers, reduces the rate of bone resorption and stimulates the rate of bone formation [61].

What evidence indicates that reducing urine calcium excretion improves bone health? In the studies by Sebastian et al., the improvement in phosphorus balance correlated with that in calcium; on a molar basis of comparison, the slope of the relation was approximately 1.0, suggesting 1 mole of phosphorus retained per mole of calcium. Because the phosphorus:calcium ratio in hydroxyapatite is less than 1.0 (6:10), adequate phosphorus was retained to have permitted calcium retention as hydroxyapatite. That is, the ratio of change in calcium to phosphorus balance (Ca_{10}/P_{10}) was sufficient for 100% of the retained calcium to have been stored as hydroxyapatite (Ca_{10}/P_6). Lemann et al. [90] and Maurer et al. [91] likewise demonstrated significant improvement in calcium and phosphorus balances when the diet net acid load was neutralized during potassium bicarbonate administration in healthy humans. In another study by Pak et al. [92] in 19 men and 5 women with excessive renal calcium excretion and nephrolithiasis, decreasing urinary calcium excretion with potassium citrate also improved bone mineral density over time. RNAE also declined in these subjects as urinary citrate levels increased.

Thus, two lines of evidence indicate that chronic low-level, diet-induced acidosis imposes a chronic drain on bone: (1) stability of blood acid–base equilibrium in the face of continuing retention of acid, and (2) amelioration of negative calcium and phosphorus balances, reduction of bone resorption, and stimulation of bone formation attendant to neutralization of the dietary acid load. To date there have been no reports of the effects on bone of *chronic* neutralization of the diet acid load or of the effects of chronic net base loading.

CROSSING THE NEUTRAL ZONE

It is well-known from the *in vitro* studies of Bushinsky and co-workers [18,93], and other investigators, that metabolic acidosis leads to resorption of bone, in part by physicochemical dissolution of bone mineral, and in part by stimulating active resorption of bone by osteoclasts and suppressing active formation of bone by osteoblasts. More recently, Bushinsky reported that, conversely, metabolic alkalosis reduces calcium efflux from bone and both suppresses osteoclastic bone resorption and stimulates osteoblastic bone formation (Fig. 3) [94]. Because these effects were linear functions of medium pH above 7.40 (as increased by increasing medium bicarbonate concentration), it was evident that even minimal degrees of metabolic alkalosis were effective. Bushinsky concluded that "[t]hese findings indicate that alkalosis can inhibit bone resorption and stimulate bone formation through alterations in bone cell function." It may be added that these findings also suggest the possibility that inducing and sustaining a low-grade metabolic alkalosis with sufficient dietary base might amplify the anti-osteoporotic effects of simply neutralizing the net acid load of the diet with smaller amounts of base. Administration of alkalosis-producing amounts of base might also support bone formation through renal conservation of calcium, as reduction in urinary calcium excretion produced by alkali loading is a linear function of the alkali load over a broad range of net acid and base inputs (unpublished observations).

These considerations have potential implications not only for treatment but also for prevention of osteoporosis. After peak bone mass is achieved in young adulthood, bone mass begins to decline progressively because bone formation fails to keep pace with bone resorption during the repeated cycles of resorption and formation (bone remodeling) that occur throughout adulthood in response to ever-changing mechanical loads and load-distributions on bone. A small reduction in the rate of osteoclastic bone resorption accompanied by a small increase in the rate of osteoclastic bone formation, such as might be achieved with low-grade alkali-loading metabolic alkalosis, might be just enough to equalize the unfavorable resorption–formation coupling relationship and prevent bone mass from declining.

Although experiments in humans to test the effects of chronic low-grade alkali induced metabolic alkalosis on age-related changes in bone mass have not been carried out, some hints may be taken from observations made on the skeletal remains of Stone Age humans. Ruff et al. [95] observed increased cortical thickness relative to body mass, and strength or rigidity, in femurs of ancestral *Homo* species, using morphometric techniques and biomechanical models. Using densitometry techniques and measures of cortical thickness, Nelson [96] found that prehistoric hunter–gatherer femoral bone was denser than that of prehistoric periodic agriculturalists, and that bone density in the hunter–gatherers was relatively stable with age compared to that of the agriculturalists. Perzigian [97] compared the age-related rates of loss of bone mineral content in two prehistoric populations, one a strictly hunter–gatherer population and one an agriculturalist population. The hunter–gatherer group consistently showed slower rates of bone loss with age than the agriculturalist group. Although many lifestyle factors, including levels and kinds of physical activity, may have contributed to the Stone Agers' greater skeletal robusticity, higher bone mass, and lower rates of bone mass decline with age, the potential role of dietary base input cannot be ignored.

IMPLICATIONS FOR FURTHER RESEARCH

For the past century, physiologists studying renal regulation of systemic acid–base equilibrium have directed their attention overwhelmingly to the mechanisms of urinary acidification and net acid excretion, in particular to the mechanisms of hydrogen ion secretion and bicarbonate reabsorption, and ammonia production, by the renal tubule. During human evolution those mechanisms were conserved and refined undoubtedly because of their adaptive value in responding to metabolic acidosis-producing conditions that were presumably experienced intermittently by early humans and their hominid ancestors: food shortage (starvation ketoacidosis, autoproteolytic sulfuric acidosis); meat feasting (sulfuric acidosis); feasting on certain plant foods, such as plums and cranberries, that are net acid producing (various organic acidoses); prolonged intense physical activity (lactic acidosis); and, infectious or toxic diarrhea (fecal bicarbonate wasting). Because those conditions were presumably episodic, and for some even uncommon [98], there is no reason to suppose that the renal mechanisms underlying urine acidification and net acid excretion were designed to operate *tonically* during an individual's lifetime. Rather, the conditions that prevail today are likely not those conditions that prevailed during the 5 or more million years of hominid evolution that eventuated in *Homo sapiens*, and our current perspective on what constitutes "normal" human renal physiology may well be off base.

ACKNOWLEDGMENTS

The authors would like to acknowledge the General Clinical Research Center (GCRC) of the University of California San Francisco under a grant from the National Institutes of Health (NCRR grant M01 0079).

REFERENCES

1. Madias, N.E., Adrogue, H.J., Horowitz, G.L., Cohen, J.J., and Schwartz, W.B. (1979). A redefinition of normal acid–base equilibrium in man: carbon dioxide as a key determinant of normal plasma bicarbonate concentration. *Kidney Int.* 16: 612–618.
2. Lemann, J., Jr., Lennon, E.J., Goodman, A.D., Litzow, J.R., and Relman, A.S. (1965). The net balance of acid in subjects given large loads of acid or alkali. *J. Clin. Invest.* 44: 507–517.
3. Schwartz, W.B. and Cohen, J.J. (1978). The nature of the renal response to chronic disorders of acid–base equilibrium. *Am. J. Med.* 64: 417–428.
4. Arruda, J.A.L. and Kurtzman, N.A. (1978). Relationship of renal sodium and water transport to hydrogen ion secretion. *Ann. Rev. Physiol.* 40: 43–66.

5. Tannen, R.L. (1980). Control of acid excretion by the kidney. *Ann. Rev. Med.* 31: 35–49.

6. Narins, R.G. and Emmett, M. (1980). Simple and mixed acid–base disorders: a practical approach. *Medicine (Baltimore)* 59: 161–187.

7. Kurtz, I., Maher, T., Hulter, H.N., Schambelan, M., and Sebastian, A. (1983). Effect of diet on plasma acid–base composition in normal humans. *Kidney Int.* 24: 670–680.

8. Lennon, E.J., Lemann, J., Jr., and Litzow, J.R. (1966). The effect of diet and stool composition on the net external acid balance of normal subjects. *J. Clin. Invest.* 45: 1601–1607.

9. Lemann, J., Jr. (1999). Relationship between urinary calcium and net acid excretion as determined by dietary protein and potassium: a review. *Nephron* 81(suppl. 1): 18–25.

10. Relman, A.S. (1978). Lactic acidosis, in *Contemporary Issues in Nephrology*, Brenner, B.M. and Stein, J.H., Eds. Churchill-Livingstone, New York.

11. Stanbury, J.B. *et al.*, Eds. (1983). *The Metabolic Basis of Inherited Disease*, 5 ed., McGraw-Hill, New York.

12. Hammeke, M., Bear, R., Lee, R., Goldstein, M., and Halperin, M. (1978). Hyperchloremic metabolic acidsois in diabetes mellitus: a case report and discussion of the pathophysiologic mechanism. *Diabetes* 27: 16–20.

13. Lemann, J., Jr. and Relman, A.S. (1959). The relation of sulfur metabolism to acid–base balance and electrolyte excretion: the effects of DL-methionine in normal man. *J. Clin. Invest.* 38: 2215–2223.

14. Coe, F.L., Firpo, J.J.J., Hollandsworth, D.L., Segil, L., Canterbury, J.M., and Reiss, E. (1975). Effect of acute and chronic metabolic acidosis on serum immunoreactive parathyroid hormone in man. *Kidney Int.* 8: 262–272.

15. Frassetto, L., Morris, R.C., Jr., and Sebastian, A. (1996). Effect of age on blood acid–base composition in adult humans: role of age-related renal functional decline. *Am. J. Physiol.* 271: 1114–1122.

16. Relman, A.S., Lennon, E.J., and Lemann, J., Jr. (1961). Endogenous production of fixed acid and the measurement of net balance of acid in normal subjects. *J. Clin. Invest.* 40: 1621–1630.

17. Frassetto, L.A., Nash, E., Morris, R.C., Jr., and Sebastian, A. (2000). Comparative effects of potassium chloride and bicarbonate on thiazide-induced reduction in urinary calcium excretion. *Kidney Int.* 58: 748–752.

18. Bushinsky, D.A. (1998). Acid–base imbalance and the skeleton, in *Nutritional Apsects of Osteoporosis*, Burckhardt, P., Dawson-Hughes, B., and Heaney, R.P., Eds. Serono Symposia/ Springer-Verlag, New York.

19. Barzel, U.S. (1995). The skeleton as an ion exchange system: implicaitons for the role of acid–base imbalance in the genesis of osteoporosis. *J. Bone Mineral Res.* 10: 1431–1436.

20. Kraut, J.A., Mishler, D.R., Singer, F.R., and Goodman, W.G. (1986). The effects of metabolic acidosis on bone formation and bone resorption in the rat. *Kidney Int.* 30: 694–700.

21. Bergstrom, W.H. and Wallace, W.M. (1954). Bone as a sodium and potassium reservoir. *J. Clin. Invest.* 33: 867–873.

22. Post, M. and Shoemaker, W. (1962). Bone electrolyte response to intravenous acid loads. *Surg. Gynecol. Obstetr.* 115: 749–756.

23. Bettice, J.A. and Gamble, J.L., Jr. (1975). Skeletal buffering of acute metabolic acidosis. *Am. J. Physiol.* 229: 1618–1624.

24. Bushinsky, D.A., Levi-Setti, R., and Coe, F.L. (1986). Ion microprobe determination of bone surface elements: effects of reduced medium pH. *Am. J. Physiol.* 250: F1090–F1097.

25. Bushinsky, D.A., Gavrilov, K., Chabala, J.M., Featherstone, J.D., and Levi-Setti, R. (1997). Effect of metabolic acidosis on the potassium content of bone. *J. Bone Mineral Res.* 12: 1664–1671.

26. Bettice, J.A. (1984). Skeletal carbon dioxide stores during metabolic acidosis. *Am. J. Physiol.* 247: F326–F330.

27. Burnell, J.M. (1971). Changes in bone sodium and carbonate in metabolic acidosis and alkalosis in the dog. *J. Clin. Invest.* 50: 327–331.
28. Lemann, J., Jr., Litzow, J.R., and Lennon, E.J. (1966). The effects of chronic acid loads in normal man: further evidence for participation of bone mineral in the defense against chronic metabolic acidosis. *J. Clin. Invest.* 45: 1608–1614.
29. Bushinsky, D.A. and Lechleider, R.J. (1987). Mechanism of proton-induced bone calcium release: calcium carbonate dissolution. *Am. J. Physiol.* 253: F998–F1005.
30. Bushinsky, D.A., Lam, B.C., Nespeca, R., Sessler, N.E., and Grynpas, M.D. (1993). Decreased bone carbonate content in response to metabolic, but not respiratory, acidosis. *Am. J. Physiol.* 265: F530–F536.
31. Bushinsky, D.A. (1989). Internal exchanges of hydrogen ions: bone, in *The Regulation of Acid–Base Balance*, Seldin, D.W. and Giebisch, G., Eds. Raven Press, New York.
32. Lemann, J., Jr., Litzow, J.R., and Lennon, E.J. (1967). Studies of the mechanism by which chronic metabolic acidosis augments urinary calcium excretion in man. *J. Clin. Invest.* 46: 1318–1328.
33. Yoshimura, H., Fujimoto, M., Okumura, O., Sugimoto, J., and Kuwada, T. (1961). Three-step-regulation of acid–base balance in body fluid after acid load. *J. Clin. Invest.* 40: 109–125.
34. Eiam-Ong, S. and Kurtzman, N.A. (1994). Metabolic acidosis and bone disease. *Mineral Electrolyte Metab.* 20: 72–80.
35. Litzow, J.R., Lemann, J., Jr., and Lennon, E.J. (1967). The effect of treatment of acidosis on calcium balance in patients with chronic azotemic renal disease. *J. Clin. Invest.* 46: 280–286.
36. Bushinsky, D.A., Chabala, J.M., Gavrilov, K.L., and Levi-Setti, R. (1999). Effects of *in vivo* metabolic acidosis on midcortical bone ion composition. *Am. J. Physiol* 277: F813–F819.
37. Wachman, A. and Bernstein, D.S. (1968). Diet and osteoporosis. *Lancet* 1: 958–959.
38. Breslau, N.A., Brinkley, L., Hill, K.D., and Pak, C.Y.C. (1988). Relationship of animal protein-rich diet to kidney stone formation and calcium metabolism. *J. Clin. Endocrinol. Metab.* 66: 140–146.
39. Gafter, U., Kraut, J.A., Lee, D.B.N., Silis, V., Walling, M.W., Kurokawa, K., Haussler, M.R., and Coburn, J.W. (1980). Effect of metabolic acidosis on intestinal absorption of calcium and phosphorus. *Am. J. Physiol.* 239: G480–G484.
40. Bushinsky, D.A., Wolbach, W., Sessler, N.E., Mogilevsky, R., and Levi-Setti, R. (1993). Physicochemical effects of acidosis on bone calcium flux and surface ion composition. *J. Bone Mineral Res.* 8: 93–102.
41. Bushinsky, D.A., Lam, B.C., Nespeca, R., Sessler, N.E., and Grynpas, M.D. (1993). Decreased bone carbonate content in response to metabolic, but not respiratory, acidosis. *Am. J. Physiol.* 265: F530–F536.
42. Adams, N.D., Gray, R.W., and Lemann, J., Jr. (1979). The calciuria of increased fixed acid production in humans: evidence against a role for parathyroid hormone and 1:25(OH)$_2$-vitamin D. *Calcif. Tissue Int.* 28: 233–238.
43. Weber, H.P., Gray, R.W., Dominguez, J.H., and Lemann, J., Jr. (1976). The lack of effect of chronic metabolic acidosis on 25-OH-vitamin D metabolism and serum parathyroid hormone in humans. *J. Clin. Endocrinol. Metab.* 43: 1047–1055.
44. Barzel, U.S. and Jowsey, J. (1969). The effects of chronic acid and alkali administration on bone turnover in adult rats. *Clin. Sci.* 36: 517–524.
45. Barzel, U.S. (1969). The effect of excessive acid feeding on bone. *Calcif. Tiss. Res.* 4: 94–100.
46. Delling, G. and Donath, K. (1973). Morphometric, electron microscopic and physico-chemical investigation in experimental osteoporosis induced by chronic acidosis in the rat. *Virchows Arch. Abt. A Path. Anat.* 358: 321–330.
47. Barzel, U.S. (1976). Acid-induced osteoporosis: an experimental model of human osteoporosis. *Calcif. Tiss. Res.* 21(suppl.): 417–422.

48. Myburgh, K.H., Noakes, T.D., Roodt, M., and Hough, F.S. (1989). Effect of exercise on the development of osteoporosis in adult rats. *J. Appl. Physiol.* 66: 14–19.

49. Upton, P.K. and L'Estrange, J.L. (1977). Effects of chronic hydrochloric and lactic acid administrations on food intake, blood acid–base balance and bone composition of the rat. *Q. J. Exp. Physiol.* 62: 223–235.

50. Jaffe, H.L., Bodansky, A., and Chandler, J.P. (1932). Ammonium chloride decalcification, as modified by calcium intake: the relation between generalized osteoporosis and osteitis fibrosa. *J. Exp. Med.* 56: 823–834.

51. Newell, G.K. and Beauchene, R.E. (1975). Effects of dietary calcium level, acid stress, and age on renal, serum, and bone responses of rats. *J. Nutr.* 105: 1039–1047.

52. Kraut, J.A., Mishler, D.R., and Kurokawa, K. (1984). Effect of colchicine and calcitonin on calcemic response to metabolic acidosis. *Kidney Int.* 25: 608–612.

53. Krieger, N.S., Sessler, N.E., and Bushinsky, D.A. (1992). Acidosis inhibits osteoblastic and stimulates osteoclastic activity *in vitro. Am. J. Physiol.* 262: F442–F448.

54. Bushinsky, D.A. (1995). Stimulated osteoclastic and suppressed osteoblastic activity in metabolic but not respiratory acidosis. *Am. J. Physiol.* 268: C80–C88.

55. Arnett, T.R. and Dempster, D.W. (1986). Effect of pH on bone resorption by rat osteoclasts *in vitro. Endocrinology* 119: 119–124.

56. Goldhaber, P. and Rabadjija, L. (1987). H + stimulation of cell-mediated bone resorption in tissue culture. *Am. J. Physiol.* 253: E90–E98.

57. Blair, H.C., Teitelbaum, S.L., Ghiselli, R., and Gluck, S. (1989). Osteoclastic bone resorption by a polarized vacuolar proton pump. *Science* 245: 855–857.

58. Teti, A., Blair, H.C., Schlesinger, P., Grano, M., Zambonin-Zallone, A., Kahn, A.J., Teitelbaum, S.L., and Hruska, K.A. (1989). Extracellular protons acidify osteoclasts, reduce cytosolic calcium, and promote expression of cell-matrix attachment structures. *J. Clin. Invest.* 84: 773–780.

59. Ross, F.P. and Teitelbaum, S.L. (2001). Osteoclast biology, in *Osteoporosis,* Marcus, R., Feldman, D., and Kelsey, J., Eds. Academic Press, San Diego, CA.

60. Bernstein, D.S., Wachman, A., and Hattner, R.S. (1970). Acid–base balance in metabolic bone disease, in *Osteoporosis,* Barzel, U.S., Ed. Grune & Stratton, New York.

61. Sebastian, A., Harris, S.T., Ottaway, J.H., Todd, K.M., and Morris, R.C., Jr. (1994). Improved mineral balance and skeletal metabolism in postmenopausal women treated with potassium bicarbonate [see comments]. *New Engl. J. Med.* 330: 1776–1781.

62. Bushinsky, D.A. (1987). Effects of parathyroid hormone on net proton flux from neonatal mouse calvariae. *Am. J. Physiol.* 252: F585–F589.

63. Bushinsky, D.A., Chabala, J.M., and Levi-Setti, R. (1989). Ion microprobe analysis of bone surface elements: effects of $1:25(OH)_2D_3$. *Am. J. Physiol.* 257: E815–E822.

64. Ro, H.-K., Tembe, V., Kurg, T., Yang, P.-Y.J., Bushinsky, D.A., and Favus, M.J. (1990). Acidosis inhibits $1:25-(OH)_2D_3$ but not cAMP production in response to parathyroid hormone in the rat. *J. Bone Miner. Res.* 5: 273–278.

65. Bushinsky, D.A., Favus, M.J., Schneider, A.B., Sen, P.K., Sherwood, L.M., and Coe, F.L. (1982). Effects of metabolic acidosis on PTH and $1:25(OH)_2D_3$ response to low calcium diet. *Am. J. Physiol.* 243: F570–F575.

66. Alpern, R.J. (1995). Trade-offs in the adaptation to acidosis. *Kidney Int.* 47: 1205–1215.

67. Alpern, R.J. and Sakhaee, S. (1997). The clinical spectrum of chronic metabolic acidosis: homeostatic mechanisms produce significant morbidity. *Am. J. Kid. Dis.* 29: 291–302.

68. Krapf, R., Seldin, D.W., and Alpern, R.J. (2000). Clinical syndromes of metabolic acidosis, in *The Kidney: Physiology and Pathophysiology,* Seldin, D.W. and Giebisch, G., Eds. Lippincott, Williams & Wilkins, Philadelphia, PA.

69. Gordon, E.E. (1963). Effect of acute metaoblic acidosis and alkalosis on acetate and citrate metabolism in the rat. *J. Clin. Invest.* 42: 137–142.
70. Sakhaee, K., Williams, R.H., Oh, M.S., Padalino, P., Adams-Huet, B., Whitson, P., and Pak, C.Y. (1993). Alkali absorption and citrate excretion in calcium nephrolithiasis. *J. Bone Mineral Res.* 8: 789–794.
71. Krapf, R., Vetsch, R., Vetsch, W., and Hulter, H.N. (1992). Chronic metabolic acidosis increases the serum concentration of 1:25-dihydroxyvitamin D in humans by stimulating its production rate: critical role of acidosis-induced renal hypophosphatemia. *J. Clin. Invest* 90: 2456–2463.
72. Garibotto, G., Russo, R., Sofia, A., Sala, M.R., Sabatino, C., Moscatelli, P., Deferrari, G., and Tizianello, A. (1996). Muscle protein turnover in chronic renal failure patients with metabolic acidosis or normal acid–base balance. *Mineral Electrolyte Metab.* 22: 58–61.
73. May, R.C., Kelly, R.A., and Mitch, W.E. (1986). Metabolic acidosis stimulates protein degradation in rat muscle by a glucocorticoid-dependent mechanism. *J. Clin. Invest.* 77: 614–621.
74. Williams, B., Layward, E., and Walls, J. (1991). Skeletal muscle degradation and nitrogen wasting in rats with chronic metabolic acidosis. *Clin. Sci.* 80: 457–462.
75. Mitch, W.E., Medina, R., Grieber, S., May, R.C., England, B.K., Price, S.R., Bailey, J.L., and Goldberg, A.L. (1994). Metabolic acidosis stimulates muscle protein degradation by activating the adenosine triphosphate-dependent pathway involving ubiquitin and proteasomes. *J. Clin. Invest.* 93: 2127–2133.
76. May, R.C., Kelly, R.A., and Mitch, W.E. (1987). Mechanisms for defects in muscle protein metabolism in rats with chronic uremia. Influence of metabolic acidosis. *J. Clin. Invest.* 79: 1099–1103.
77. Lotspeich, W.D. (1965). Renal hypertrophy in metabolic acidosis and its relation to ammonia excretion. *Am. J. Physiol.* 208: 1135–1142.
78. Nath, K.A., Hostetter, M.K., and Hostetter, T.H. (1985). Pathophysiology of chronic tubulo-interstitial disease in rats: interactions of dietary acid load, ammonia, and complement component C3. *J. Clin. Invest.* 76: 667–675.
79. Clark, E.C., Nath, K.A., Hostetter, M.K., and Hostetter, T.H. (1990). Role of ammonia in tubulointerstitial injury. *Mineral Electrolyte Metab.* 16: 315–321.
80. Tolins, J.P., Hostetter, M.K., and Hostetter, T.H. (1987). Hypokalemic nephropathy in the rat: role of ammonia in chronic tubular injury. *J. Clin. Invest.* 79: 1447–1458.
81. Nath, K.A., Salahudeen, A.K., Clark, E.C., Hostetter, M.K., and Hostetter, T.H. (1992). Role of cellular metabolites in progressive renal injury. *Kidney Int. Suppl.* 38: S109–S113.
82. Gennari, F.J., Cohen, J.J., and Kassirer, J.P. (1982). Normal acid–base values, in *Acid–Base*, Cohen, J.J. and Kassirer, J.P., Eds. Little, Brown & Co., Boston.
83. Oh, M.S. (1991). Irrelevance of bone buffering to acid–base homeostasis in chronic metabolic acidosis. *Nephron* 59: 7–10.
84. Oh, M.S. and Carroll, H.J. (2000). External balance of electrolytes and acids and alkali, in *The Kidney: Physiology and Pathophysiology*, Seldin, D.W. and Giebisch, G., Eds. Lippincott, Williams & Wilkins, Philadelphia, PA.
85. Alaimo, K., McDowell, M.A., Briefel, R.R, Bischof, A.M., Caughman, C.R., Loria, C.M., and Johnson, C.L. (1988–1991; 1994). *Dietary Intake of Vitamins, Minerals, and Fiber of Persons Ages 2 Months and Over in the United States: Third National Health and Nutrition Examination Survey, Phase 1, 1988–1991*, Advance Data No. 258, Advance Data Reports from the National Health Survey and the National Health and Nutrition Examination Survey, U.S. Department of Public Health.
86. Heaney, R.P., Recker, R.R., and Saville, P.D. (1977). Calcium balance and calcium requirements in middle-aged women. *Am. J. Clin. Nutr.* 30: 1603–1611.

87. Recker, R.R. and Heaney, R.P. (1985). The effect of milk supplements on calcium metabolism, bone metabolism and calcium balance. *Am. J. Clin. Nutr.* 41: 254–263.
88. Lewis, N.M., Marcus, M.S.K., Behling, A.R., and Greger, J.L. (1989). Calcium supplements and milk: effects on acid–base balance and on retention of calcium, magnesium, and phosphorus. *Am. J. Clin. Nutr.* 49: 527–533.
89. Harvey, J.A., Zobitz, M.M., and Pak, C.Y.C. (1985). Calcium citrate: reduced propensity for the crystallization of calcium oxalate in urine resulting from induced hypercalciuria of calcium supplementation. *J. Clin. Endocrinol. Metab.* 61: 1223–1225.
90. Lemann, J., Jr., Gray, R.W., and Pleuss, J.A. (1989). Potassium bicarbonate, but not sodium bicarbonate, reduces urinary calcium excretion and improves calcium balance in healthy men. *Kidney Int.* 35: 688–695.
91. Maurer, M., Riesen, W., Muser, J., Hulter, H.N., and Krapf, R. (2003). Neutralization of Western diet inhibits bone resorption independently of K intake and reduces cortisol secretion in humans. *Am. J. Physiol. Renal Physiol.* 284: F32–F40.
92. Pak, C.Y., Peterson, R.D., and Poindexter, J. (2002). Prevention of spinal bone loss by potassium citrate in cases of calcium urolithiasis. *J. Urol.* 168: 31–34.
93. Bushinsky, D.A. and Frick, K.K. (2000). The effects of acid on bone. *Curr. Opin. Nephrol. Hypertens.* 9: 369–379.
94. Bushinsky, D.A. (1996). Metabolic alkalosis decreases bone calcium efflux by suppressing osteoclasts and stimulating osteoblasts. *Am. J. Physiol.* 271: F216–F222.
95. Ruff, C.B., Trinkaus, E., Walker, A., and Larsen, C.S. (1993). Postcranial robusticity in *Homo*. I. Temporal trends and mechanical interpretation. *Am. J. Phys. Anthropol.* 91: 21–53.
96. Nelson, D. (2000). Bone density in three archaeological populations. *Am. J. Phys. Anthropol.* 63: 198.
97. Perzigian, A.J. (1973). Osteoporotic bone loss in two prehistoric Indian populations. *Am. J. Phys. Anthropol.* 39: 87–95.
98. Cordain, L., Miller, J., and Mann, N. (1999). Scant evidence of periodic starvation among hunter-gatherers. *Diabetologia* 42: 383–384.

CHAPTER 23

Effect of Various Classes of Foodstuffs and Beverages of Vegetable Origin on Bone Metabolism in the Rat

ROMAN C. MÜHLBAUER

Bone Biology Group, Department Clinical Research, University of Bern, Bern, Switzerland

ABSTRACT

Osteoporosis is a major health issue in aging populations. From a medical and economical view it would, therefore, be desirable if low bone mass leading to osteoporotic fractures could be prevented. A nutritional approach would be an inexpensive means to achieve this goal. As the effects of the nutritional strategies recommended today are rather modest, research into novel strategies preventing bone loss is needed. The effect on bone resorption was measured with the urinary excretion of tritium released from bone of 9-week-old rats prelabeled with tritiated tetracycline from weeks 1 to 6. The effect on bone mass was assessed with pQCT. So far we found 25 out of 53 items with inhibitory activity. Activity appears to be restricted to the categories of vegetables, salads, herbs, mushrooms, and fruits (24 out of 35 items effective). From the categories of beans, nuts and seeds, carbohydrate sources, and beverages, only the red wine residue was effective. To date, compounds responsible for the inhibition of resorption are only known for some herbs rich in essential oils, for which we have recently

Nutritional Aspects of Osteoporosis, Second Edition

identified monoterpenes as active components. Furthermore, onions and pine oil were studied as to their effect on bone mass. Onions increased trabecular bone mineral density (BMD) in growing rats, and pine oil blunted the loss of trabecular BMD in aged, ovariectomized rats. Finally, as assessed in a similar experimental design with various doses of a mixture of active items, we determined 170 mg (dry items) per rat per day as the minimal effective dose. This dose corresponds to 6.2 g of fresh active items per kg body weight, possibly suggesting that the amount of active items consumed by way of a regular Western diet with two to three servings a day of 80 g each of fruits and vegetables might be too low to elicit a protective effect in humans. Although it is difficult to change nutritional habits in humans, the international campaign "Take Five" (initiated for the chemoprevention of certain forms of cancer) shows that it is possible to increase the daily number of servings, at least of fruits and vegetables, from three to five. Whether five daily servings of the active items we have identified in rats are capable to inhibit bone resorption in humans must now be established with clinical intervention studies.

INTRODUCTION

Bone mass in adult humans decreases with age, leading to an increased risk of fractures [1]. Osteoporotic fractures, besides causing suffering to the patient, are a major burden to health care as the direct expenditure for osteoporosis and associated fractures is around US$ 17 billion/year in the United States [2], exceeds US$ 10 billion/year in Europe [3], and is around US$ 1 billion/year in Switzerland alone [4]. From a medical and economical view it would, therefore, be desirable to prevent low bone mass. A nutritional approach would be an inexpensive means to achieve this goal; however, the effects of the nutritional strategies recommended today are rather modest. Indeed, even the effect of calcium in milk on the relative risk of hip fractures seems to be restricted to the 10% of the female population with the lowest intake of calcium [5]. Thus, research into novel nutritional strategies preventing bone loss is needed.

Osteoporosis occurs most frequently in postmenopausal women following the decrease of estrogen levels. Hormone-replacement therapy (HRT) is effective in the prevention of bone loss, but compliance with HRT is low because of side effects. This has stimulated research of alternatives to the classical HRT (e.g., the use of phytoestrogens to prevent bone loss). It has been suggested that the high consumption of soy products providing 30 to 60 mg of the estrogenic isoflavones genistein and daidzein per day in the traditional Japanese diet may contribute to the low prevalence of postmenopausal osteoporosis in Japan [6]. Indeed, treatment with soy-protein-containing isoflavones inhibits bone loss in an animal model for postmenopausal osteoporosis (i.e., the ovariectomized rat) [7]. Treatment of perimenopausal and postmenopausal women with 40 g/day of a soy-protein isolate providing 80 or 90 mg of isoflavones per day, respectively, attenuated the loss of bone mineral density (BMD) in the spine but not at other sites; lower doses were ineffective [8,9]. In a randomized double-blind, placebo-controlled study it was found recently that in early postmenopausal women genistein at the dose of 54 mg/day was as effective as HRT in preventing bone loss in the spine and in the femoral neck [10]. Thus, genistein appears to be a promising pharmacologically active agent; however, the doses required for this effect are beyond nutritional possibilities. Indeed, to achieve an intake of 54 mg of genistein from soy products, for example, about 200 g of tofu should be consumed daily[11].

A nutritional strategy based on soy products would imply a fundamental modification of Western nutritional habits which is hardly feasible, a fact that was predictable some 10 years ago. As we found previously that components other than soy from a rat chow inhibited bone resorption [12], we have chosen not to investigate the effect of phytoestrogens but we have investigated whether some components of our Western diet also display bone-modulating activities.

MATERIALS AND METHODS

ANIMALS

Wistar Hanlbm rats were kept in standard animal facilities that comply with the Swiss and U.S. National Institutes of Health guidelines for care and use of experimental animals. The experiments performed were approved by the State Committee for the Control of Animal Experimentation. Nine-week-old male rats prelabeled with tritiated tetracycline were used to measure bone resorption. For the effect on bone mass either 9-week-old females or 1-year-old ovariectomized retired breeder rats were used as the osteoporosis model.

Monitoring of Bone Resorption

The urinary excretion of ^{3}H-labeled tetracycline ([^{3}H]-Tc) from chronically prelabeled rats, an extensively validated method, was used to monitor bone resorption [13–16]. As this technique is labor intensive, only limited numbers of rats can be handled, thus for each experiment 3 Wistar Hanlbm dams with 12 three-day-old male pups each were purchased (RCC, Ltd., Füllinsdorf, Switzerland). The 36 pups were injected from the first week of life twice a week for 6 weeks with increasing amounts of [^{3}H]-Tc [13]. [^{3}H]-Tc is deposited into bone and is released when bone is resorbed [13]. After discontinuation of labeling, the rats were transferred to metabolic cages. After 10 days of acclimatization, baseline bone resorption was monitored by measuring the daily urinary [^{3}H] excretion. After 10 days of baseline measurement, the 10-day dietary intervention was started in 26 rats that were homogeneously assigned to the groups; that is, the baseline [^{3}H] urinary excretion of all rats was ranked and to each treatment group one animal with a similar rank was assigned until the number of animals per group was completed. Using this protocol, the mean [^{3}H] excretion was similar for all groups at the start of the dietary intervention. ^{3}H in urine was determined by liquid scintillation counting. Aliquots of 1 mL urine were counted in 10 mL of Irga-Safe Plus^{TM} scintillator (Packard International, Zürich, Switzerland) and the result (dpm) was multiplied by the 24-hr urine volume.

Assessment of Bone Mass

Total bone mineral content (BMC) and/or trabecular bone mineral density (BMD) were measured in the proximal metaphysis of the left tibia by quantitative computed tomography (XCT Research SA, software version 5.40; Stratec Medizintechnik, Pforzheim, Germany), as previously described [17,18]. A cross-section starting 5 mm distal to the joint space was evaluated, using a threshold for trabecular bone of 400 mg/cm^3.

FEEDING AND DIETS

From the time when the rats were housed in the metabolic cages, they were given demineralized water to drink and the diets were given in a stainless steel crucible as wet food to minimize spillage in the cage; thus, deionized water was added to batches of food powder to give a dough-like consistency conducive to making food balls. During the 10 days of treatment, the rats were fed the semipurified diet 2160 (Kliba-Mühlen, Kaiseraugst, Switzerland) in order to mimic a typical Western diet with large proportions of refined components as well as to avoid any interference on bone resorption from natural components of a "normal" diet [19]. In order to make the rats insensitive to the content of Ca and P in the food items to be tested, a semipurified diet with a high content of Ca and P (1.1 g/100 g and 1.2 g/100 g, respectively) was used. The rats were trained to consume 23 g of wet food per day (13.1 g dry matter). If not stated differently, for the treatment 1 g/day of the dry additives was mixed with the semipurified diet. Appropriate amounts of the items to be investigated were added to batches of wet food sufficient for 10 days of dietary intervention. These diets were then aliquoted into daily portions and kept frozen at $-20°C$ until use.

Processing of Foodstuffs and Beverages for the Various Additions to the Diets

Fresh vegetables, salads, and herbs were purchased locally, carefully washed with tap water, minced, air-dried at about $50°C$, and ground to a fine powder. Nine vegetables (broccoli; Brussels sprouts; cauliflower; Chinese, white, and red cabbage; French beans; dry kidney beans; and potatoes) were cooked in water (as customary for human nutrition) and mashed in a blender together with the water before freeze drying. Ready-to-use frozen spinach was freeze-dried before grinding. The moisture was removed from commercially available dried onion flakes, Italian parsley, garlic powder, and heat-inactivated white hylum soybeans by adsorption over silica gel before grinding. Plums, oranges, bananas, and apples were carefully washed and the stone (plums) or peel (orange and banana) was discarded; the fruit was then cut and freeze dried before grinding. Before grinding, the moisture was removed by adsorption over silica gel from commercially available, dried, farmed mushrooms—shiitake and field agaric (*Lentinus edodes* and *Agaricus hortensis*, respectively)—and from the locally harvested wild mushroom yellow boletus (*Boletus edulis*), which was air dried at about $50°C$. The shell was removed from roasted peanuts before grinding. Linseed and kernels of Brazil nuts were purchased from a local retailer and ground without prior treatment. Parboiled steamed rice was freeze dried, and dark bread without crust, made from wheat flour type 1050, was air dried at about $50°C$ before grinding. Prior to freeze-drying, fresh eggs were whipped slightly and fresh meat (beef) was minced. Skimmed milk was purchased from a local retailer. A mixture of 15.1 parts glucose, 12.9 parts fructose, and 17.2 parts sucrose ("sugars"), similar to that contained in dry onion [20], was prepared from analytical-grade sugars. Regular instant coffee and soluble cocoa powder were used as purchased, while black and green tea were ground prior to use. Normal cola was freeze dried because a pilot experiment revealed that, after a few days, rats given cola in liquid form had a much higher liquid intake compared to the control rats given demineralized water (fluid intake increased from 28 ± 5 mL/day in control rats to 88 ± 3 mL in rats drinking cola). As the rats on cola also consumed all the food, this led to a gain in body weight of 43 ± 7 g as compared to 7 ± 1 g in control rats during the same time period. To overcome these difficulties, the dry residue from cola was added to the diet. To avoid a similar problem with beer and red wine, the alcohol was removed under reduced pressure at 60°C (Rotovapor; Büchi, Flawil, Switzerland) and the remnant was freeze dried. All these items were high-vacuum packed and stored at 4°C until use.

Essential Oils

Oil of cumin (oleum carvi, rect.), oil of eucalyptus (oleum eucalypti, >80% Ph. Eur.), oil of fennel (oleum foeniculi), oil of juniper berries (oleum juniperi e baccis, purum), pine oil (oil of fir; oleum *Pini sibiricum*), dwarf-pine oil (oleum *Pini pumilionis*), oil of rosemary (oleum rosmarini, DAB) and sage oil (oleum salviae, Dalmatian) were purchased from Carl Roth, Inc. (Reinach, Switzerland). Sweet orange-peel oil from Hänseler, Inc. (Herisau, Switzerland) was purchased at a local drugstore.

Monoterpenes

Thujone (mixture of isomers), eucalyptol (99%, purum), (+)-camphor (>99%), Borneol (>98%, mixture of isomers), menthol (>98%, Chinese), (–)-α-pinene (>97%), and β-pinene (depur) were purchased from Carl Roth (Reinach, Switzerland), thymol (puriss.) from E. Merck (Darmstadt, Germany); (–)-bornylacetate (97%) and (S)-*cis*-verbenol were purchased from Aldrich (Buchs, Switzerland).

STATISTICAL METHODS

The significance of differences of means were evaluated with the Student's T-test.

RESULTS AND DISCUSSION

EFFECT OF FOODS ON BONE RESORPTION

Effect of Vegetables, Salads, and Herbs on Bone

When 1 g of dried onion was added to the daily diet we found an increase of total bone mineral content in growing rats (Fig. 1). This effect was associated with an inhibition of bone resorption. Subsequent experiments showed that not only onion but also other members of the same botanical family such as garlic, wild garlic, and leek were inhibitory. From the cabbage family,

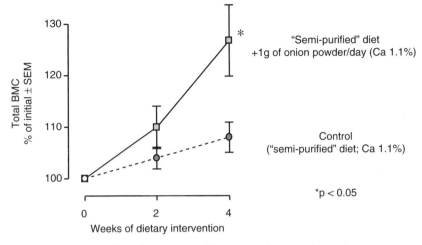

FIGURE 1   Effect of onion on total bone mineral content in growing rats.

broccoli, Chinese cabbage, and red cabbage were active. Furthermore, arrugula, cucumber, dill, lettuce, both forms of parsley—namely, common (crisp) parsley and Italian parsley—as well as tomato significantly inhibited bone resorption [21]. Later, we found that herbs rich in essential oils, such as rosemary, sage, and thyme, also significantly inhibited bone resorption [22]. Because some vegetables, such as carrot, cauliflower, endive, potato, and soy, given at the 1-g dose did not significantly inhibit bone resorption [21], it cannot generally be stated that the consumption of vegetables is beneficial to bone. This prompted us recently to perform a survey of activity of different classes of foodstuffs of vegetable origin. We found that additionally fennel, French beans, and celeriac but not spinach and red pepper significantly inhibited bone resorption [23]. Because 9 out of 29 vegetables, salads, and herbs investigated had no significant effect, the question is open as to whether a significant effect could have been obtained with larger doses. The dose of 1 g dry foodstuff per day per 250 g rat corresponds to 8% of the daily intake of dry matter and is, therefore, already a high but still realistic dose of an individual food item which precludes higher doses to be used.

Effect of Fruits on Bone Resorption

In this group, four items were investigated. We found that prunes and oranges significantly inhibited bone resorption but not banana and apple [23]. Prunes at a very high dose (25% of daily intake) have been shown by others to inhibit bone loss in rats, the rationale for the study with prunes being their abundant polyphenol content, thought to protect bone by scavenging free radicals [24]. As discussed below, we have no basis to conclude that polyphenols in general inhibit bone resorption.

Effect of Nuts, Beans (Dry Kernels) and Seeds on Bone Resorption

Brazil nuts, peanuts, kidney beans, and linseed were investigated in this group. None of them displayed significant activity [23]. We have previously also not found a significant effect with soy at the dose of 1 g/rat/day [21]; however, the lack of effect of soy might be due not only to too low of a dose, but also possibly to the model we have used.

Effect of Mushrooms on Bone Resorption

The Chinese farmed mushroom shiitake was devoid of activity, while the farmed field agaric and the wild growing yellow boletus significantly inhibited bone resorption [23]. This exemplifies once more that, as long as the active compounds are not known, generalizations cannot be made.

Effect of Carbohydrate Sources on Bone Resorption

Parboiled rice, dark bread, and sugars were all devoid of activity [23]. As we found no effect for bread made of dark wheat flour containing 5.2% dietary fiber [20], it appears likely that no effect on bone resorption is to be expected from flours with a lower fiber content commonly used to make white bread and many kinds of pasta. Because potato also does not display significant inhibitory activity [21], it appears that the major carbohydrate sources of the human diet are devoid of activity.

EFFECT OF BEVERAGES ON BONE RESORPTION

Finally, of the beverages tested, only the residue from red wine significantly inhibited bone resorption, but not beer, green and black tea, instant coffee, cola, or cocoa [23]. Tea was given at a lower dose because a pilot experiment showed that green tea given at the dose of 1 g was not well tolerated as it reduced food intake and body weight. Green and black tea were therefore administered at the dose of 0.25 g/rat/day. Instant coffee was administered at the dose of 0.1 g/rat/day. The doses of coffee and of tea still correspond to about 14 cups/day if extrapolated to a 70-kg human.

As outlined above, prunes at a very high dose (25% of daily intake) have been shown by others to inhibit bone loss in rats, the rationale for the study with prunes being their abundant polyphenol content, thought to protect bone by scavenging free radicals [24]. We found a significant effect with prunes at a dose corresponding to 8% of the daily intake. If polyphenols in general were responsible for the effect observed, other foodstuffs containing large amounts of polyphenols could also be inhibitory. However, from the beverages tested, only red wine inhibits bone resorption, despite the fact that some beverages have a large content of polyphenols. The daily polyphenol content provided per rat with the additions we have used, calculated from published data [25], was within a range of 2.4 to 3.9 mg for beer, 40 to 161 mg for red wine, 55 to 82 mg for black tea, 50 to 87 mg for green tea, and 120 to 180 mg for cocoa. Thus, it appears unlikely that from polyphenols in general an effect on bone resorption can be expected.

A significant effect on bone by beer could possibly have been expected, considering the carryover of the estrogenic humulone from the beer ingredient hop [26]. As intact male rats were used, the lack of effect might be due not only to too low of a dose but possibly also to the fact that the model we have used to assess effects on bone resorption is not tailored to be exquisitely sensitive to phytoestrogens. Accordingly, we have previously also not found a significant effect with soy at the dose of 1 g/rat/day [21]; for an effect, larger doses of 2.5 g/rat/day were necessary (unpublished observation). We have chosen this model that is sensitive to inhibitors of bone resorption in general [27] because bone loss occurs in old age in both sexes.

Coffee, tea, cola, and cocoa are rich in caffeine. Caffeine intake is a risk factor for bone loss in humans because it increases the urinary excretion of calcium. The risk appears, however, to be modifiable as it can be offset by moderate milk consumption [28]. We have used a high calcium diet throughout these studies to make the rats insensitive to the content of calcium in the food items to be tested, which makes it plausible that we could not see a stimulation of bone resorption by caffeine-rich food items.

In order to make sure that freeze–dried cola corresponded to native cola in terms of acid content we have compared the two items. For this, freeze–dried cola was reconstituted to its original volume with demineralized water and the pH as well as the titratable acid were measured as done previously [29]. The pH of reconstituted cola was 2.55 as compared to 2.52 for control cola. The consumption of 0.01 mol/L NaOH to titrate 1 mL of reconstituted cola to pH 7.4 was 0.88 ± 0.1 mL ($\pm$SD), while for control cola 1.10 ± 0.1 mL were needed. Thus, reconstituted cola appears to have a 20% lower titratable acid as compared to native cola. Nevertheless, rats receiving 1 g/day of cola powder had received a conspicuous load of noncarbonic acid because 1 g of cola powder still corresponds to 2.2 L for a 70-kg human when the 20%

loss of titratable acid is taken into account. Bone resorption was not significantly different from control, possibly because young rats with intact renal function can excrete large amounts of acid into the urine so that the buffering by bone is not required [29]; this might well explain why cola did not stimulate bone resorption in our animal model.

Summarized, the activity on bone resorption cannot be associated with a single category of food items but rather is distributed among various categories. Of the 50 food items of vegetable origin studied, 25 are inhibitory. Of the 36 items studied in the categories vegetables, salads, herbs, mushrooms, and fruits, 25 inhibit bone resorption, while 13 out of 14 items studied in the categories of nuts, beans (dried kernels) and seeds, carbohydrate sources, and beverages are devoid of activity.

IS THE EFFECT OF VEGETABLES ON BONE RESORPTION DUE TO THEIR BASE EXCESS?

Dietary protein rich in the sulfur-containing amino acids methionine and cystine metabolically generate sulfuric acid, and it is held that this acid load is in part buffered by bone mineral, leading to bone dissolution [30]. Fruits and vegetables rich in potassium citrate [31], however, metabolically generate base, thus buffering the acid produced by protein-rich animal foodstuffs; therefore, it is thought that they protect bone [32,33]. We have shown that while some common vegetables, salads, and herbs inhibit bone resorption in the rat, foodstuffs of animal origin rich in protein, such as egg, meat, and skimmed milk, do not [21]. This evidence was interpreted by others to reflect the mechanism outlined above [34].

Onion was chosen for in-depth *in vivo* investigations concerning the acid–base metabolism. Addition of 7% onion to the semipurified-diet slightly increased urinary pH and slightly decreased both titratable acid and ammonium excretion. Altogether, the treatment with onion led to a decrease of the cumulative proton excretion by $17 \pm 3\%$ $(P < 0.01)$. Bone resorption decreased by $18 \pm 2\%$ $(P < 0.001)$. Thus, the effect of onion on bone resorption is of similar magnitude as the effect on proton excretion; however, no causal relationship is warranted unless the experiment is done. To mimic the base excess of onion, rats receiving the semipurified-diet were given potassium citrate at a dose buffering the metabolic acid load from the semipurified-diet (with casein as the sole protein source). A daily dose of 252 mg of potassium citrate mixed with food fulfills this requirement. When this dose of potassium citrate was added to the semipurified-diet, we found no effect on bone resorption. Furthermore, the effect of onion or a mixture of 14 active vegetables on bone resorption was not diminished in rats when 252 mg of potassium citrate was added to the food. Thus, we demonstrated that, although the inhibitory effect of vegetables on bone resorption correlates with their base excess, the two phenomena are independent, at least in the rat. The effect of vegetables, salads, and herbs, which inhibit bone resorption in the rat, is therefore not mediated by their base excess but possibly by pharmacologically active compounds [29].

EFFECT OF ESSENTIAL OILS AND MONOTERPENES ON BONE

As outlined above, when 1 g of powdered leaves from sage, rosemary, and thyme, herbs rich in essential oils, was fed to rats, bone resorption was inhibited. We have therefore hypothesized that possibly essential oils are inhibitors of bone resorption. The essential oils extracted from rosemary, sage, and thyme (Fig. 2) indeed inhibited bone resorption, as do pine oil, dwarf-pine oil, the related medicinal turpentine, oil of juniper, and eucalyptus. Sage oil, pine oil, and turpentine inhibited bone resorption in a dose-dependent fashion, pine oil being the most potent. Thus, from the 11 essential oils investigated, 8 inhibited bone resorption in the rat while oil of cumin, oil of fennel, and sweet orange peel oil were found to be devoid of significant activity.

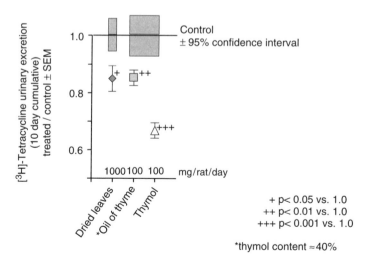

FIGURE 2 Effect of thyme, essential oil of thyme, and thymol on bone resorption in rats.

Pure components of the essential oils were then studied. A mixture of the four major monoterpenes occurring in 200 mg of sage oil [35] (80 mg thujone, 24 mg eucalyptol, 14 mg camphor, and 10 mg borneol) was nearly as effective as 200 mg of sage oil, suggesting that these four monoterpenes are the active components. When tested singly at the above doses, thujone, eucalyptol, and camphor were effective inhibitors. At a higher dose of 100 mg/day, borneol appeared to be more potent than eucalyptol and camphor. α-Pinene, β-pinene, and bornylacetate, the major components of the pine oil used, were also potent inhibitors of resorption. This was also the case for menthol and thymol. Thus, nine monoterpenes, components of the active herbs or essential oils, inhibit bone resorption. A mixture of equal parts of these monoterpenes was also active, suggesting that their effect is additive. Thus, essential oils and monoterpenes are efficient inhibitors of bone resorption.

As the incidence of osteoporosis in humans is much more frequent in women, with bone turnover (resorption > formation) increasing after menopause, an animal model of osteoporosis, the aged ovariectomized (OVX) rat in which a marked decrease in trabecular bone mineral density (BMD) and bone mineral content (BMC) occurs [36], has been used to study the effect of pine oil. Pine oil protects the animals from the loss of both trabecular BMD (by 70%; $P < 0.05$) (Fig. 3) and total BMC (by 60%; not significant) [22].

To date we have identified nine monoterpenes contained in the essential oils of sage, rosemary, and thyme and other plants as inhibitors of bone resorption. We also showed that the activity from onion is extractable with water or with ethanol/water, inhibits resorption *in vivo* and *in vitro* [37], and prevents bone loss in an osteoporosis model [38]. The solubility of this activity is, therefore, different from that of the

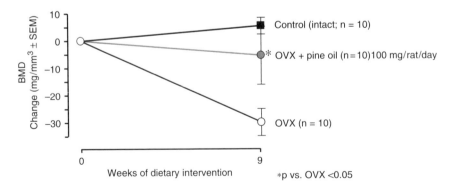

FIGURE 3   Effect of pine oil on trabecular bone mineral density in aged OVX rats.

highly lipophilic monoterpenes, suggesting at least two different classes of active molecules.

EFFECT OF FRUITS AND VEGETABLES ON BONE MINERAL DENSITY IN HUMANS

Epidemiological data have shown that the consumption of fruit and vegetables is associated with greater bone mineral density in humans [32,33,39]. Our results in rats can possibly confirm and explain the effects of fruits and vegetables on bone mineral density observed in the human studies and expand bone-resorption-inhibitory food items to the categories salads, herbs, mushrooms, and red wine. Our interpretation of the effect, however, contrasts with the interpretation from human studies, where it has been claimed that the base excess of fruits and vegetables buffers noncarbonic metabolic acid that would otherwise be buffered by bone mineral, leading to bone dissolution [32,33]. If the acid hypothesis were correct, we should have found foodstuffs that stimulate bone resorption, which we did not find. What we found, however, was that the inhibitory effect of 14 foodstuffs of vegetable origin on bone resorption is not mediated by their base excess but possibly by pharmacologically active compounds [29]. Thus, based on the results from our dietary intervention studies in rats, we conclude that components of the human diet are either bone-resorption-inhibitory food items or inert. As a consequence, a model that implies a high rate of bone resorption that can be opposed by inhibitory food items can be envisaged.

WHAT SHOULD WE EAT?

To minimize stimulation of bone resorption by calcium depletion, the recommended daily intake of calcium for women and men over 65 years of age is 1500 mg/day [40]. The preferred source of calcium is through calcium-rich food such as dairy products [40]; however, the effect of this strategy might be rather modest [5]. As the effect of bone-resorption-inhibitory food items occurs in our rat model despite a high calcium diet, our findings suggest that an abundant consumption of bone-resorption-inhibitory food items, together with a sufficient mineral supply, might offer an additional benefit to the consumer.

The minimal effective dose of bone-resorption-inhibitory food items we established recently is 170 mg/rat as assessed with a mixture of equal parts of arrugula, broccoli, cucumber, Chinese cabbage, red cabbage, dill, garlic, wild garlic, leek, lettuce, onion, Italian parsley, common parsley, and tomato [41]. This dose corresponds to 6.2 g of fresh bone-resorption-inhibitory food items per kilogram body weight, indicating that the amount of bone-resorption-inhibitory food items consumed by way of a regular Western diet might not be sufficient to elicit a protective effect in humans. However, other compounds occurring in plant-derived foodstuffs, such as vitamins (K and C) and the phytoestrogen genistein, have been identified to be potentially important for bone health as they support bone formation [10,42,43]. Our methodology does not allow us to make conclusions as to the effect of foodstuffs on bone formation. Notwithstanding this limitation, it can be summarized that the evidence available today suggests that foodstuffs of vegetable origin offer a variety of activities (possibly secondary plant products, although the nature of many are still unknown) that either stimulate bone formation and/or are bone-resorption-inhibitory food items, which, when present in our diet in sufficient amounts, in concerted action could slow down bone loss.

If the high incidence of osteoporosis in Western societies is taken as evidence that the amount of such activities consumed by way of the typical two to three servings of fruits and vegetables per day in the Western diet is not sufficient to elicit a protective effect, the strategy to increase the number of servings should be recommended. Although it is difficult to change nutritional habits in humans, the international campaign "Take Five" shows that it is possible to increase the daily number of servings, at least of fruits and vegetables, from three to five servings of 80 g each [44]. The campaign "Take Five" was started as a result of the overwhelming epidemiological evidence that a generous consumption of fruits and vegetables is associated with a reduced risk for certain forms of cancer [45]. A higher consumption of fruits and vegetables seems to reduce the risk for another condition associated with age—low bone mass [32,33,39], the main risk factor for osteoporotic fractures. It will, therefore, be of interest to assess bone mass in persons who have increased their fruit and vegetable intake to five servings per day for cancer prevention.

Our work shows that not all fruits and vegetables are effective and that bone-resorption-inhibitory food items are widely distributed among vegetable components of the human diet. Thus, regular consumption of bone-resorption-inhibitory food items shown on Fig. 4 could be an efficient alternative to ingest sufficient amounts of bone protective activities. However, before such a recommendation can be given, the amounts necessary to obtain an effect in humans must be established in a clinical intervention study.

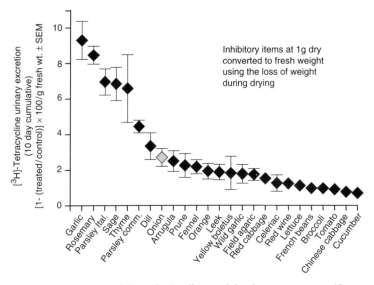

FIGURE 4 Relative potency of fresh foodstuffs to inhibit bone resorption. (© Roman C. Mühlbauer, 2003. Reproduced with permission.)

REFERENCES

1. Lindsay, R. and Cosman, F. (1992). Primary osteoporosis, in *Disorders of Bone and Mineral Metabolism*, Coe, F.L. and Favus, M.J., Eds. Raven Press, New York, pp. 831–888.
2. Melton, L.J. and Heaney, R.P. (2003). Too much medicine? Or too little? *Bone* 32: 327–331.
3. White, P. and Compston, J. (1998). *Osteoporosis: Clinical and Commercial Perspectives*, Carter Mill, London.
4. Lippuner, K., von Overbeck, J., Perrelet, R., Bosshard, H., and Jaeger, P. (1997). Incidence and direct medical costs of hospitalizations due to osteoporotic fractures in Switzerland. *Osteoporosis Int.* 7: 414–425.
5. Kanis, J.A. (1999). The use of calcium in the management of osteoporosis. *Bone* 24: 279–290.
6. Fujita, T. (1991). Osteoporosis: east and west. *Calcif. Tissue Int.* 48: 151–152.
7. Harrison, E., Adjei, A., Ameho, C., Yamamoto, S., and Kono, S. (1998). The effect of soybean protein on bone loss in a rat model of postmenopausal osteoporosis. *J. Nutr. Sci. Vitaminol. (Tokyo)* 44: 257–268.
8. Alekel, D.L., Germain, A.S., Peterson, C.T., Hanson, K.B., Stewart, J.W., and Toda, T. (2000). Isoflavone-rich soy protein isolate attenuates bone loss in the lumbar spine of perimenopausal women. *Am. J. Clin. Nutr.* 72: 844–852.
9. Potter, S.M., Baum, J.A., Teng, H., Stillman, R.J., Shay, N.F., and Erdman, J.W., Jr. (1998). Soy protein and isoflavones: their effects on blood lipids and bone density in postmenopausal women. *Am. J. Clin. Nutr.* 68(suppl.): 1375S–1379S.
10. Morabito, N., Crisafulli, A., Vergara, C., Gaudio, A., Lasco, A., Frisina, N., D'Anna, R., Corrado, F., Pizzoleo, M.A., Cincotta, M., Altavilla, D., Ientile, R., and Squadrito, F. (2002). Effects of genistein and hormone-replacement therapy on bone loss in early

postmenopausal women: a randomized double-blind placebo-controlled study. *J. Bone Mineral Res.* 17: 1904–1912.

11. Coward, L., Barnes, N.C., Setchell, K.D.R., and Barnes, S. (1993). Genistein, daidzein, and their β-glycoside conjugates: antitumor isoflavones in soybean foods from American and Asian diets. *J. Agric. Food Chem.* 41: 1961–1967.

12. Mühlbauer, R.C. and Fleisch, H. (1996). Natural components in rat diet have potent effects on bone resorption. *J. Bone Mineral Res.* 11: S188 (abstract #S395).

13. Mühlbauer, R.C. and Fleisch, H. (1990). A method for continual monitoring of bone resorption in rats: evidence for a diurnal rhythm. *Am. J. Physiol.* 259: R679–R689.

14. Egger, C.D., Mühlbauer, R.C., Felix, R., Delmas, P.D., Marks, S.C., and Fleisch, H. (1994). Evaluation of urinary pyridinium crosslink excretion as a marker of bone resorption in the rat. *J. Bone Mineral Res.* 9: 1211–1219.

15. Mühlbauer, R.C. and Fleisch, H. (1995). The diurnal rhythm of bone resorption in the rat: effect of feeding habits and pharmacological inhibitors. *J. Clin. Invest.* 95: 1933–1940.

16. Antic, V.N., Fleisch, H., and Mühlbauer, R.C. (1996). Effect of bisphosphonates on the increase in bone resorption induced by a low calcium diet. *Calcif. Tissue Int.* 58: 443–448.

17. Mühlbauer, R.C., Schenk, R.K., Chen, D., Lehto-Axtelius, D., and Hakanson, R. (1998). Morphometric analysis of gastrectomy-evoked osteopenia. *Calcif. Tissue Int.* 62: 323–326.

18. Li, F. and Mühlbauer, R.C. (1999). Food fractionation is a powerful tool to increase bone mass in growing rats and to decrease bone loss in aged rats: modulation of the effect by dietary phosphate. *J. Bone Mineral Res.* 14: 1457–1465.

19. Brown, N.M. and Setchell, K.D.R. (2001). Animal models impacted by phytoestrogens in commercial chow: implications for pathways influenced by hormones. *Lab. Invest.* 81: 735–747.

20. Souci, S.W., Fachmann, W., and Kraut, H. (1989). *Food Composition and Nutrition Tables 1989/90*, Wissenschaftliche Verlagsgesellschaft mbH, Stuttgart.

21. Mühlbauer, R.C. and Li, F. (1999). Effect of vegetables on bone metabolism. *Nature* 401: 343–344.

22. Mühlbauer, R.C., Lozano, A., Palacio, S., Reinli, A., and Felix, R. (2003). Common herbs, essential oils, and monoterpenes potently modulate bone metabolism. *Bone* 32: 372–380.

23. Mühlbauer, R.C., Reinli, A., and Lozano, A. (2003). Human foodstuffs and beverages inhibiting bone resorption: a survey. 30th European Symposium on Calcified Tissues, Rome, Italy, 8–12 May, 2003. *Calcif. Tissue Int.* 72: 413 (abstract #P-320).

24. Arjmandi, B.H., Lucas, E.A., Juma, S., Soliman, A., Stoecker, B.J., Khalil, D.A., Smith, B.J., and Wang, C. (2001). Dried plums prevent ovariectomy-induced bone loss in rats. *JANA* 4: 50–56.

25. Bravo, L. (1998). Polyphenols: chemistry, dietary sources, metabolism, and nutritional significance. *Nutr. Rev.* 56: 317–333.

26. Tobe, H., Muraki, Y., Kitamura, K., Komiyama, O., Sato, Y., Sugioka, T., Maruyama, H.B., Matsuda, E., and Nagai, M. (1997). Bone resorption inhibitors from hop extract. *Biosci. Biotechnol. Biochem.* 61: 158–159.

27. Mühlbauer, R.C. (1994). Biochemical assessment of bone metabolism in rodents, in *Sex Steroids and Bone*, Ziegler, R., Pfeilschifter, J., and Bräutigam, M., Eds. Springer-Verlag, Berlin, pp. 191–202.

28. Barrett-Connor, E., Chang, J.C., and Edelstein, S.L. (1994). Coffee-associated osteoporosis offset by daily milk consumption: the Rancho Bernardo Study. *JAMA* 271: 280–283.

29. Mühlbauer, R.C., Lozano, A., and Reinli, A. (2002). Onion and a mixture of vegetables, salads and herbs affect bone resorption in the rat by a mechanism independent of their base excess. *J. Bone Mineral Res.* 17: 1230–1236.

30. Barzel, U.S. (1995). The skeleton as an ion exchange system: implications for the role of acid–base imbalance in the genesis of osteoporosis. *J. Bone Mineral Res.* 10: 1431–1436.
31. Frassetto, L.A., Todd, K.M., Morris, R.C., Jr., and Sebastian, A. (1998). Estimation of net endogenous noncarbonic acid production in humans from diet potassium and protein contents. *Am. J. Clin. Nutr.* 68: 576–583.
32. Tucker, K.L., Hannan, M.T., Chen, H., Cupples, L.A., Wilson, P.W., and Kiel, D.P. (1999). Potassium, magnesium, and fruit and vegetable intakes are associated with greater bone mineral density in elderly men and women. *Am. J. Clin. Nutr.* 69: 727–736.
33. New, S.A., Robins, S.P., Campbell, M.K., Martin, J.C., Garton, M.J., Bolton-Smith, C., Grubb, D.A., Lee, S.J., and Reid, D.M. (2000). Dietary influences on bone mass and bone metabolism: further evidence of a positive link between fruit and vegetable consumption and bone health? *Am. J. Clin. Nutr.* 71: 142–151.
34. Osterweil, N. (1999). An onion a day keeps the orthopedist away: vegetables inhibit bone loss in animal models for osteoporosis. *Medcast Med. News* 23–29, electronic citation, Sept. 23, 1999.
35. Wagner, H. (1993). *Pharmazeutische Biologie: Drogen und ihre Inhaltsstoffe*, Gustav Fischer, Verlag, Stuttgart.
36. Wronski, T.J., Walsh, C.C., and Ignaszewski, L.A. (1986). Histologic evidence for osteopenia and increased bone turnover in ovariectomized rats. *Bone* 7: 119–123.
37. Mühlbauer, R.C., Li, F., and Guenther, H.L. (1998). Common vegetables consumed by humans potently modulate bone metabolism *in vitro* and *in vivo*. *Bone* 23: S387 (abstract #W391).
38. Ingold, P., Kneissel, M., Mühlbauer, R.C., and Gasser, J.A. (1998). Extracts from onion prevent tibial cortical and cancellous bone loss induced by a high phosphate/low protein diet in aged retired breeder rats. *Bone* 23: S387 (abstract #W388).
39. Tucker, K.L., Chen, H., Hannan, M.T., Cupples, L.A., Wilson, P.W., Felson, D., and Kiel, D.P. (2002). Bone mineral density and dietary patterns in older adults: the Framingham Osteoporosis Study. *Am. J. Clin. Nutr.* 76: 245–252.
40. NIH Consensus conference. (1994). Optimal calcium intake. NIH Consensus Development Panel on Optimal Calcium Intake. *JAMA* 272: 1942–1948.
41. Mühlbauer, R.C., Lozano, A., Reinli, A., and Wetli, H. (2003). Various selected vegetables, fruits, mushrooms and red wine residue inhibit bone resorption in rats. *J. Nutr.* 133: 3592–3597.
42. Feskanich, D., Weber, P., Willett, W.C., Rockett, H., Booth, S.L., and Colditz, G.A. (1999). Vitamin K intake and hip fractures in women: a prospective study. *Am. J. Clin. Nutr.* 69: 74–79.
43. Heaney, R.P. (1996). Nutrition and risk for osteoporosis, in *Osteoporosis*, Marcus, R., Feldman, D., and Kelsey, J., Eds., Academic Press, San Diego, CA, pp. 483–509.
44. Cox, D.N., Anderson, A.S., Reynolds, J., McKellar, S., Lean, M.E., and Mela, D.J. (1998). Take Five, a nutrition education intervention to increase fruit and vegetable intakes: impact on consumer choice and nutrient intakes. *Br. J. Nutr.* 80: 123–131.
45. Willett, W.C. (1994). Diet and health: what should we eat? *Science* 264: 532–537.

CHAPTER 24

A Role for Fruit and Vegetables in Osteoporosis Prevention?

Susan A. New

Centre for Nutrition and Food Safety, School of Biomedical and Molecular Sciences, University of Surrey, Guildford, Surrey, United Kingdom

As noted by Kraut and Coburn [1], the famous words by Mencken in the early 20th century about the meaning of life and death may also apply to the struggle of the healthy skeleton against the deleterious effects of retained acid: "Life is a struggle, not against sin, not against the money power, not against malicious animal magnetism, but against hydrogen ions."

—Henry Louis Mencken (1919)

ABSTRACT

The role that the skeleton plays in acid–base homeostasis has been gaining great interest in the scientific literature and media. Interestingly, theoretical considerations of the role alkaline bone mineral may play in the defense against acidosis date as far back as the late 19th century. Pioneering work in the mid-1960s showed that natural, pathological, and experimental states of acid loading/acidosis have been associated with hypercalciuria and negative calcium balance. At the cellular level, a reduction in extracellular pH has been shown to have a direct enhancement on osteoclastic activity. Population-based studies have demonstrated a beneficial effect of fruit and vegetable/potassium intake on axial and peripheral bone mass and bone metabolism in men and women across all age ranges, and the results of the DASH (dietary approaches to stopping hypertension) and DASH–sodium intervention trials provide further support for a fruit and vegetable/bone

Nutritional Aspects of Osteoporosis, Second Edition

health link. There is now an urgent requirement for intervention trials centered specifically on fruit and vegetables as the supplementation vehicle and assessing a wide range of bone health indices including fracture risk.

INTRODUCTION

The health-related benefit of a high consumption of fruit and vegetables on a variety of diseases has been gaining increasing prominence in the literature for a number of years (Fig. 1) [2]. A number of observational, experimental, clinical, and intervention studies over the last decade have suggested a positive link between fruit and vegetable consumption and the skeleton. This chapter will review the strength of the evidence supporting a link between alkaline-forming foods and bone health, including the key theoretical considerations and practical implications.

IMPORTANCE OF ACID–BASE HOMEOSTASIS TO OPTIMUM HEALTH

Acid–base homeostasis is vital for optimum health, with the extracellular fluid pH remaining between 7.35 and 7.45. A major requirement of the body is to ensure that hydrogen ion concentrations are maintained between 0.035 and 0.045 meq/L [3]. The body's adaptive response involves three specific mechanisms: (1) buffer systems, (2) exhalation of CO_2, and

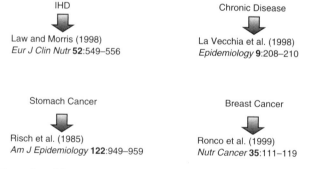

FIGURE 1   Examples of the importance of fruit and vegetables to the prevention of ischemic heart disease (IHD), cancer and other health outcomes. (With thanks to Dr. Veroniqne Coxam (Aprifel, France) (2003) for assistance with information.)

(3) kidney excretion. On a daily basis, humans eat substances that both generate and consume protons; hence, humans on a typical Western diet generate approximately 1 mEq per kg body weight of acid per day. In considering systemic acidosis, the more acid precursors a diet contains, the greater the degree of systemic acidity; as we age, our overall renal function declines, including the ability to excrete acid [4]. As shown by Frassetto and Sebastian [5], with each advancing year, humans become slightly but significantly more acidic.

A LINK BETWEEN ACID–BASE MAINTENANCE AND SKELETAL INTEGRITY?

THEORETICAL AND EXPERIMENTAL CONSIDERATIONS OF ACID–BASE AND BONE

Theoretical considerations of the role that alkaline bone mineral may play in the defense against acidosis date back as far as the late 1880s and early 20th century, with the fundamental concepts being established in the late 1960s and early 1970s [6]. A number of studies published during this period provided evidence that in natural (*e.g.*, starvation), pathological (*e.g.*, diabetic acidosis), and experimental (*e.g.*, ammonium chloride ingestion) states of acid loading and acidosis, an association exists with both hypercalciuria and negative calcium balance. The pioneering work of Lemann *et al.* [7] and Barzel [8] showed extensively the effects of acid from the diet on bone mineral in both man and animal.

DIETARY ACIDITY AND BONE: SIZE OF THE EFFECT?

In 1968, Wachman and Bernstein [9] put forward a hypothesis linking the daily diet to the development of osteoporosis based on the role of bone in acid–base balance. When the extent of loss is considered, if 2 mEq/kg per body weight of calcium per day is required to buffer about 1 mEq/kg per body weight of fixed acid per day, over 10 years (and assuming a total body calcium of approximately 1 kg), this would account for 15% loss of inorganic bone mass in an average individual. Thus, it is important to note that the effect of dietary acidity on the skeleton needs only to be relatively small to have a large impact over time.

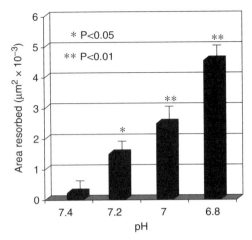

FIGURE 2   Increase in osteoclastic activity with a reduction in extracellular pH. Mean values were significantly different from that at pH 7.4: $*P < 0.05$, $**P < 0.01$. (From Ref. 10.)

Mechanisms for a Deleterious Effect of Acid on Bone

There are clear mechanisms for the deleterious effect of acid on bone. A direct enhancement of osteoclastic activity, independent of parathyroid hormone, follows a reduction in extracellular pH (Fig. 2) [10]. There is evidence that a small drop in pH, close to the physiological range, causes a tremendous burst in bone resorption [11,12], and metabolic acidosis has also been shown to stimulate resorption by activating mature osteoclasts already present in calvarial bone rather than by inducing formation of new osteoclasts [13].

ACIDITY OF FOODS AND SKELETAL HEALTH: CONCEPT OF POTENTIAL RENAL ACID LOADS

A topic of recent debate has been the potentially deleterious effect of specific foods on the skeleton [14–17]. Important work in this area by Remer and Manz [18] examining the potential renal acid loads (PRALs) of a variety of foods have shown many grain products and some cheeses have a high PRAL level (Table I). Because many of these foods are consumed in abundance by lactoovovegetarians, this may provide some of the reasons why there is a lack of a positive effect on bone health indices in studies comparing vegetarians versus omnivores [19].

TABLE I   Potential Renal Acid Load (PRAL) Values of a Variety of Foods and Food Groups

Food/Food Group	PRAL (mEq/100 g Edible Portion)	Food/Food Group	PRAL (mEq/100 g Edible Portion)
Fruits and Fruit Juices		**Milk, Dairy Products, and Eggs**	
Apples	-2.2	Milk (whole, pasteurized)	0.7
Bananas	-5.5	Yogurt (whole milk, plain)	1.5
Raisins	-21.0	Cheddar cheese (reduced fat)	26.4
Grape Juice	-1.0	Cottage cheese	8.7
Lemon Juice	-2.5	Eggs (yolk)	23.4
Vegetables		**Meat, Meat Products, and Fish**	
Spinach	-14.0	Beef (lean only)	7.8
Broccoli	-1.2	Chicken (meat only)	8.7
Carrots	-4.9	Pork (lean only)	7.9
Potatoes	-4.0	Liver sausage	10.6
Onions	-1.5	Cod (fillets)	7.1
Grain Products		**Beverages**	
Bread (white wheat)	3.7	Coca Cola®	0.4
Oat flakes	10.7	Coffee (infusion)	-1.4
Rice (brown)	12.5	Tea (Indian infusion)	-0.3
Spaghetti (white)	6.5	White wine	-1.2
Cornflakes	6.0	Red wine	-2.4

Source: Remer, T. and Manz, F. (1995). *J. Am. Diet. Assoc.* 95: 791–797.

POSITIVE LINK BETWEEN FRUIT AND VEGETABLES, ALKALI, AND BONE HEALTH: A REVIEW OF CURRENT EVIDENCE

CLINICAL STUDIES

Extensive work in this area has been undertaken by Lemann (at the subject level) [20–23] and Bushinsky (at the cellular level) [24–27]. Pioneering work on the effect of normal endogenous acid production on bone by Sebastian and colleagues in 1994 [28] demonstrated that short-term potassium bicarbonate administration resulted in a decrease in urinary calcium and phosphorus, with overall calcium balance becoming more positive (or less negative). Changes were also seen in markers of bone metabolism, with a reduction in urinary excretion of hydroxyproline (bone resorption) and an increased excretion of serum osteocalcin (bone formation) (Table II). No studies have yet addressed the long-term impact of alkali administration on skeletal integrity, and work is urgently required in this area. Little information is available on the direct effect of dietary modification on calcium and bone metabolism. In an interesting study by

320   Nutritional Aspects of Osteoporosis

TABLE II   Clinical Application—KHCO₃ Supplementation Study

	Before KHCO₃	During KHCO₃	Change
Ca Balance (mg/day/60 kg)	−180 ± 124	−124 ± 76	+56 ± 76
P balance (mg/day/60 kg)	−208 ± 127	−161 ± 92	+47 ± 64
Serum OC (ng/ml)	5.5 ± 2.8	6.1 ± 2.8	+0.6 ± 0.48
Urinary HP (mg/day)	28.9 ± 12.3	26.7 ± 10.8	−2.2 ± *
NRAE (mmol/day)	70.9 ± 10.1	12.8 ± 21.8	−58.1 ± *

Sebastion, A. *et al., N. Engl. J. Med.*, 330, 1776–1781, 1994. With permission.

Buclin and colleagues [29], an acid-forming diet increased urinary calcium excretion by 74% and bone resorption, as measured by C-terminal peptide excretion, by 19% compared to the alkali-forming diet, both at baseline and after an oral calcium load. Further studies are urgently required to address the impact of dietary alkalinity and acidity on skeletal integrity, both in the short and long term.

Intervention Studies

There are currently no specific intervention studies examining directly the effect of fruit and vegetable consumption or alkali administration on markers of bone health, but several are currently underway, and their results are awaited with great interest. However, the results of the DASH (dietary approaches to stopping hypertension) and DASH–sodium intervention trials have important implications for bone. In the DASH study, diets rich in fruit and vegetables were associated with a significant fall in blood pressure compared with baseline measurements; however, of particular interest to the bone field was the finding that increasing fruit and vegetable intake from 3.6 to 9.5 daily servings decreased the urinary calcium excretion from 157 mm/day to 110mg/day [30]. The authors suggested this was due to the "high fibre content of the diet possibly impeding calcium absorption." However, a more likely explanation, put forward by Barzel [31], was a reduction in the acid load with the fruit and vegetable diet compared to the control diet. The findings of the DASH–sodium trial demonstrate a further important finding for bone health. As reported by Lin *et al.* [32], the impact of two dietary patterns on indices of bone metabolism were examined. The DASH diet emphasizes fruits, vegetables, and low-fat dairy products and reduces the intake of red meats; in this second DASH II trial, three levels of sodium intake were investigated (50, 100, and 150 nmol/L). Subjects consumed the control diet at the level of 150 mmol sodium intake per day for

2 weeks and then were randomly assigned to eat either the DASH diet or the control diet at all three sodium levels for a further 4 weeks in random order. The DASH diet, compared with the control diet, was found to significantly reduce both bone formation (by measurement of the marker osteocalcin) by 8 to 10% and bone resorption (by measurement of the marker CTx) by 16 to 18% (Dr. F. Ginty, personal communication). This finding is of critical importance to the bone field concerning dietary alkali and its potential benefit on bone, and clearly paves the way for the justification of further work in this area

OBSERVATIONAL STUDIES

As shown in Table III, a number of population-based studies published in the last decade have shown a beneficial effect of fruit and vegetable/potassium intake on indices of bone health in all of these age groups: young boys and girls, premenopausal women, perimenopausal women, postmenopausal women, and elderly men and women [33–46]. A recent systematic review on over 4500 subjects suggests a small ($\sim$0.9%) but significant effect on bone health (New and Torgerson, unpublished data). Work is now needed to determine which particular types of fruit and vegetables (including or excluding potatoes) have the most direct impact on the skeleton.

CONCEPT OF NEAP AND ITS POTENTIAL IMPACT ON THE SKELETON

To quantify further the link between acid–base balance and skeletal health, determination of the acid–base content of diets consumed by individuals and populations is a useful way forward. Pioneering work by Sebastian [47] and colleagues has shown us that, on a daily basis, humans eat substances that both generate and consume protons; as a result, consumption of a normal Western diet is associated with chronic, low-grade metabolic acidosis. The severity of the associated metabolic acidosis is determined, in part, by the net rate of endogenous noncarbonic acid production that varies with diet. Frassetto et al. [48], from Sebastian's group, proposed a simple algorithm to determine the rate of net endogenous noncarbonic acid production (NEAP) from considerations of the acidifying effect of protein (via sulfate excretion) and the alkalizing effect of potassium (via provision of salts of weak organic acids). They have found that the protein-to-potassium ratio predicts net acid excretion and, in turn, net renal acid excretion predicts

TABLE III Impact of Fruit and Vegetables on Bone: A Review of Population-Based Studies Showing a Positive Link

Author	Year	Source	Details	Findings
Eaton-Evans et al.	1993	Proc. Nutr. Soc. 52: 44A	77 females, 46–56 years old	Vegetables
Michaelsson et al.	1995	Calcified Tissue Int. 57: 86–93	175 females, 28–74 years old	K intake
New et al.	1997	Am. J. Clin. Nutr. 65: 1831–1839	994 females, 45–49 years old	K, Mg, fiber, vitamin C; past intake of fruits and vegetables
Tucker et al.	1999	Am. J. Clin. Nutr. 69: 727–736	229 males, 349 females, 75 years old	K, Mg, fruits and vegetables
New et al.	2000	Am. J. Clin. Nutr. 72: 142–151	62 females, 45–54 years old	K, Mg, fiber, vitamin C; past intake of fruit and vegetables
Jones et al.	2001	Am. J. Clin. Nutr. 73: 839–844	215 boys, 115 girls, (ages unknown)	K, urinary K
Chen et al.	2001	J. Bone Mineral Res. 16: S386	668 females (ages unknown)	Fruit
Miller et al.	2001	J. Bone Mineral Res. 16: S395	Males, 50–91 years old (number unknown)	K, Mg
Stone et al.	2001	J. Bone Mineral Res. 16: S388	1075 males, 65 years old and over	K, lutein
New et al.	2002	Osteoporosis Int. 13: S77	164 females, 55–87 years old	K, fruits and vegetables

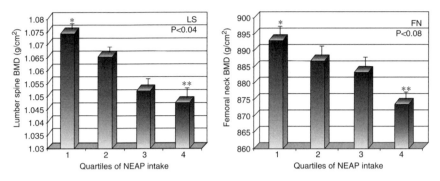

FIGURE 3   Association between net endogenous non-carbonic acid production (NEAP) and BMD in 994 women; Baseline values are shown for the lumbar spine and femoral neck BMD from Study 1 of the Aberdeen Prospective Osteoporosis Screening Study (APOSS).

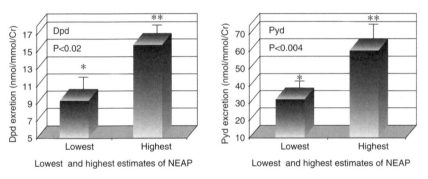

FIGURE 4   Association between net endogenous non-carbonic acid production (NEAP) and bone resorption in 62 women; Baseline values are show for the lumbar spine and femoral neck BMD from Study 2 of the Aberdeen Prospective Osteoporosis Screening Study (APOSS).

calcium excretion. Estimations of NEAP have been calculated from the Aberdeen Prospective Osteoporosis Screening Study (APOSS) baseline and longitudinal datasets. In the APOSS baseline, women with the lowest estimate of NEAP were found to have higher lumbar spine and femoral neck bone mineral density (Fig. 3) and significantly lower urinary pyridinium cross-link excretion (Fig. 4) [49]. Findings for bone resorption were mirrored in APOSS longitudinal studies. In 2323 women, adjusting for the key confounding factors, women with the lowest estimate of NEAP were found to have significantly lower pyridinoline and deoxypyridinoline excretion [50]. Further studies are now required to examine the effect of NEAP on indices of bone health in other age groups.

CALCIUM/ALKALI SUPPLEMENTS AND OPTIMUM BONE HEALTH

There is growing recognition that calcium may play a critical role in the relationship between the balance of a beneficial versus detrimental effect of protein on the skeleton [51–53]; hence, while it has yet to be proved, it is possible that calcium supplements may be favorable to bone, not just through the additional mineral that they supply but also through their provision of additional alkali salts [54]. Thus, it would be sensible to suggest reanalysis of existing nutrition and bone health datasets to focus specifically on the effect of protein-to-potassium ratios and protein-to-calcium ratios on indices of bone health. One possible hypothesis is that in the absence of sufficient dietary alkali to neutralize the protein-derived acid, net calcium loss ensues and the anabolic drive of dietary protein on the bone matrix is ineffective in maintaining bone mineral density.

FRUIT AND VEGETABLES AND BONE: EXPLORING OTHER IMPORTANT FACTORS

Exciting work by Muhlbauer and colleagues suggests that vegetables, herbs, and salads commonly consumed in the human diet affect bone resorption in the rat by a mechanism that is not mediated by their base excess [55] but possibly through pharmacologically active compounds which are currently being explored [56]. These data suggest that the positive associations found between fruit and vegetable consumption and bone may be due to some other, yet unidentified dietary component rather than alkali-excess effect [57] and is clearly an area for further research.

CONCLUDING REMARKS

The role that the skeleton plays in acid–base homeostasis has been gaining increasing prominence in the literature, and a number of observational, experimental, clinical, and intervention studies over the last decade have indicated a positive link between fruit and vegetable consumption and bone [58]. This is an exciting area for bone health research; work should now focus specifically on fruit and vegetables as the supplementation vehicle and should assess a wide range of bone health indices, including fracture risk. Also needed are experimental studies (at the cellular, animal, and human level) to determine other aspects of fruit and vegetables that are beneficial to bone metabolism, including key micronutrients and phytoestrogens.

ACKNOWLEDGMENTS

The author would like to pay special tribute to Professor Anthony Sebastian, Professor of Medicine and Co-Director of the General Clinical Research Center, University of California, San Francisco, California, for inspiring us all with his pioneering work, ideas, and dedication to the field of acid–base homeostasis and the skeleton.

REFERENCES

1. Kraut, J.A. and Coburn, J.W. (1994). Bone, acid and osteoporosis. New Engl. J. Med. 330: 1821–1822.
2. New, S.A. (2003). Intake of fruit and vegetables: implications for bone health. Proc. Nutr. Soc. 62: 889–899.
3. Green, J. and Kleeman, R. (1991). Role of bone in regulation of systematic acid–base balance [editorial review]. Kidney Int. 39: 9–26.
4. Frassetto, L.A., Morris, R.C., Jr., and Sebastian, A. (1996). Effect of age on blood acid–base composition in adult humans: role of age-related renal functional decline. Am. J. Physiol. (Renal Fluid Electrolyte Physiol.) 271: F1114–F1122.
5. Frassetto, L.A. and Sebastian, A. (1996). Age and systemic acid–base equilibrium: analysis of published data. J. Gerontol. 51A, B91–B99.
6. Barzel, U.S. (1995). The skeleton as an ion exchange system: implications for the role of acid–base imbalance in the genesis of osteoporosis. J. Bone Mineral Res. 10: 1431–1436.
7. Lemann, J., Jr., Litzow, J.R., and Lennon, E.J. (1966). The effects of chronic acid loads in normal man: further evidence for the participation of bone mineral in the defense against chronic metabolic acidosis. J. Clin. Invest. 45: 1608–1614.
8. Barzel, U.S. (1969). The effect of excessive acid feeding on bone. Calcified Tissue Res. 4: 94–100.
9. Wachman, A. and Bernstein, D.S. (1968). Diet and osteoporosis. Lancet I: 958–959.
10. Arnett, T.R. and Dempster, D.W. (1986). Effect of pH on bone resorption by rat osteoclasts in vitro. Endocrinology 119: 119–124.
11. Arnett, T.R. and Spowage, M. (1996). Modulation of the resorptive activity of rat osteoclasts by small changes in extracellular pH near the physiological range. Bone 18: 277–279.
12. Bushinsky, D.A. (1996). Metabolic alkalosis decreases bone calcium efflux by suppressing osteoclasts and stimulating osteoblasts. Am. J. Physiol. (Renal Fluid Electrolyte Physiol.), 271: F216–F222.
13. Meghji, S., Morrison, M.S., Henderson, B., and Arnett, T.R. (2001). pH dependence of bone resorption: mouse calvarial osteoclasts are activated by acidosis. Am. J. Physiol., Endocrinol. Metab. 280: E112–E119.
14. Fox D. (2001). Hard cheese. New Scientist Dec. 15, 42–45.
15. New, S.A., Macdonald, H.M., Reid, D.M., and Dixon, A.St.J. (2002). Hold the soda. New Scientist 2330: 54–55.
16. Plant, J. and Tidey, J. (2003). Understanding, Preventing and Overcoming Osteoporosis. Virgin Books, London.

17. New, S.A. and Francis, R. (2003). Book review. *Sci. Parliament. J.* 60(4): 21.

18. Remer, T. and Manz, F. (1995). Potential renal acid load of foods and its influence on urine pH. *J. Am. Diet. Assoc.* 95: 791–797.

19. New, S.A. (2001). Impact of food clusters on bone, in *Nutritional Aspects of Osteoporosis '2000: 4th International Symposium on Nutritional Aspects of Osteoporosis, Switzerland, 1997*, Dawson-Hughes, B., Burckhardt, P., and Heaney, R.P., Eds. Ares-Serono Symposia/Academic Press, San Diego, CA, pp. 379–397.

20. Lemann, J., Jr., Litzow, J.R., and Lennon, E.J. (1967). Studies of the mechanisms by which chronic metabolic acidosis augments urinary calcium excretion in man. *J. Clin. Invest.* 46: 1318–1328.

21. Lemann, J., Jr., Gray, R.W., Maierhofer, W.J., and Cheung, H.S. (1986). The importance of renal net acid excretion as a determinant of fasting urinary calcium excretion. *Kidney Int.* 29: 743–746.

22. Lemann, J., Jr., Gray, R.W., and Pleuss, J.A. (1989). Potassium bicarbonate, but not sodium bicarbonate, reduces urinary calcium excretion and improves calcium balance in healthy men. *Kidney Int.* 35: 688–695.

23. Lemann, J., Jr., Pleuss, J.A., Gray, R.W., and Hoffmann, R.G. (1991). Potassium administration increases and potassium deprivation reduces urinary calcium excretion in healthy adults. *Kidney Int.* 39: 973–983.

24. Bushinsky, D.A., Kreiger, N.S., Geisser, D.I., Grossman, E.B., and Coe, F.L.(1983). Effects of bone calcium and proton fluxes *in vitro*. *Am. J. Physiol.* 245: F204–F209.

25. Bushinsky, D.A. and Sessler, N.E. (1992). Critical role of bicarbonate in calcium release from bone. *Am. J. Physiol. (Renal Fluid Electrolyte Physiol.)* 263: F510–F515.

26. Bushinsky, D.A. Lam, B.C. Nespeca, R., Sessler, N.E., and Grynpas, M.D. (1993). Decreased bone carbonate content in response to metabolic, but not respiratory, acidosis. *Am. J. Physiol. (Renal Fluid Electrolyte Physiol.)* 265: F530–F536.

27. Bushinsky, D.A. (1997). Decreased potassium stimulates bone resorption. *Am. J. Physiol. (Renal Fluid Electrolyte Physiol.)* 272: F774–780.

28. Sebastian, A., Harris, S.T., Ottaway, J.H., Todd, K.M., and Morris, R.C., Jr. (1994). Improved mineral balance and skeletal metabolism in postmenopausal women treated with potassium bicarbonate. *New Engl. J. Med.* 330: 1776.

29. Buclin, T., Cosma, M., Appenzeller, M., Jacquet, A.F., Decosterd, L.A., Biollaz, J., and Burckhardt, P. (2001). Diet acids and alkalis influence calcium retention on bone. *Osteoporosis Int.* 12: 493–499.

30. Appel, L.J., Moore, T.J., Obarzanek, E., Vallmer, W.M., Svetkey, L.P., Sacks, F.M., Bray, G.A., Vogt, T.M., and Cutler, J.A. (1997). A clinical trial of the effects of dietary patterns on blood pressure. *New Engl. J. Med.* 336: 1117–1124.

31. Barzel, U.S. (1997). Dietary patterns and blood pressure [letter]. *New Engl. J. Med.* 337: 637.

32. Lin, P., Ginty, F., Appel, L., Svetky, L., Bohannon, A., Barclay, D., Gannon, R., and Aickin, M. (2001). Impact of sodium intake and dietary patterns on biochemical markers of bone and calcium metabolism. *J. Bone Mineral Re.* 16(suppl. 1): S511.

33. Eaton-Evans, J., McIlrath, E.M., Jackson, W.E., Bradley, P., and Strain, J.J. (1993). Dietary factors and vertebral bone density in perimenopausal women from a general medical practice in Northern Ireland [abstract]. *Proc. Nutr. Soc.* 52: 44A.

34. Michaelsson, K., Holmberg, L., Maumin, H., Wolk, A., Bergstrom, R., and Ljunghall, S. (1995). Diet, bone mass and osteocalcin: a cross-sectional study. *Calcified Tissue Int.* 57: 86–93.

35. New, S.A., Bolton-Smith, C., Grubb, D.A., and Reid, D.M. Nutritional influences on bone mineral density: a cross-sectional study in premenopausal women. *Am J Clin Nutr* (1997). 65: 1831–1839.

36. Tucker, K. L., Hannan, M.T., Chen, H., Cupples, A., Wilson, P.W.F., and Kiel, D.P. (1999). Potassium and fruit and vegetables are associated with greater bone mineral density in elderly men and women. *Am. J. Clin. Nutr.* 69: 727–736.

37. New, S.A., Robins, S.P., Campbell, M.K., Martin, J.C., Garton, M.J., Bolton-Smith, C., Grubb, D.A., Lee, S.J., and Reid, D.M. (2000). Dietary influences on bone mass and bone metabolism: further evidence of a positive link between fruit and vegetable consumption and bone health? *Am. J. Clin. Nutr.* 71: 142–151.

38. Chen, Y., Ho, S.C., Lee, R., Lam, S., and Woo, J. (2001). Fruit intake is associated with better bone mass among Hong Kong Chinese early postmenopausal women. *J. Bone Mineral Res.* 16(suppl. 1), S386.

39. Miller, D.R., Krall, E.A., Anderson, J.J., Rich, S.E., Rourke, A., and Chan, J. (2001). Dietary mineral intake and low bone mass in men: the VALOR Study. *J. Bone Mineral Res.* 16(suppl. 1), S395.

40. Stone, K.L., Blackwell, T., Orwoll, E.S., Cauley, J.C., Barrett-Connor, E., Marcus, R., Nevitt, M.C., and Cummings, S.R. (2001). The relationship between diet and bone mineral density in older men. *J. Bone Mineral Res.* 16(suppl. 1), S388.

41. Jones, G., Riley, M.D., and Whiting, S. (2001). Association between urinary potassium, urinary sodium, current diet, and bone density in prepubertal children. *Am. J. Clin. Nutr.* 73: 839–844.

42. New, S.A., Smith, R., Brown, J.C., and Reid, D.M. (2002). Positive associations between fruit and vegetable consumption and bone mineral density in late postmenopausal and elderly women. *Osteoporosis Int.* 13: S77.

43. Macdonald, H.M., New, S.A., Grubb, D.A., and Reid, D.M. (2002). Higher intakes of fruit and vegetables are associated with higher bone mass in perimenopausal Scottish women. *Proc. Nutr. Soc.* 60: 202A.

44. Whiting, S. (2002). *J. Nutr.*

45. Macdonald, H.M., New, S.A., Fraser, W.D., and Reid, D.M. (2002). Increased fruit and vegetable intake reduces bone turnover in early postmenopausal Scottish women. *Osteoporosis Int.* 13: S97.

46. Tylvasky, F., Holliday, K., Danish, R., Womack, C., Norwood, J., and Carbone, L. (2004). Fruit and vegetable intakes are an independent predictor of bone size in early pubertal children. *Am. J. Clin. Nutr.* 79: 311–317.

47. Kurtz, I., Maher, T., Hulter, H.N., Schambelan, M., and Sebastian, A. (1983). Effect of diet on plasma acid–base composition in normal humans. *Kidney Int.* 24: 670–680.

48. Frassetto, L., Todd, K., Morris, R.C., Jr., and Sebastian, A. (1998). Estimation of net endogenous noncarbonic acid production in humans from dietary protein and potassium contents. *Am. J. Clin. Nutr.* 68: 576–583.

49. New, S.A., MacDonald, H.M., Campbell, M.K., Martin, J.C., Garton, M.J., Robins, S.P., and Reid, D.M. (2004). Lower estimates of net endogenous noncarbonic acid production (NEAP) are positively associated with indices of bone health in pre/peri-menopausal women. *Am. J. Clin. Nutr.* 79: 131–138.

50. Macdonald, H.M., New, S.A., Fraser, W.D., and Reid, D.M. (2002). Estimates of NEAP are associated with increased bone turnover in early postmenopausal women: findings from APOSS longitudinal. *J. Bone Mineral Res.* 17: 1131.

51. Heaney, R.P. (1998). Excess dietary protein may not adversely affect bone. *J. Nutr.* 128: 1054–1057.

52. Dawson-Hughes, B. and Harris, S.S. (2002). Calcium intake influences the association of protein intake with rates of bone loss in elderly men and women. *Am. J. Clin. Nutr.* 75: 773–779.

53. Heaney, R.P. (2002). Protein and calcium: antagonists or synergists? *Am. J. Clin. Nutr.* 75: 609.

54. New, S.A. and Millward, D.J. (2003). Calcium, protein and fruit and vegetables as dietary determinants of bone health [letter]. *Am. J. Clin. Nutr.* 77: 1340–1341.
55. Muhlbauer, R.C., Lozano, A.M., Reinli, A. (2002). Onion and a mixture of vegetables, salads and herbs affect bone resorption in the rat by a mechanism independent of their base excess. *J. Bone Mineral Res.* 17: 1230–1236.
56. Muhlbauer, R.C., Felix, R., Lozano, A., Palacio, S., and Reinli, A. (2003). Common herbs, essential oils and monoterpenes potently modulate bone metabolism. *Bone* (in press).
57. Oh, M.S. and Uribarri, J. (1996). Bone buffering of acid: fact or fancy? *J. Nephrol.* 9: 261–262.
58. New, S.A. (2002). The role of the skeleton in acid–base homeostasis: the 2001 Nutrition Society Medal Lecture. *Proc. Nutr. Soc.* 61: 151–164.

PART VIII

Acid Load From Food—Second Part

The Ovine Model for the Study of Dietary Acid Base, Estrogen Depletion and Bone Health

JENNIFER M. MACLEAY,[1] D.L. WHEELER,[2] and A.S. TURNER[1]

[1]College of Veterinary Medicine and Biomedical Sciences; [2]College of Engineering, Colorado State University, Fort Collins, Colorado

ABSTRACT

The study of dietary-induced metabolic acidosis is a growing and important area of research with respect to achievement of peak bone mineral density and the development of osteoporosis. The development of an animal model in which to study dietary acidosis and bone health is essential to fully understand both the pathophysiology and the interplay of other factors such as estrogen depletion or exercise with dietary acidosis. Our laboratory has found *Ovis aries* (sheep) to be an excellent model. We have found that sheep are sensitive to dietary-induced metabolic acidosis and that the changes in bone at a histologic and biomechanical level are similar to those seen in human osteoporosis. This chapter is a summary of our research data to date. Ongoing and future studies will focus on the impact of dietary-induced metabolic acidosis on osteocalcin, vitamin D, cortisol, and parathyroid hormone concentrations in addition to bone static and dynamic histomorphology and mechanical testing in both mature and juvenile sheep.

Nutritional Aspects of Osteoporosis, Second Edition
Copyright © 2004 by Elsevier Science (USA)
All rights of reproduction in any form reserved.

331

INTRODUCTION

Postmenopausal osteoporosis is a multifactorial disease influenced by genetics, lifestyle, geography, living arrangements (vitamin D status), and dietary factors. Recognizing that all factors contributing to osteoporosis are important areas of research, our laboratory is particularly interested in the influence of diet on the development and treatment of osteoporosis. Recent studies support that consumption of a diet rich in anions relative to cations (i.e., dietary cation–anion difference, or DCAD; potential renal acid load of foods) leads to metabolic acidosis [21]. The body responds to chronic metabolic acidosis by mobilizing calcium as a physiologic buffer. This ultimately leads to a total body depletion of calcium that is at least partially independent of the calcium content of the diet. The proposed mechanism through which this occurs is by increasing the body's sensitivity to parathyroid hormone as well as a consistent, non-pulsatile hyperparathyroidism [14]. Moderate hyperparathyroidism has been described in type 1 osteoporosis in the elderly. Therefore, these two mechanisms may be similar and possibly additive in their affect on bone, ultimately leading to severe bone mineral loss.

Several excellent reviews concerning the influence of dietary acid–base exist in the literature of both human and veterinary medicine [10,21,22,24]; however, many questions remain unanswered with respect to how strong an influence dietary acid–base has on the development of osteoporosis. Our laboratory is advocating the use of the ewe as an ideal model to study this affect. The purpose of this chapter is to provide some review of the veterinary use of dietary acid–base and the profound affect we have seen in the ewe as we investigate the influence of dietary acid–base metabolism.

BACKGROUND AND SIGNIFICANCE

A true non-primate, postmenopausal osteoporosis model has been an elusive target for researchers. Most animal species when ovariectomized maintain bone mineral density in the face of estrogen depletion. Sheep have many advantages that make them an excellent model in which to study osteoporosis. Sheep are seasonally polyestrous and have been shown to lose bone mineral density after ovariectomy [37]. Because they are housed in groups they are very inexpensive to house and are a readily available large animal model. The single drawback in using sheep as a model for studying osteoporosis has been the inability to achieve levels of bone loss comparable to those seen in human postmenopausal osteoporosis with ovariectomy alone. One reason that may be contributing to the scientific community's inability to find an adequate animal model for osteoporosis may be neglect of the confounding factors, other than estrogen depletion, that contribute to the development of osteoporosis. One such important confounding factor is diet. Non-primate mammalian diets are rich in alkalinizing foods that do not induce metabolic acidosis as modern human diets do; therefore, diet may account for at least some of the interspecies variation we see with respect to loss of bone in older mammals.

In human beings, osteoporosis is a multifactorial disorder being influenced by genetics, environment, lifestyle, and dietary factors. Several authors have strongly implicated chronic, dietary metabolic acidosis as being a major factor in the development of osteoporosis in patients from Western societies [5]. We hope to use this animal model to investigate more deeply the relationship between the combined effect of diet on metabolic acid–base.

A true animal model of postmenopausal osteoporosis has been elusive to researchers. Primates are the only non-human mammal to experience a natural menopause; however, research using primates is costly and has public policy concerns. The ovariectomized mature rat has also been studied, but its major drawback is the lack of secondary remodeling in bone. In addition, studies of dietary-induced metabolic acidosis and bone physiology in the rat may not be ideal as rats have not been found to show a negative calcium balance under conditions of high protein feeding, and therefore may not be the model of choice for studying protein-induced hypercalciuruia [40]. A large animal model of postmenopausal osteoporosis used successfully by our laboratory and others is the mature, ovariectomized ewe. The sheep has secondary remodeling of the skeleton, has an estrous cycle that is similar to humans 6 months of the year, and has shown sensitivity to estrogen depletion [16,25,33–38]. In addition, the ewe is an economic and practical large animal model compared to the primate and remarkably comparable in cost to small mammals such as the pig or rabbit.

THE INFLUENCE OF DIETARY STRONG IONS

The affects of dietary strong ions on acid–base physiology and subsequently calcium metabolism are profound. Dietary strong ions are absorbed from the intestinal tract into the blood stream and there exert a direct affect on the body's acid–base status. According to Stewart's theories, acid–base state is determined by three independent variables; the strong ions (or strong ion difference), total protein, and plasma carbon dioxide (P_{CO2}) [29]. In the absence of pathology, dietary strong ions are the major influence on the body's acid–base status. A mild metabolic acidosis ensues when anions predominate in the diet and this is referred to as a diet low in cation–anion difference (low DCAD); other common used terminology includes potential renal acid load and acid/alkaline ash diets. The mammalian body responds to chronic dietary metabolic acidosis by mobilizing calcium from bone to act as a buffer in order to maintain relative electroneutrality. The kidney then excretes the mobilized calcium and the excess dietary ions in the urine [7,8,19,26,28,39,40].

Dietary anthropologists have proposed that the present day human diet is dramatically different from that of humans 10 to 90,000 years ago [4]. During ancient times, humans were primarily hunter-gatherers who existed on a high-calorie diet consisting largely of fruits, vegetables, and lean game. This diet has overall a low acid load to an alkalinizing load for the body. Over the last 10,000, years humans have consumed increasingly larger proportions of cultivated grains such that grains now comprise the majority of our caloric intake on a daily basis. In addition, the nutrient demands of the modern human are similar to those of ancient humans. But, because of decreased activity, our total caloric intake is typically less and therefore our total mineral intake is less than ancient humans. This lower overall intake of minerals may be suboptimal for long-term health. While the implications, pros, and cons of the modern human diet compared to that of ancient humans may be weighed against each other on many levels, our laboratory and others have focused on one particular aspect of this modernization of the human diet. Compared to the ancient diets, modern humans now typically consume foods that are rich in proteins (which are high in sulfur-containing amino acids) and relatively low in potassium. This leads to a state of low grade, dietary-induced metabolic acidosis.

Long-term dietary-induced metabolic acidosis does not appear to be immediately detrimental to health, but researchers are now hypothesizing that this subtle change in diet is contributing to the onset of osteoporosis because it causes long-term leaching of calcium from bone [4,5,7,23,26]. The affect of a diet that overall is low in DCAD has become more important with the progress of modern medicine and the inherently longer, postmenopausal lifespan of modern women and men. The shift from a relatively high-potassium and low-protein diet to the converse shifts the strong ion intake such that the diet's influence on blood pH becomes more acidifying than alkalinizing. The longer life span of humans also appears to be a confounder. With age, the ability of the human kidney to excrete acid declines. This further exacerbates the acidifying affect of modern diets [11,26].

The major ionic buffer utilized by the mammalian body to combat metabolic acidosis is calcium that is recruited primarily from bone. This occurs through several mechanisms: (1) recruitment of calcium from the fluid around bone, (2) direct stimulation of osteoclasts in the face of acidosis, and (3) an increase in the sensitivity of bone to parathyroid hormone (PTH). The increased sensitivity to PTH is interesting, as it is a similar mechanism proposed to occur in women during the rapid phase of bone loss occurring in the months and early years after menopause [2].

Bone is a unique organ in that it is constantly being remodeled. Bone turnover is characterized by two opposite activities: the formation of new bone by osteoblasts and the resorption of old bone by osteoclasts. Metabolic acidosis induces mobilization of the soluble calcium pool in the bone milieu and stimulates osteoclasts while inhibiting osteoblasts, thereby releasing calcium from hydroxyapatite crystals into the circulation [6,7]. Over time, increased intestinal absorption of calcium appears to occur as well but does not overcome the calcium loss. Based on our and others' preliminary data, the mammalian body does not appear to override osteopenia with enhanced calcium retention. That is, in the face of ongoing chronic metabolic acidosis, the body will largely continue wasting skeletal calcium despite progressive osteopenia. In older mammals decreased kidney function is a common consequence to aging. In humans, this age-related decrease in renal function compounds dietary-induced metabolic acidosis as the kidney becomes less able to excrete dietary acids [10,26].

It has been assumed that, provided total dietary calcium intake is adequate, a mild metabolic acidosis would not adversely affect bone health. Research has revealed that this assumption is invalid. Studies in humans and rodents and our data for sheep all support that, despite being provided what would typically be considered sufficient calcium intake, long-term mild or severe metabolic acidosis leads to overall loss of bone mineral and contributes to the onset of osteopenia and osteoporosis [1,3,8,9,11,12,14,15,17,19,22,23,27,28,30–32,39,40].

The effect of alkalinizing diets has been less well studied; however, it has been proposed that alkalinizing diets may offset the loss of bone by astronauts [9]. In addition, studies have been performed to investigate if dietary alkalinization can improve calcium balance [26]. Daily oral intake of potassium bicarbonate has been experimentally implemented in humans with the goal of neutralizing consumed acids or endogenous acid production. The investigators observed a 27% reduction in urinary calcium loss and a 31% increase in positive calcium balance. They also observed significant decreases in urinary hydroxyproline, a biomarker of bone resorption, and increases in serum osteocalcin, a biomarker of bone formation. The results from several similar studies suggest that $KHCO_3$, other potassium salts, or alkalinizing salts of other cations may be used to similarly improve calcium balance. This evidence points to the possibility that manipulation of DCAD in postmenopausal women with abnormal bone turnover could be beneficial [26].

Certainly, research using a large animal model would further our knowledge concerning the influence of diet on acid–base balance and ultimately bone health. A significant advantage of using a large animal model is that we are able to more fully elucidate the effects of diet on bone using large bone sampling, biomarkers of bone turnover, bone biomechanical testing, bone histomorphometry, and microcomputerized tomography.

DETERMINATION OF DIETARY ACID LOAD

Different equations have been used in the literature to determine the potential for a particular diet to induce metabolic acidosis. All ions consumed from food have the potential to contribute to the acid–base balance of the individual. Researchers have investigated the intricacies of the relationship among all ions in the diet and have formulated several equations to accurately reflect the overall cation–anion difference of the diet. The formulation of the equations depends on the strong ions that the researcher is interested in investigating and may reflect the intestinal absorption of the nutrient.

In veterinary medicine, the ability of a diet to lead to metabolic acidosis or alkalosis has been described by several equations, including:

$$DCAD \ (mEq) = (Na + K + Ca + Mg) - (Cl + S + P)$$

$$DCAD \ (mEq) = (Na + K + (0.38 \times Ca) + (0.30 \times Mg)) - (Cl + (0.6 \times S) + (0.5 \times P))$$

$$DCAD \ (mEq) = (Na + K + (0.15 \times Ca + (0.15 \times Mg) - (Cl + 0.2 \times S + 0.3 \times P)$$

$$Strong \ ion \ difference \ (mEq) = (Na + K) - (Cl)$$

$$DCAD \ (mEq) = (Na + K) - (Cl + S)$$

The final equation has been found to be both highly correlated to the incidence of periparturient hypocalcemia in dairy cows and simple to calculate for the average veterinary nutritionist, and it has become the *de facto* standard for calculating the DCAD of a diet for dairy cattle [22]. Convention is that the dietary DCAD value is expressed as milliequivalents per kilogram of dietary dry matter. One drawback of this equation is that it does not take into account the total dietary intake of cations and anions which is related to the total caloric intake (body weight) of the individual.

In human medicine, the following equations have been proposed in the literature:

$$mEq = Organic \ acids + sulfuric \ acids - base$$

$$RNAE = (Cl + P + SO_4 + \text{organic acids}) - (Na - K - Ca - Mg)$$

$$\text{Inorganic cation} - \text{anion difference (mEq)} = (Na + K + Ca + Mg) - (Cl + P)$$

$$RNAE = 62.1 \times (\text{protein}/K) - 17.9 \text{ (energy adjusted)}$$

$$RNAE = (0.91 \times \text{protein}) - (0.57 \times K) + 21 \text{ (non-energy adjusted)}$$

$$RNAE = (0.94 \times \text{protein}) - (0.61 \times K) + 22 \text{ (energy adjusted)}$$

$$NEAP = 86.745 - (0.669 \times K) + (0.469 \times \text{Protein})$$

where RNAE is renal net acid excretion, and NEAP is net endogenous acid production.

There are advantages and disadvantages for each equation listed above, and it is likely that no single equation would be best suited for both human and animal studies. In animal studies, the rations can be exactly controlled such that the exact intake of sulfur can be determined, whereas in human studies the amino acid composition of different proteins varies such that the sulfur content of the total diet is often estimated. In addition, the human diet contains relatively large quantities of table salt as $NaCl$ such that the contributions of sodium and chloride to the overall cation–anion balance of the diet is less than it is in composed animal rations. Therefore, it may be more acceptable to omit sodium and chloride from human dietary equations than it would be when calculating DCAD for an experimental animal's ration. When the diet is shifted to induce metabolic acidosis, the cause in humans is likely due to reduced potassium intake and increased intake of sulfur. When altering the ration for experimental animals, the easiest way to induce metabolic acidosis is by decreasing potassium intake and increasing chloride intake by adding ammonium chloride. Convention in veterinary medicine is to discuss the potential acidifying affect of the diet as milliequivalents per kilogram of dry matter of feed or total ration. This does not take into account the total amount consumed by animals of varying body weight. In human studies, the acid load for a particular diet and for a given caloric intake on a per-day basis is more commonly used.

In general, non-primate mammalian calcium intake is quite large in comparison to human intake. A typical ration of hay for sheep provides 10 g of calcium per day, and our metabolic-acidosis-induction diet contained approximately 8 g of calcium per day. While the experimental diet contained 6 g less of calcium per day, both values are well in excess of the recommended intake for humans of comparable weight.

THE DAIRY CONNECTION

While the influence of dietary strong ions exists in all mammals, the influence of strong ions consumed in the diet has been extensively studied and exploited in the modern feeding and management of dairy cows [13]. Post-parturient hypocalcemia is a common and potentially lethal consequence to calving for present-day dairy cows that are bred for excessive milk production. Immediately postpartum, the genetically superior dairy cow rapidly produces large quantities of milk. Large quantities of milk contain large quantities of calcium and the amount of calcium secreted into the milk outstrips the cow's relatively quiescent physiologic mechanisms to mobilize calcium. The increased calcium demand initiates the mobilization of calcium through increased intestinal absorption, decreased renal excretion, and increased mobilization from bone. It takes several days for physiologic mechanisms to become fully active, especially those responsible for increased mobilization of calcium from bone. Research has shown that placing a cow on a low DCAD diet at least 4 to 7 days prepartum greatly reduces the incidence of post-parturient hypocalcemia. This primes the mechanisms responsible for inducing increased bone turnover prior to the onset of increased calcium demand and is far more effective than simply increasing dietary calcium intake alone [13,14]. After calving, the cow is moved to a high-calcium diet that is high in DCAD for the remainder of her milking period; therefore, dairy cows are only exposed to low DCAD diets for the 1 to 4 weeks prior to calving, and long-term effects of low DCAD diets have not been investigated in non-human mammals. It does appear that sheep respond similarly to cattle with respect to dietary cation–anion differences based on a series of studies that were performed by Takagi et al. [30–32].

PRELIMINARY STUDIES

The interaction of diet and acid–base status and progressive bone loss is a newer field of study with regard to osteoporosis. Research using a large animal model has not been reported to any significant degree in the literature. While research in the rat is often useful with regard to bone, the rat does not appear to be as useful in the study of diet, acid–base, and osteoporosis as it lacks secondary remodeling of the skeleton to any large degree and appears to adapt quickly to dietary-induced metabolic acidosis [40]. Substantial amounts of information need to be acquired to fully understand the interplay and the impact of long-term metabolic acidosis as influenced by diet on bone health. We need to examine the predominant factors in the development of osteoporosis to begin to understand how they interact to induce bone loss and how this bone loss compares to that seen in humans.

Our laboratory has completed two preliminary studies examining the effect of dietary strong ions on the development of osteoporosis using the postmenopausal model, the mature ovariectomized sheep. The studies examined sheep consuming an acidifying diet for up to a year. Our studies indicate that osteoporosis can be induced by a diet sufficient in calcium but low in cation–anion difference regardless of ovariectomy. The metabolic acidosis induced by these diets caused significant increases in calcium wasting in the urine, decreased bone mineral density, and increased bone fragility. The data suggest that the decrease in bone mineral density and increased fragility are at least partially synergistic between ovariectomy and the low DCAD diet.

EFFECT OF A DIET LOW IN CATION–ANION BALANCE ON BONE MINERAL DENSITY IN MATURE OVARIECTOMIZED EWES

Our laboratory has conducted several studies and has additional studies ongoing that examine the affect of dietary acid–base on bone metabolism [18,20]. In the first, short-term study, we examined the bone mineral density of the lumbar spine in two groups of sheep. In both groups, we saw a significant affect of the metabolic-acidosis-inducing diet to cause bone loss at the lumbar spine at 3 and 6 months. Ovariectomy (OVX) alone led to bone loss, but overall bone mineral density was not significantly lower compared to control sheep at 6 months. This finding is similar to that of previous studies [38]. We saw a tendency for the combination of OVX and dietary metabolic acidosis to increase bone mineral density loss as an additive affect (Fig. 1). Mean decreases in bone mineral density were 1 to 2 standard deviations below age-matched controls. A T-score to compare bone mineral densities to individuals of peak bone mineral density could not be performed, as the age of and the value of peak bone mineral density in sheep are unknown. Details of the diet consumed are presented in Table I.

Mandibles recovered at necropsy at 6 months had a similar pattern of bone mineral density loss as measured by dual-energy x-ray absorptiometry (DEXA). When mandibles were examined by DEXA 12 months after OVX and consuming the metabolic acidosis diet we saw significantly greater loss of bone mineral density in sheep consuming the metabolic acidosis diet (Figs. 2 and 3). Consistent with human osteoporosis, the greatest decreases

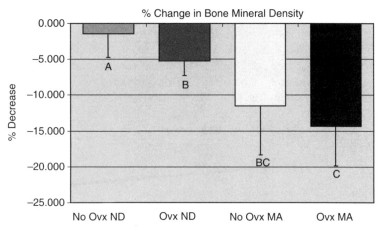

% Change in Bone Mineral Density

Group: Mean of 6 sheep per group at 6 months compared to baseline with
Standard Deviation shown.

FIGURE 1   Percent change in bone mineral density. OVX, ovariectomy; ND, normal diet;
MA, metabolic-acidosis-inducing diet. Unlike letters are significantly different from one another
at $P \leq 0.05$.

in bone mineral density were seen in bones rich in cancellous bone versus
cortical bone (Figs. 4 and 5).

Bone markers, serum bone alkaline phosphatase and urine deoxypyridinoline, were increased in sheep consuming the metabolic acidosis diet and that
had been ovariectomized; however, compared to the DEXA results, no
additive affect between OVX and dietary-induced metabolic acidosis was seen.
Urinary fractional excretion of calcium and phosphorus was greatly increased
in sheep consuming the metabolic-acidosis-inducing diet compared to
controls and sheep that had been ovariectomized alone.

Vertebral body strength was found to be significantly decreased in sheep
consuming the metabolic acidosis diet compared to control sheep and
sheep that were ovariectomized but consumed a normal diet (Figs. 6
and 7). Similar to the BMD findings, there was a trend towards an additive
affect between diet and OVX with respect to increasing weakness. Bone
histology revealed increased void star volume and thinner trabeculae in
sheep consuming the metabolic acidosis diet compared to controls (Fig. 5).
Biomechanical data supported that the significant decrease in bone mineral
density loss was associated with a significant decrease in bone strength
and modulus. Bone strength was least in the metabolic acidosis/OVX group,
supporting a potential synergy between these two modalities in inducing
osteoporosis.

TABLE 1 Total Amount Consumed per Day (Assuming an Intake of Approximately 3000 kcal per Day per 80-kg Sheep)

	Na g (mEq)	K g (mEq)	S g (mEq)	Cl g (mEq)	Mg g (mEq)	P g (mEq)	Ca g (mEq)	Crude Protein (g)	Acid Load (mEq)
ND	0.41 (17)	44.8 (1145)	3.5 (218)	6.2 (176)	4 (329)	3.5 (203)	10.8 (536)	208	1011
MA	5.95 (258)	31 (800)	14.5 (903)	27.25 (769)	8.4 (691)	5.58 (324)	7.9 (390)	304	174

Note: ND, normal dietary cation difference; MA, low dietary cation–anion difference, metabolic acidosis inducing diet. Acid load is computed as $(Na + K + [0.15 \times Ca] + [0.15 \times Mg]) - ([Cl + (0.2 \times S] + [0.3 \times P])$.

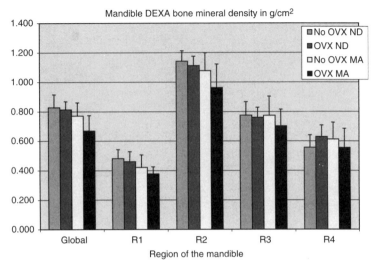

FIGURE 2 Mandibular dual x-ray absorptiometry (DEXA) for differing regions of the mandible at 6 months. OVX, ovariectomy; ND, normal diet; MA, metabolic-acidosis-inducing diet; global, whole mandible; R1, caudal to molar teeth; R2, molar teeth region; R3, interdental space; R4, incisors.

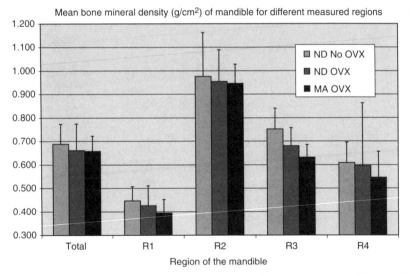

FIGURE 3 Mandibular dual x-ray absorptiometry (DEXA) for differing regions of the mandible at 12 months. Group sizes were 21 ND/OVX, 18 ND/no OVX, and 23 MA/OVX. MA/no OVX were not available for comparison. OVX, ovariectomy; ND, normal diet; MA, metabolic-acidosis-inducing diet; global, whole mandible; R1, caudal to molar teeth; R2, molar teeth region; R3, interdental space; R4, incisors.

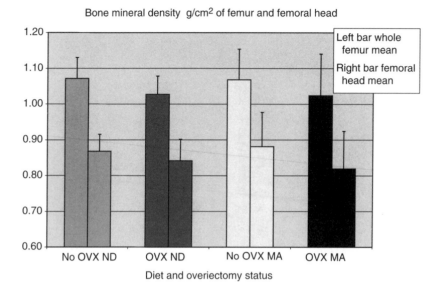

FIGURE 4   Bone mineral density (g/cm^2) of the femur and femoral head for 4 groups of 6 sheep at 6 months.

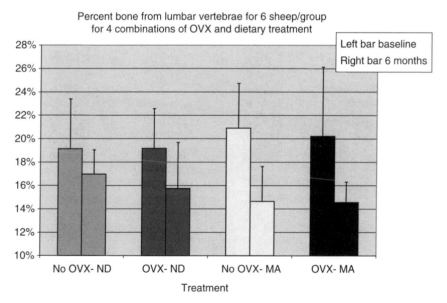

FIGURE 5   Histological analysis; percent bone from lumbar vertebrae for 6 sheep per group at baseline and 6 months. OVX, ovariectomy; ND, normal diet, MA, metabolic-acidosis-inducing diet.

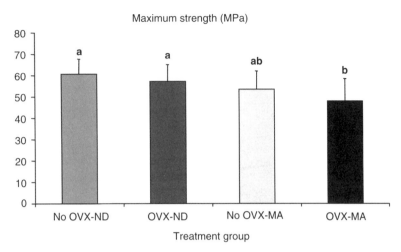

FIGURE 6   Maximum strength of L3 and L5 whole vertebral bodies; mean of 6 sheep per group at 6 months.

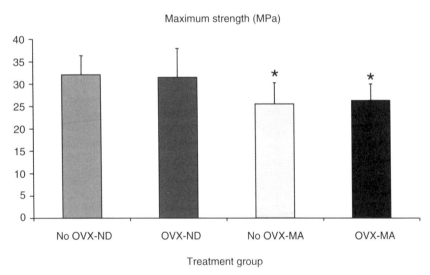

FIGURE 7   Maximum trabecular cube strength of L7. Mean of 6 sheep per group at 6 months. No OVX/ND, OVX/ND > no OVX/MA, OVX/MA ($P < 0.05$).

When histological sections of lumbar vertebrae were analyzed, we found a significant decrease in percent bone (Fig. 5). An analysis of variance (ANOVA) found the metabolic acidosis/no OVX group to be significantly lower at 6 months compared to time zero ($P = 0.0099$), and the metabolic acidosis/OVX group was also significantly lower at 6 months compared to time zero ($P = 0.048$). There was not a significant difference in the other two groups. Further histological analyses including star volume, trabecular thickness, and dynamic histomorphometry (including mineralizing surface, mineral apposition rate, and bone formation rate) are currently being performed.

These findings are similar to that seen in type 1, estrogen-depletion-associated osteoporosis in humans. Supportive of this conclusion was the finding that BMD of the femoral head was not significantly decreased in the sheep examined (Fig. 4). A significant decrease in femoral head BMD is more associated with type 2 or senile osteoporosis in humans. In this case, it may simply reflect sites of rapid (vertebral) versus slow (femoral head/neck) bone loss tied to and independent of areas of high cortical versus trabecular bone content.

CONCLUSION

A true non-primate postmenopausal osteoporosis model has been an elusive target for researchers. Certainly, in human beings osteoporosis is a multifactorial disorder being influenced by genetics, environment, lifestyle, as well as dietary factors. By examining the combined effect of diet and estrogen depletion we hope to move the sheep forward as a more useful animal model. In addition, we hope to shed light on the interaction between diet and estrogen depletion as a potential cause for why estrogen depletion has an apparent different effect on bone mineral density loss and strength in different groups of women. In addition, the study of metabolic alkalosis as a potential tool in preventing, treating, or offsetting the effects of estrogen depletion has not heretofore been investigated in a large animal model. Additional answers concerning the methods by which dietary acidosis increases bone turnover by investigating changes in vitamin D status and parathyroid hormone are areas of future investigation.

ACKNOWLEDGMENTS

The studies described here were conducted at the Colorado State University's Small Ruminant Comparative Orthopaedic Research Laboratory and were supported with funding from the CSU College Research Council, Stryker Biotech, Inc., and the National Institutes of Health (Grant R01 AR47434-01).

REFERENCES

1. Barzel, U. (1995). The skeleton as an ion exchange system: implications for the role of acid–base imbalance in the genesis of osteoporosis. *J. Bone Mineral Res.* 10: 1431–6.
2. Bilezikian, J. and Silverberg, S. (2001). The role of parathyroid hormone and vitamin D in the pathogenesis of osteoporosis, in *Osteoporosis*, Vol. 2, Marcus, R., Feldman, D., and Kelsey, J., Eds. Academic Press, San Diego, pp. 71–84.
3. Bogert, J. *et al.* (1922). The effects of acid-forming and base forming diets upon calcium and magnesium metabolism. *J. Biol. Chem.* 54: 375–386.
4. Boyd Eaton, S. and Cordain, L. (1997). Evolutionary aspects of diet: old genes, new fuels. *World Rev. Nutr. Diet* 81: 26–37.
5. Brown, S. and Jaffe, R. (2000). Acid–alkaline balance and its effect on bone health. *Int. J. Integrative Med.* 2(6): 1–12.
6. Bushinsky, D. (1996). Metabolic alkalosis decreases bone calcium efflux by suppressing osteoclasts and stimulating osteoblasts. *Am. J. Physiol.* 271: F216–F222.
7. Bushinsky, D. (2001). Chronic acidosis: calcium release. *Eur. J. Nutr.* 40: 240–244.
8. El-Maraghi, N., Platt, B., and Stewart, R. (1965). The effect of interaction of dietary protein and calcium on the growth and maintenance of the bone of young adult and aged rats. *Br. J. Nutr.* 19: 491–509.
9. Fettman, M.J. (2000). Dietary instead of pharmacological management to counter the adverse effects of physiological adaptations to space flight. *Pflügers Arch. Eur. J. Physiol.* 441(suppl.): R15–R20.
10. Frassetto, L., Morris, R.J., Sellmeyer, D., Todd, K., and Sebastian, A. (2001). Diet, evolution and aging: the pathophysiolgic effects of post-agricultural inversion of the potassium-to-sodium and base-to-chloride ratios in the human diet. *Eur. J. Nutr.* 40: 200–213.
11. Frassetto, L., Todd, K., Morris, R.J., and Sebastian, A. (1998). Estimation of net endogenous noncarbonic acid production in humans from diet potassium and protein contents. *Am. J. Clin. Nutr.* 68: 576–583.
12. Givens, M. (1917). Studies in calcium and magnesium metabolism: the effects of base and acid. *J. Biol. Chem.* 31: 421–433.
13. Goff, J.P. (1987). The pathophysiology and prevention of milk fever. *Vet. Med.* 82: 943–950.
14. Goff, J.P., Horst, R.L., and Mueller, F.J. (1991). Addition of chloride to a prepartal diet high in cations increases 1,25-dihydroxyvitamin D response to hypocalcemia preventing milk fever. *J. Dairy Sci.* 74: 3863–3871.
15. Hu, J., Zhao, X., Parpia, B., and Campbell, T. (1993). Dietary intakes and urinary excretion of calcium and acids: a cross sectional study of women in China. *Am. J. Clin. Nutr.* 58: 398–406.
16. Lill, C.A., Fluegel, A.K., and Schneider, E. (2000). Sheep model for fracture treatment in osteoporotic bone: a pilot study about different induction regimens. *J. Orthop. Trauma* 14: 559–565.
17. MacLeay, J., Les, C., Toth, C., Wheeler, D., and Turner, A.S. (2002). Effect of a diet low in cation–anion balance on bone mineral density in mature ovariectomized ewes. *J. Vet. Int. Med.* 16: 338.
18. MacLeay, J., Olson, J.D., Toth, C., Wheeler, D., and Turner, A.S. (2003). Effect of an acidifying diet on bone mineral density, bone alkaline phosphatase and urine deoxypyridinoline in mature ovariectomized ewes, in Proceedings of the 49th Orthopedic Research Society, New Orleans, p. 380.
19. Margen, S., Chu, J., Kaufmann, N., and Calloway, D. (1974). Studies in calcium metabolism. 1. The calciuretic effect of dietary protein. *Am. J. Clin. Nutr.* 27: 584–589.

20. Millets, J., MacLeay, J., Turner, A.S., and Wheeler, D. (2003). Skeletal fragility associated with a low cation–anion difference diet in mature ewes, in Proceedings of the 49th Orthopedic Research Society, New Orleans, p. 54.
21. New, S. (2002). The role of the skeleton in acid–base homeostasis. *Proc. Nutr. Soc.* 61: 151–164.
22. Oetzel, G.R. (1993). Use of anionic salts for prevention of milk fever in dairy cattle. *The Compendium* 15: 1138–1145.
23. Remer, T. *et al.* (1995). Potential renal acid load of foods and its influence on urine pH. *J. Am. Diet. Assoc.* 95.
24. Riond, J. (2001). Animal nutrition and acid base balance. *Eur. J. Nutr.* 40: 245–254.
25. Rubin, C., Turner, A.S., Mallinckrodt, C., and McLeod, K. (2001). Anabolism: low mechanical signals strengthen bone. *Nature* 412: 603–604.
26. Sebastian, A., Harris, S., Ottaway, J., Todd, K., and Morris, R.J. (1994). Improved mineral balance and skeletal metabolism in postmenopausal women treated with potassium bicarbonate. *New Engl. J. Med.* 23: 1776–1781.
27. Sherman, H. (1912). The balance of acid-forming and base forming elements in foods, and its relation to ammonia metabolism. *J. Biol. Chem.* 11.
28. Spencer, H., Krammer, L., Osis, D., and Norris, R. (1978). Effect of high protein (meat) intake on calcium metabolism in man. *Am. J. Clin. Nutr.* 31: 2167–2180.
29. Stewart, P. (1983). Modern quantitative acid–base chemistry. *Can. J. Physiol. Pharmacol.* 61: 1444–1461.
30. Takagi, H. and Block, E. (1991). Effects of manipulating dietary cation–anion balance on macromineral balance in sheep. *J. Dairy Sci.* 74: 4202–4214.
31. Takagi, H. and Block, E. (1991). Effects of reducing dietary cation–anion balance on calcium kinetics in sheep. *J. Dairy Sci.* 74: 4225–4237.
32. Takagi, H. and Block, E. (1991). Effects of various dietary cation–anion balances on response to experimentally induced hypocalcemia in sheep. *J. Dairy Sci.* 74: 4215–4224.
33. Turner, A.S. (2001). Animal models of osteoporosis: necessity and limitations. *Eur. Cells Mater.* 1: 66–81.
34. Turner, A.S. (2001). Research in orthopedic surgery, in *Surgical Research*, Souba, W. and Wilmore, D., Eds., Academic Press, San Diego, pp. 80-1 to 80-64.
35. Turner, A.S. (2002). The sheep as a model for osteoporosis in humans. *Vet. J.* 163: 1–8.
36. Turner, A.S., Alvis, M., Mallinckrodt, C., and Bryant, H. (1995). Dose response effects of estradiol on bone mineral density in ovariectomized ewes. *Bone* 17(suppl.): 421S–427S.
37. Turner, A.S., Alvis, M., Mallinckrodt, C., and Bryant, H. (1995). Dual-energy x-ray absorptiometry in sheep: experiences with *in vivo* and *in vitro* studies. *Bone* 17(suppl.): 381S–387S.
38. Turner, A.S., Alvis, M., Myers, W., Stevens, M.L., and Lundy, M.W. (1995c). Changes in bone mineral density and bone-specific alkaline phosphatase in ovariectomized ewes. *Bone* 17(suppl.): 395S–402S.
39. Whiting, S. and Draper, H. (1980). The role of sulfate in the calciuria of high protein diets in adult rats. *J. Nutr.* 110, 212–222.
40. Whiting, S.J., and HH, D. (1981). Effect of chronic high protein feeding on bone composition in the adult rat. *J. Nutr.* 111: 178–183.

CHAPTER 26

The Natural Dietary Potassium Intake of Humans: The Effect of Diet-Induced Potassium-Replete, Chloride-Sufficient, Chronic Low-Grade Metabolic Alkalosis, or Stone Age Diets for the 21st Century

LYNDA A. FRASSETTO, R. CURTIS MORRIS, JR., and ANTHONY SEBASTIAN
Department of Medicine and General Clinical Research Center, University of California, San Francisco, California

ABSTRACT

Our preagricultural hominid ancestors ate diets consisting of uncultivated and relatively unprocessed animal and plant foods readily available in the environment. Such diets contain abundant potassium and scant sodium and chloride. In contrast, typical diets in industrialized countries today contain much less potassium and much more sodium and chloride. Because potassium in foods exists largely as salts of organic acids, such as potassium citrate or malate, which the body metabolizes to potassium bicarbonate, today's typical diet supplies relatively small amounts of potential

Nutritional Aspects of Osteoporosis, Second Edition
Copyright © 2004 by Elsevier Science (USA)
All rights of reproduction in any form reserved.

bicarbonate. Our preagricultural ancestors' potassium-rich diet, therefore, likely contained much larger quantities of potential bicarbonate than our contemporary diet.

Hypothesizing a large variety of possible preagricultural hominid diets based on nutritional anthropological criteria, we estimated the range of likely intakes of potassium and bicarbonate precursors by ancestral hominids and early humans. Within paleoanthropologically accepted bounds of animal-to-plant food ratios and animal fat densities of ancestral diets, ancestral hominid potassium intakes ranged from 295 to 542 mEq/day—4 to 7 times greater than the third National Health and Examination Survey (NHANES III) average of 76 mEq/day. Net endogenous acid production (NEAP) averaged −88 ± 82 mEq/day; the negative value is indicative of net bicarbonate production, sufficient to sustain a mild metabolic alkalosis. In contrast, contemporary diets yield positive values for NEAP and sustain a mild metabolic acidosis.

Accordingly, we suggest that the natural, and therefore presumably optimal, potassium and acid–base state of humans is a potassium-rich, chloride-sufficient, chronic-low-grade metabolic alkalosis. Assuming that all organisms are best fitted to the environment that prevailed when the genes of their ancestors were naturally selected, contemporary humans live in a nutritional potassium and acid–base environment mismatched to their genetically conditioned metabolism and physiology. That mismatch has implications for bone health.

ANCESTRAL DIETARY PATTERNS

Human ancestry can be traced back more than 5 million years before encountering an ancestor who also was an ancestor of humanity's nearest living relatives, the pongids (e.g., chimpanzees, gorillas). Homo sapiens emerged from hominid ancestors sometime during the last 5% of that period. Homo sapiens' hominid ancestors lived as hunter–gatherers, eating a diverse, plant-based diet with variable amounts of meat in increasing proportion as hunting technology progressed, particularly with the emergence of Homo sapiens [1,2]. The nutrient content of that diet was a major feature of the environment influencing the genetic evolution of the hominid lineage leading to the emergence of Homo sapiens.

With the emergence of Homo sapiens during the past 100,000 to 200,000 years, the hunter–gatherer lifestyle continued, until the invention of agriculture about 10,000 years ago, when the composition of the human diet underwent a revolutionary change with major acid–base implications. The Upper Paleolithic period, beginning about 40,000 years ago and ending about 10,000 years ago, is the last period in history before agriculture in which *Homo sapiens* habitually ate exclusively a hunter–gatherer diet similar to the one to which they had become fitted by their genes. The last 10,000 years of human history are believed to be too short a time on an evolutionary scale for major genetic adaptations to have occurred in response to the profound changes in the nutrient composition of the diet that resulted from the switch to the modern agriculturalist diet. From a nutritional point of view [8–10] and incidentally also from a psychological [11] and socio-biological [12] point of view, contemporary humans are genetically Stone Age hunter–gatherers.

In comparison with the diet habitually ingested by preagricultural *Homo sapiens* living in the Upper Paleolithic period, the diet of contemporary *Homo sapiens* is rich in saturated fat, simple sugars, sodium, and chloride and poor in fiber, magnesium, and potassium [4,9]. These and numerous other post-agricultural dietary compositional changes have been implicated as risk factors in the pathogenesis of diseases of civilization, including athero-sclerosis, hypertension, type 2 diabetes, osteoporosis, and certain types of cancer [13–15].

One characteristic of the contemporary human diet for which no quantitative comparison has been made with the inferred ancestral preagricultural diet is its imbalance of nutrient precursors of hydrogen and bicarbonate ions, resulting in the body's net production of noncarbonic acid, ranging over an order of magnitude from 10 to 150 mEq/day among diets [16–19]. Although multiple homeostatic mechanisms operate to mitigate the resulting deviations in systemic acid–base equilibrium, on average blood acidity remains increased and plasma bicarbonate concentra-tions decreased in proportion to the magnitude of the daily net acid load [17,18]. Increasing evidence suggests that such persisting, albeit low-grade, acidosis and the relentless operation of responding homeostatic mechanisms result in numerous injurious effects on the body, including dissolution of bone, muscle wasting, kidney stone formation, and damage to the kidney [20–23].

ESTIMATION OF THE DIET NET ACID LOAD
OF THE ANCESTRAL HUMAN DIET

From extensive data on the diets of existing hunter–gatherer societies and from inferences about the nature of the Paleolithic environment, Eaton and Konner [4] reconstructed the Paleolithic diet and estimated the probable daily nutrient intakes of Paleolithic humans. In an estimated 3000-kilocalorie diet, meat constituted 35% of the diet by weight and plant foods, 65%. Total protein intake was estimated as 251 g/day, of which animal protein was 191 g, and plant proteins, 60 g. By contrast, contemporary humans consume less than one-half that amount of animal protein, and only about one-third that amount of plant protein per kilocalorie of diet consumed [24]. Sodium (Na) intake was estimated at about 29 mEq per day and potassium intake in excess of 280 mEq per day. By contrast, contemporary humans consume between 100 and 300 mEq of sodium per day and about 80 mEq of potassium per day. That is, in the switch to the modern diet, the K/Na ratio was reversed, from 1:10 to more than 3:1. Because food sodium is largely in the form of chloride (Cl) salts and food potassium largely in the form of bicarbonate-generating (HCO_3) organic acid salts, the $Cl:HCO_3$ ratio of the diet correspondingly has become reversed.

In computing the potential net acid (or base) load of the Paleolithic diet, three factors must be taken into consideration that determine diet composition: (1) animal-to-plant food energy intake ratio, (2) animal food fat energy density, and (3) distribution of plant food energies among plant food groups. The potential net acid load of lean meats varies little by animal source [25], presumably reflecting the similarity of protein composition of skeletal muscle across vertebrate species. However, the potential net base load of plant foods varies greatly among the differing plant species [25,26], with some foods supplying substantial amounts of net base a day per gram of protein (e.g., carrots, bananas) and some substantially smaller amounts (e.g., potatoes, beans), while some supply a net acid load (e.g., wheat, rice) (Table I). Both Sherman and Gettler [27] in 1912 and Hu et al. [28] in 1993 reported that rice increased NEAP as reflected in renal net acid excretion (RNAE) rates. Analyzing the data presented by Blatherwick [26], where subjects ate a baseline diet and had large amounts of one food item added

TABLE I   Comparison of Net Acid Loads from Various Plant Food Groups

Plant Food Group	Net Acid Load (mEq/10,460 kJ)
Cereal grains	56
Nuts	6
Legumes	−77
Fruit	−92
Tubers	−102
Roots	−414
Leafy greens	−536

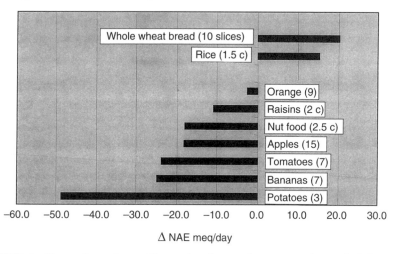

FIGURE 1   Changes in renal net acid excretion after supplementation of a standard diet with a single food item. (Adapted from Blatherwick [26].)

while measuring NEAP, demonstrated that both wheat and rice increased daily RNAE (Fig. 1).

So, while all plant foods contain protein, in those plant foods that are net base-producing, the content of potassium-associated bicarbonate precursors (*e.g.*, potassium citrate) exceeds their content of hydrogen ion precursors from the accompanying plant protein, though of differing degree among different species of plants. Accordingly, one cannot predict the potential net acid (or base) load of the diet from knowledge of its total animal and vegetable content alone.

DIET DATABASE

For the primary data, we assembled a nutrient database of 53 food items from among the major food groups most likely to have been consumed by Paleolithic humans: 9 lean meats (including 4 wild game meats) and 44 plant foods assigned either to one of 6 groups (roots, nuts, tubers, fruit, leafy green vegetables, and vegetable fruit) or to one of 4 groups (roots and tubers, leafy green vegetables, nuts, and fruit) depending on which of the diet-selection strategies were being implemented (see above). When used, the category vegetable fruit included fruit that is more commonly referred to as a vegetable, such as tomatoes, pumpkin, zucchini, cucumbers, eggplant, and okra. Cereal grains and legumes were excluded because of their late (mostly postagricultural) incorporation into the human diet [29–31]. Eligible food items were selected if included in *McCance and Widdowson's The Composition of Foods* [32], the major nutrient database reporting values for all the inorganic cations and anions required to compute NEAP (see below). The components of NEAP were first calculated for individual food items and then were averaged by food group (Tables II and III).

TABLE II   Potassium Content of Various Food Groups

Food Group	Items per Group	K (mmol per 100 kcal)	Examples
Vegetable fruits	6	35.7	Tomatoes, cucumbers, zucchini, eggplant, pumpkin
Leafy greens	5	34.9	Spinach, lettuce, cabbage, kale
Roots	5	25.0	Carrots, radishes, turnips, rutabaga, onions
Beans and peas	6	13.4	Kidney beans, peas, green beans, chick peas, soybeans
Fruits	14	11.3	Apples, oranges, bananas, apricots, grapes, strawberries
Tubers	3	10.4	Potatoes, sweet potatoes, yams
Milk and yogurt	3	8.7	Skimmed milk, whole milk, yogurt
Meats	10	6.0	Beef, lamb, pork, poultry, fish, rabbit
Nuts	10	3.1	Walnuts, cashews, almonds, Brazil nuts, hazelnuts
Eggs	1	2.5	Chicken eggs
Cereal grains	5	2.2	Wheat, rice, oats, rye
Cheese	4	1.1	Edam, Stilton, cottage, cheddar

TABLE III   Examples of Food Group Calculations for NEAP

Group Name	N	Pro (g/d)	S-BIC (mEq/gp)	UA (mEq/gp)	OAE (mEq/d)	NEAP (mEq/d)
Meat	9	178	67	4		
Nuts	10	7	−1	9		
Beans	5	30	−84	167		
Vegetable fruit	6	24	−64	117		
Tubers	3	6	−20	31		
Roots	5	10	−51	82		
Fruit	15	5	−26	39		
Totals	53	260	−178	450	100	−78

Note: Animal-to-plant ratio, 35%:65%; animal-fat energy, 26%. N = number of food items in group; Pro = dietary protein (g/day); S-BIC = dietary sulfur minus calculated bicarbonate (mean mEq for each food group); UA = dietary unmeasured anion content (mean mEq for each food group); OAE = daily organic acid excretion, calculated from OAE = 0.15 × UA + 32.9 [37]; NEAP = daily net endogenous acid production, calculated from NEAP = S + OAE − BIC.

Because McCance and Widdowson's database includes one game meat only (deer), we added three additional game meats (buffalo, wild rabbit, and antelope) from the U.S. Department of Agriculture's *Nutrient Database for Standard Reference* [33], assuming a chloride content of 67% of sodium content (in mmol), which corresponds to that of deer and is similar to that of five lean cuts of diverse domestic meats (62%) [32].

The complete nutrient composition profiles necessary for computing net acid load, including the content of chloride and the sulfur-containing amino acids, were unavailable for wild plant foods. Although the protein content and the content of certain minerals in some comparable wild and cultivated plant food groups differ [34], the magnitude of these differences is too small to have a major effect on the net acid load from these food groups.

Computing NEAP for the contemporary diet required expanding the database to include dairy foods, eggs, cereal grains, and a food group of energy-dense, nutrient-poor foods (*e.g.*, separated fats, refined sugars, and vegetable oils) [24], the latter of which were considered to be protein and mineral free for purposes of computing NEAP (Table III).

BASIS FOR THE COMPUTATIONAL MODEL

On a daily basis, NEAP can be computed from the sum of the production rates of sulfuric acid (resulting from the metabolism of dietary sulfur-containing amino acids) and organic acids (resulting from incomplete combustion of carbohydrates and fats) minus that of bicarbonate (resulting from the combustion of dietary organic acid salts of potassium and magnesium) [35], all of which can be computed from the nutrient composition of individual foods. Sulfuric acid and bicarbonate yields can be determined individually for each food item in the diet, the former from the sulfur content calculated from cysteine and methionine [33] and the latter with use of the method of Remer and Manz [36], which is based on each item's content of major inorganic cations and anions and published data on the average fractional intestinal absorption of each of nutrient. The difference between the major inorganic cation and anion contents (expressed in milliequivalents, corrected for intestinal absorption), typically a positive value, reflects the amount of unmeasured organic acid salts available to the body for metabolism to bicarbonate and hence reflects the potential systemic bicarbonate (base) load from the food item. Rates of sulfuric acid and bicarbonate production for the entire diet can then be calculated either as the sum of the values for the individual foods or, after assignment of the individual foods to food groups, as the sum of the average values for the food groups. We used the latter procedure in the present analysis (Table III). A single value for organic acid production for the entire diet can be computed from the total unmeasured anion content of the diet, as per the method of Kleinman and Lemann [37].

RESULTS

Using a variety of plausible animal-to-plant food energy intake ratios, animal food fat energy densities, and distributions of plant food energies among plant food groups for ancestral hominids and using established computational methods for estimating systemic sulfuric and organic acid and bicarbonate yields from individual food items, adjusting for fractional intestinal absorption, we computed the diet-dependent NEAP for a series of retrojected preagricultural diets and compared those with computed and measured values for typical American diets [38]. The best fit for the data was by multiple linear regression analysis, where NEAP $= 87 + (0.47 \times$ protein$) - (0.67 \times$ potassium$)$, accounting for 99% of the variability among diets ($R^2 = 0.986$). Of the 159 ancestral diet scenarios tested, 87% (139/159) were net base producing, with NEAP averaging -88 ± 82 mEq/day (Fig. 2).

TESTING FOR BIAS IN THE COMPUTATIONAL MODEL

To test whether the computational model is biased toward generating negative NEAP values, we applied the model to an average American diet, which is known to be net acid producing [18]. Using the same computational model, we evaluated the average American diet, the composition of which was reported in the most recent U.S. National Health and Examination Survey (NHANES III) [24,39]. We used our modified version of the Remer–Manz model [36] to estimate the contribution of cereal grains to the NEAP of the average American diet. NHANES III data allow estimation of the percent of calories ingested for 10 food groups, including cereal grains as a separate group. For a reported average daily energy intake of 8983 kJ (2147 kcal), the model was net acid producing—NEAP, $+48$ mEq/day—a value remarkably similar to the average NEAP of free-living healthy American adults as estimated from their renal net acid excretion rates— 49 ± 18 mEq/day [19] and 43 ± 19 mEq/day [19,40]. Thus, in contrast to the known positive NEAP for contemporary diets [17–19,35–37], the great majority (87%) of retrojected ancestral preagricultural diets were net base producing.

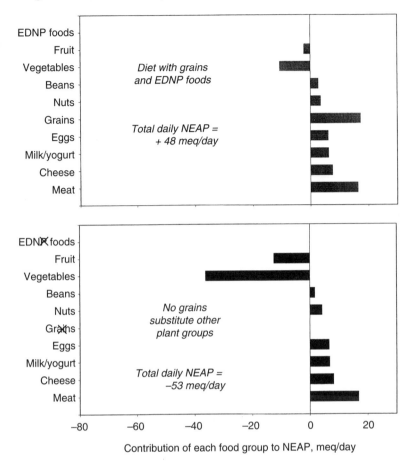

FIGURE 2   (Upper graph) Calculated daily net endogenous acid production in the American diet from NHANES III. (Lower graph) Calculated daily net endogenous acid production after substitution of energy-dense, nutrient-poor (EDNP) foods and grain with other plant foods.

Using the NHANES III database, we also calculated that 63% of calories in the modern diet comes from grains, fats and oils, and refined sugars [24]. Eliminating cereal grains and substituting fruits and vegetables eliminates the diet's net acid load (NEAP, +48 versus –4 mEq/day). Eliminating both cereal grains and energy-dense, nutrient-poor (EDNP) foods and substituting fruits and vegetables renders the diet decidedly net base producing (NEAP, –53 mEq/day) (Fig. 3).

We also evaluated the use of the multiple linear regression equation in 20 steady-state diets from studies done on a metabolic ward for which dietary protein and potassium intake were known and for which renal net

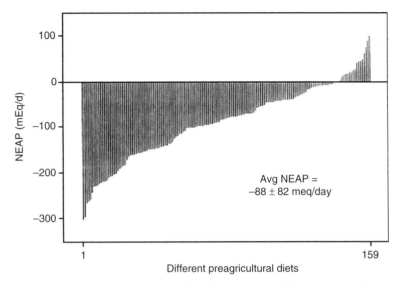

FIGURE 3   Calculated net endogenous acid production in 159 different pre-agricultural diets. NEAP is calculated as mean ± SD.

acid excretion (a marker of net endogenous acid production) had been measured [41] (Fig. 4). The measured mean net acid excretion for the 20 diets was 71 ± 41 mEq/day, while the calculated net endogenous acid production was 74 ± 25 mEq/day, a very close comparison.

In a similar evaluation, we used the multiple linear regression equation from data in the study by Maurer *et al.* [42] in 9 subjects on a metabolic ward on a defined diet and in whom RNAE was measured. Mean measured net acid excretion at baseline was 83 ± 5 mEq/day, while the calculated net endogenous acid production was 76 mEq/day. The computational model is therefore not biased toward negative NEAP values; rather, the model closely predicts the observed average value of the substantial positive net acid load from both free-living American diets and from metabolic study diets.

ANCESTRAL POTASSIUM INTAKES

Using the same standard nutrient databases, we estimated potassium contents for the retrojected ancestral diets and compared them with values for typical American diets (NHANES III survey). Within paleoanthropologically accepted bounds of animal-to-plant food ratios and animal fat densities of ancestral diets, ancestral human potassium intakes ranged

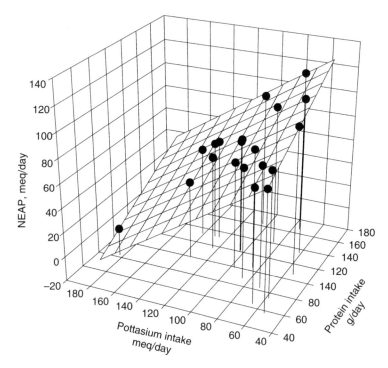

FIGURE 4   Relationship between steady-state net endogenous acid production and the known dietary contents of protein and potassium for 20 different whole-food diets using the multiple linear regression equation calculated from the 159 pre-agricultural diets. NEAP = 87 + (0.47 × protein) − (0.67 × potassium).

from 295 to 542 mEq/day—4 to 7 times greater than the NHANES III average. The transition to such a potassium-poor diet was accounted for by replacement of potassium-rich plant foods (especially roots, tubers, fruits, leafy greens, vegetable fruits) with EDNP foods (separated fats, oils, refined sugars) and with potassium-poor plant foods (especially cereal grains) introduced by agriculture (ca. 10,000 BP). These findings suggest that the natural, and therefore presumably optimal, potassium intake in humans is substantially higher than contemporary diets provide. Because potassium intake correlates positively with bone mineral density [43–45], these findings may have important implications for the pathogenesis of osteoporosis.

With the advent of agriculture, cereal grains such as rice and wheat became staples of the diet; however, compared to other plant food groups, cereal grains contain little potassium (Table I). Accordingly, unlike most plant foods, cereal grains supply little potential bicarbonate. Indeed, metabolism of cereal grains generally supplies acid precursors in excess of base producers and yields a dietary net acid load (Table II).

Among plant foods, the yield of net endogenous acid correlates inversely with potassium content:

Diet acid load (mEq/10,460 kJ) = 77.612 − (0.571 × diet potassium load (mEq/10,460 kJ); $r = 0.89$ and $n = 48$

In part because of their high fraction of cereal grain products and in part because in the modern diet high-bicarbonate-yielding plant foods have been displaced by animal foods and EDNP foods (*e.g.*, separated fats), modern diets are both low in bicarbonate precursors and high in acid precursors, leading to a positive value for net endogenous acid production.

ACID–BASE RELATIONSHIP TO BONE HEALTH AND BONE MINERAL DENSITY

Epidemiologic studies have also demonstrated a relationship between bone mineral density and calculated net acid excretion. Studies from the Framingham osteoporosis group have demonstrated that bone mineral density increases with increasing protein intake [46] and high fruits and vegetables (and also potassium) intake [47]. Studies by New *et al.* [23,48], using the ratio of protein to potassium intake in the diet to calculate net acid excretion (NAE), demonstrated that women with the highest estimated NAE had the lowest bone mineral density.

Short-term physiologic studies have demonstrated a relationship between decrease in net acid excretion and calcium or phosphate loss and bone breakdown. In the study by Maurer *et al.* [42], after stabilization on the initial diet, reduction in net acid excretion to 12 ± 3 mEq/day for 7 days was associated with a decrease in urinary calcium and phosphate excretion and a decrease in daily urinary excretion of markers of bone breakdown, pyridino-line, deoxypyridinoline, and N-telopeptide, suggesting decreasing bone breakdown. In an earlier study by Sebastian *et al.* [21], reduction in renal net acid excretion to 13 ± 22 mEq/day for 18 days was associated with a positive calcium and phosphate balance and an increase in osteocalcin levels, suggestive of increasing bone formation.

There are no long-term prospective studies comparing the effects of high net acid intake to low or negative (high base) intake; rather, the types of studies discussed above demonstrate support for the concept that higher net acid loads over time adversely affect bone. If our hominid precursors evolved on diets similar to the ones in this report, then our analysis suggests that diets relatively high in potassium (a marker for base-containing fruits and vegetables) to protein (a marker for acid-producing metabolites) intake are important for bone health and improved bone mineral density.

CONCLUSIONS

Adapting an agricultural-based diet ~10,000 years ago, *Homo sapiens* crossed the neutral zone, switching from systemic net base production to net acid production, and greatly reduced their potassium intake. The chronic low-grade metabolic acidosis and its sequelae typical of present-day humans eating contemporary diets reflect a *mismatch* between the nutrient composition of our present diets and the genetically determined nutrients we require for optimal systemic acid–base status. Neutralization of metabolic acids may mitigate the small but progressive effects of acids on bone and muscle loss, as well as other systems, but supplying a substantial net base load and increasing potassium intake may have anabolic effects on bone [49].

IMPLICATIONS FOR FURTHER RESEARCH

During human evolution, renal acid excretory mechanisms were conserved and refined undoubtedly because of their adaptive value in responding to metabolic acidosis-producing conditions that were presumably experienced intermittently by early humans and their hominid ancestors: food shortage (starvation ketoacidosis, autoproteolytic sulfuric acidosis); meat feasting (sulfuric acidosis); feasting on certain plant foods, such as plums and cranberries, that are net acid producing (various organic acidoses); prolonged intense physical activity (lactic acidosis); and, infectious or toxic diarrhea (fecal bicarbonate wasting). Because those conditions were presumably episodic, and for some even uncommon [50], there is no reason to suppose that the renal mechanisms underlying urine acidification and net acid excretion were designed to operate *tonically* during an individual's lifetime. We argue that, under the more usual day-to-day conditions of eating a typical hunter–gatherer type diet and of engaging in average levels of hunter–gatherer physical activity, early humans and their hominid ancestors were most often exposed to a net load of base and that renal regulation of systemic acid–base equilibrium over a lifetime was predominantly directed toward regulation of urinary alkalinization and net base excretion.

The ancestral human diet was net base producing because base input from plant foods exceeded acid input from animal foods. Because base-producing plant foods are rich in potassium, the diet likewise was rich in potassium. Indeed, the estimated potassium content of ancestral hominid diets is as much as three or four times greater than that of contemporary diets [4,51,52]. Although much is known about the mechanisms of adaptation to chronic potassium loads and to a lesser extent about the mechanisms of adaptation to chronic base loads, little is known about the overall physiology under the combined conditions of habitual dietary potassium and base loads at levels likely to have been supplied by the ancestral diet. Considering that those conditions prevailed during the 5 or more million years of hominid evolution that eventuated in *Homo sapiens* and that they prevailed in each generation throughout the growth and development and reproductive period of each individual, our current perspective on what constitutes normal human physiology may well require re-evaluation.

ACKNOWLEDGMENTS

The authors would like to acknowledge the General Clinical Research Center (GCRC) of the University of California, San Francisco, under a grant from the National Institutes of Health (NCRR grant M01 0079) and to thank Renee Mirriam for her help with the research and Susan New for her encouragement.

REFERENCES

1. Gaulin, S.J.C. and Konner, M. (1977). On the natural diet of primates, including humans, in *Nutrition and the Brain*, Vol. 1, Wurtman, R. and Wurtman, J. Eds. Raven Press, New York.
2. Gaulin, S.J. (1979). A Jarman/Bell model of primate feeding niches. *Human Ecol.* 7: 1–20.
3. Fogel, R.W. (2000). *The Last Great Awakening and the Future of Egalitarianism*, The University of Chicago Press, Chicago, IL.
4. Eaton, S.B. and Konner, M. (1985). Paleolithic nutrition: a consideration of its nature and current implications. *New Engl. J. Med.* 312: 283–289.
5. Boyd, R. and Silk, J.B. (2000). *How Humans Evolved*, 2 ed. W.W. Norton & Co., New York.
6. Cordain, L., Miller, J.B., Eaton, S.B., Mann, N., Holt, S.H., and Speth, J.D. (2000). Plant–animal subsistence ratios and macronutrient energy estimations in worldwide hunter–gatherer diets [see comments]. *Am J. Clin. Nutr.* 71: 682–692.
7. Mann, N. (2000). Dietary lean red meat and human evolution. *Eur. J. Nutr.* 39: 71–79.
8. Eaton, S.B. and Cordain, L. (1997). Evolutionary aspects of diet: old genes, new fuels. Nutritional changes since agriculture. *World Rev. Nutr. Diet.* 81: 26–37.
9. Eaton, S.B., Eaton III, S.B., and Konner, M.J. (1999). Paleolithic nutrition revisited, in *Evolutionary Medicine*, Trevathan, W.R., Smith, E. O., and McKenna, J.J., Eds. Oxford University Press, New York.

10. Eaton, S.B., Konner, M., and Shostak, M. (1988). Stone agers in the fast lane: chronic degenerative diseases in evolutionary perspective. *Am. J. Med.* 84: 739–749.

11. Cosmides, L., Tooby, J., and Barkow, J.H. (1992). *The Adapted Mind: Evolutionary Psychology and the Generation of Culture*, Oxford University Press, New York.

12. Greenhaff, P.L., Gleeson, M., and Maughan, R.J. (1988). The effects of a glycogen loading regimen on acid–base status and blood lactate concentration before and after a fixed period of high intensity exercise in man. *Eur. J. Appl. Physiol Occup. Physiol.* 57: 254–259.

13. American Institute for Cancer Research (1997). *Food, Nutrition and the Prevention of Cancer: A Global Perspective.* American Institute for Cancer Research, Washington, D.C.

14. WHO (1990). *Diet, Nutrition, and the Prevention of Chronic Diseases: Report of a WHO Study Group.* World Health Organization, Geneva.

15. Committee on Diet and Health, Food and Nutrition Board, Commission on Life Sciences, and National Research Council (1989). *Diet and Health: Implications for Reducing Chronic Disease Risk.* National Academy Press, Washington, D.C.

16. Lemann, Jr., J. and Lennon, E.J. (1972). Role of diet, gastrointestinal tract and bone in acid base homeostasis. *Kidney Int.* 1: 275–279.

17. Kurtz, I., Maher, T., Hulter, H.N., Schambelan, M., and Sebastian, A. (1983). Effect of diet on plasma acid–base composition in normal humans. *Kidney Int.* 24: 670–680.

18. Frassetto, L., Morris, R. C., Jr., and Sebastian, A. (1996). Effect of age on blood acid-base composition in adult humans: Role of age-related renal functional decline. *Am. J. Physiol.* 271: 1114–1122.

19. Lemann, J., Jr. (1999). Relationship between urinary calcium and net acid excretion as determined by dietary protein and potassium: a review. *Nephron* 81(suppl. 1): 18–25.

20. Alpern, R.J. and Sakhaee, S. (1997). The clinical spectrum of chronic metabolic acidosis: homeostatic mechanisms produce significant morbidity. *Am. J. Kid. Dis.* 29: 291–302.

21. Sebastian, A., Harris, S.T., Ottaway, J.H., Todd, K.M., and Morris, R.C., Jr. (1994). Improved mineral balance and skeletal metabolism in postmenopausal women treated with potassium bicarbonate [see comments]. *New Engl. J. Med.* 330: 1776–1781.

22. Frassetto, L., Morris, R.C., Jr., and Sebastian, A. (1997). Potassium bicarbonate reduces urinary nitrogen excretion in postmenopausal women. *J. Clin. Endocrinol. Metab.* 82: 254–259.

23. New, S.A., Bolton-Smith, C., Grubb, D.A., and Reid, D.M. (1997). Nutritional influences on bone mineral density: a cross-sectional study in premenopausal women. *Am. J. Clin. Nutr.* 65: 1831–1839.

24. Smit, E., Nieto, F.J., Crespo, C.J., and Mitchell, P. (1999). Estimates of animal and plant protein intake in U.S. adults: results from the Third National Health and Nutrition Examination Survey, 1988–1991. *J. Am. Diet. Assoc.* 99: 813–820.

25. Remer, T. and Manz, F. (1995). Potential renal acid load of foods and its influence on urine pH. *J. Am. Diet. Assoc.* 95: 791–797.

26. Blatherwick, N.R. (1914). The specific role of foods in relation to the composition of the urine. *Arch. Int. Med.* 14: 409–450.

27. Sherman, H.C. and Gettler, A.O. (1912). The balance of acid-forming and base-forming elements in foods, and its relation to ammonia metabolism. *J. Biol. Chem.* 11: 323–338.

28. Hu, J.-F., Zhao, X.-H., Parpia, B., and Campbell, T.C. (1993). Dietary intakes and urinary excretion of calcium and acids: a cross-sectional study of women in China. *Am. J. Clin. Nutr.* 58: 398–406.

29. O'Dea, K. (1991). Traditional diet and food preferences of Australian aboriginal hunter–gatherers. *Philos. Trans. R. Soc. London B Biol. Sci.* 334: 233–241.

30. Harlan, J.R. (1999). Harvesting of wild-grass seed and implications for domestication, in *Prehistoire de l'Agriculture: Nouvelles Approches Experimentales et Ethnographiques*, Anderson, P.C., Ed. Centre National de la Recherche Scientifique, Paris.

31. Cordain, L. (1999). *The Late Role of Grains and Legumes in the Human Diet, and Biochemical Evidence of Their Evolutionary Discordance*, Beyond Vegetarianism (www.beyondveg.com).
32. Holland, B., Welch, A.A., Unwin, I.D., Buss, D.H., Paul, A.A., and Southgate, D.A.T. (1991). *McCance and Widdowson's The Composition of Foods*, Fifth ed. The Royal Society of Chemistry and Ministry of Agriculture, Fisheries and Food, Cambridge, U.K.
33. U.S.D.A. (2000). *Nutrient Database for Standard Reference*, Release 13. U.S.D.A Agricultural Research Service.
34. Milton, K. (1999). Nutritional characteristics of wild primate foods: do the diets of our closest living relatives have lessons for us? *Nutrition* 15: 488–498.
35. Lennon, E.J., Lemann, Jr., J., and Litzow, J.R. (1966). The effect of diet and stool composition on the net external acid balance of normal subjects. *J. Clin. Invest.* 45: 1601–1607.
36. Remer, T. and Manz, F. (1994). Estimation of the renal net acid excretion by adults consuming diets containing variable amounts of protein. *Am. J. Clin. Nutr.* 59: 1356–1361.
37. Kleinman, J.G. and Lemann, J., Jr. (1987). Acid production, in *Clinical Disorders of Fluid and Electrolyte Metabolism*, Maxwell, M.H., Kleeman, C.R., and Narins, R.G., Eds. McGraw-Hill, New York.
38. Sebastian, A., Frassetto, L.A., Sellmeyer, D.E., Merriam, R.L., and Morris, Jr., R.C. (2002). Estimation of the net acid load of the diet of ancestral preagricultural *Homo sapiens* and their hominid ancestors. *Am. J. Clin. Nutr.* 76: 1308–1316.
39. Kant, A.K. (2000). Consumption of energy-dense, nutrient-poor foods by adult Americans: nutritional and health implications. The Third National Health and Nutrition Examination Survey, 1988–1994. *Am. J. Clin. Nutr.* 72: 929–936.
40. Frassetto, L.A., Nash, E., Morris, Jr., R.C., and Sebastian, A. (2000). Comparative effects of potassium chloride and bicarbonate on thiazide-induced reduction in urinary calcium excretion. *Kidney Int.* 58: 748–752.
41. Frassetto, L.A., Todd, K.M., Morris, Jr., R.C., and Sebastian, A. (1998). Estimation of net endogenous noncarbonic acid production in humans from diet potassium and protein contents. *Am. J. Clin Nutr.* 68: 576–583.
42. Maurer, M., Riesen, W., Muser, J., Hulter, H.N., and Krapf, R. (2003). Neutralization of Western diet inhibits bone resorption independently of K intake and reduces cortisol secretion in humans. *Am. J. Physiol. Renal Physiol.* 284: F32–F40.
43. Tucker, K.L., Hannan, M.T., Chen, H., Cupples, L.A., Wilson, P.W., and Kiel, D.P. (1999). Potassium, magnesium, and fruit and vegetable intakes are associated with greater bone mineral density in elderly men and women. *Am. J. Clin. Nutr.* 69: 727–736.
44. New, S.A., Robins, S.P., Campbell, M.K., Martin, J.C., Garton, M.J., Bolton-Smith, C., Grubb, D.A., Lee, S.J., and Reid, D.M. (2000). Dietary influences on bone mass and bone metabolism: further evidence of a positive link between fruit and vegetable consumption and bone health? *Am. J. Clin. Nutr.* 71: 142–151.
45. Jones, G., Riley, M.D., and Whiting, S. (2001). Association between urinary potassium, urinary sodium, current diet, and bone density in prepubertal children. *Am. J. Clin. Nutr.* 73: 839–844.
46. Hannan, M.T., Felson, D.T., and Anderson, J.J. (1992). Bone mineral density in elderly men and women: results from the Framingham Osteoporosis Study. *J. Bone Mineral Res.* 7: 547–553.
47. Tucker, K.L., Hannan, M.T., Chen, H., Cupples, L.A., Wilson, P.W.F., and Kiel, D.P. (1999). Potassium, magnesium, and fruit and vegetable intakes are associated with greater bone mineral density in elderly men and women. *Am. J. Clin. Nutr.* 69: 727–736.
48. New, S.A., Macdonald, H.M., Grubb, D.A., and Reid, D. (2001). Positive association between net endogenous non-carbonic acid production (NEAP) and bone health: further support for the importance of the skeleton to acidbase balance [letter]. *Bone* 28(suppl.), S94.

49. Bushinsky, D.A. (1996). Metabolic alkalosis decreases bone calcium efflux by suppressing osteoclasts and stimulating osteoblasts. *Am. J. Physiol.* 271: F216–F222.
50. Cordain, L., Miller, J., and Mann, N. (1999). Scant evidence of periodic starvation among hunter–gatherers. *Diabetologia* 42: 383–384.
51. Eaton, S.B., Eaton III, S.B., and Konner, M.J. (1997). Paleolithic nutrition revisited: a twelve-year retrospective on its nature and implications [see comments]. *Eur. J. Clin Nutr.* 51: 207–216.
52. Sebastian, A., Frassetto, L.A., Sellmeyer, D.E., and Morris., Jr., R.C. (2001). The natural dietary potassium intake of humans exceeds current intakes minimally by a factor of four. *J. Am. Soc. Nephrol.* 12: 40A.

PART IX

Protein

N-Acetyl Cysteine Supplementation of Growing Mice: Effects on Skeletal Size, Bone Mineral Density, and Serum IGF-I

CHERYL L. ACKERT-BICKNELL,[1] WESLEY G. BEAMER,[1] and CLIFFORD J. ROSEN[1,2]

[1]The Jackson Laboratory, Bar Harbor, Maine; [2]The Maine Center for Osteoporosis Research and Education, St. Joseph Hospital, Bangor, Maine

ABSTRACT

Bone mineral density (BMD) has been correlated to serum insulin-like growth factor I (IGF-I) levels in humans and mice, although the precise relationship between these two variables is unknown. Under certain conditions, supplementation of mice lacking γ-glutamyl transpeptidase (GGTP) with N-acetylcysteine (NAC) has shown to significantly increase body weight, rescue serum IGF-I, and enhance femoral BMD. Based on these data, we hypothesized that cysteine was an important regulator of hepatic IGF-I expression and, as such, might contribute to acquisition of peak growth and bone acquisition; hence, we examined the effect of NAC treatment on young, growing, normal female mice from three inbred strains: C57BL/6JBm, C3H/HeJ, and 129/SvJ. Female mice at 4 weeks of age were treated for 4 weeks with either acidified water (acidified with HCl, pH 2.8–3.2) or acidified water supplemented with 10 g/L of NAC. Mice treated with NAC gained less weight than control mice, within each strain ($P < 0.01$). No reduction in food consumption was observed in the NAC-treated mice. Femur length,

Nutritional Aspects of Osteoporosis, Second Edition

femoral BMD, and serum IGF-I were all noticeably reduced as compared to controls within a given strain ($P < 0.05$, $P < 0.01$, and $P < 0.01$, respectively). In this study, NAC supplementation had a profoundly negative effect on bone growth and serum IGF-I. Given the recent popularity of NAC as a dietary supplement, caution must be exercised when considering the use of NAC supplementation in children and adolescents.

INTRODUCTION

Many factors influence the acquisition of bone size and bone mineral density (BMD) during puberty and adolescence in humans, and it is thought that the amount and size of bone accrued during adolescence affects future fracture risk in the elderly [1]. Insulin-like growth factor I (IGF-I) is a ubiquitous growth factor that is thought to act both under the influence of, and independently of, growth hormone on skeletal growth and development [2–7]. IGF-I is both an endocrine hormone acting on bone and an autocrine/paracrine factor produced by osteoblasts [2–4]. Transgenic mice with reduced serum IGF-I show reduced femur length, periosteal circumference, and total BMD. The effect of low serum IGF-I on bone worsens in severity as serum IGF-I levels are reduced [3].

Treatment with N-acetylcysteine (NAC) has been shown to increase serum IGF-I levels and stimulate skeletal growth and bone acquisition in mice deficient in γ-glutamyl transpeptidase [8]. NAC is a thiol compound for which L-cysteine, inorganic sulfites, and glutathione appear to be the main metabolites [9–11]. It is these metabolites that are thought to be responsible for the majority of the biological activity of NAC [11]. NAC has been used for at least three decades as a mucolytic [11] and more recently in the treatment of acute acetaminophen overdose [9,10]. Of late, NAC is showing potential in the treatment of cancer, cardiovascular disease, human immunodeficiency virus (HIV) infection, Sjögren syndrome, influenza, hepatitis C, and myoclonus epilepsy, as well as aiding in smoking cessation and offering protection from second-hand smoke [9–11]. NAC is widely available as a dietary supplement without a prescription and is being advertised in the popular press as a curative of many more common ailments.

Increases in weight have been reported in wild-type mice treated with NAC from a young age through adulthood [12] and, as noted, NAC supplementation improved (but not totally restored) vertebral BMD and bone size in GGTP-deficient mice [8]. Despite the long history of use of NAC, there is very little in the literature about the effect of NAC in otherwise health children. In healthy adult humans, the use of NAC in conjunction with anaerobic exercise has been shown to result in a greater weight loss than that resulting from anaerobic exercise alone [13], but the effect of NAC on bone growth has not been studied. The aim of this study was to investigate the effects of NAC on serum IGF-I levels and bone growth in healthy young mice, outside of possible influences by genetic background.

MATERIALS AND METHODS

ANIMAL

All mice used in this study were raised at the Jackson Laboratory and all studies were approved by the animal research committee of the Jackson Laboratory. Mice were maintained in groups of 2 to 5 in polycarbonate boxes (130 cm^2) on bedding of sterilized white pine shavings under conditions of 14 hours of light and 10 hours of darkness. Mice were fed pasteurized pellet diet (National Institutes of Health 31 diet: 18% protein, 6% fat) *ad libitum*. Twenty female mice from each of C57BL/6JBm, C3H/HeJ, and 129/SvJ were used in this study. Ten mice from each strain were given acidified water (acidified with HCl, pH 2.8–3.2) *ad libitum*, and the remaining 10 mice where given acidified water supplemented with 10 g/L of NAC (Sigma, St. Louis, MO) *ad libitum*. All mice were obtained at 4 weeks of age, and treatment was continued for 4 weeks. Body weights were taken at baseline, at 2 weeks of treatment, and at 4 weeks of treatment. Blood was collected at baseline and at 4 weeks. After 4 weeks of treatment, the animals were sacrificed and femurs were collected and preserved in 95% ethanol.

MEASUREMENT OF SERUM IGF-I

Serum IGF-I was measured by radioimmunoassay (RIA) using a polyclonal antibody to IGF-I (ALPCO, Windham, NH) as has been previously described [4]. Binding proteins were acid dissociated from the IGF-I. The sample was neutralized in the presence of excess IGF-II to prevent the binding proteins from re-complexing with IGF-I. The assay sensitivity was 0.01 ng/mL, and there was no antibody cross reactivity with IGF-II. The interassay confidence value (CV) was 5.3%.

BONE DENSITY AND MORPHOLOGY MEASUREMENTS

Bone mineral density and femur length was measured as previously described [4,14]. Briefly, the density of isolated right femora was assessed by peripheral quantitative computed tomography (pQCT; Stratec XCT 960M; Norland Medical Systems, Ft. Akinson, WI). A threshold of 1.300 attenuation units differentiated bone from non-calcified tissues such as adipose and muscle tissue; a threshold of 2.000 differentiated high-density cortical bone from low-density bone. Precision of the XCT 960M for repeated measurement of the same femur was 1.2%. Femoral lengths were determined by digital calipers to the nearest 0.01 mm.

STATISTICAL ANALYSIS

Statistical analyses were preformed using StatView, version 4.5, software (SAS Institute, Cary, NC). Unpaired Student's *t*-tests were used to compare IGF-I, weight gain at all time points, and femoral length and bone mineral density within a strain between treatment groups. All values are reported as the mean ± SEM.

RESULTS

BODY WEIGHT

Body weights of all mice were taken at baseline, at 2 weeks, and at 4 weeks of treatment. As was expected there were differences in body weight between the three strains of mice used at baseline but not among the mice within any given strain. As can be seen in Fig. 1, significantly less weight was gained in the NAC-treated mice as compared to the controls, regardless of strain, and this can be observed as early as 2 weeks of treatment. Other reagent grades and production lots of NAC were tried to account for a possible bad lot of the NAC, but the same results were observed regardless (data not shown). Mice treated with NAC showed no gross physical anomalies at necropsy. Mice treated with NAC were not noticeably lethargic or distressed and did not have a wasted appearance. Measurements of daily food consumption showed that NAC mice were eating approximately 3 g of chow a day (data not shown). This is consistent for C57BL/6J mice (www.jax.org/phenome).

BONE DENSITY AND MORPHOLOGY

Treatment with NAC during the post pubertal growth phase affected all aspects of long bone growth, regardless of genetic background. Mice treated with NAC had shorter femurs (Table I) with reduced bone mineral

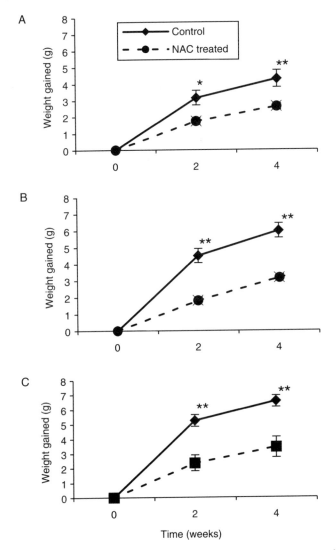

FIGURE 1 Weight gained in C57BL/6JBm (A), C3H/HeJ (B), and 129/SvJ (C) over the course of a 4-week treatment with NAC. *$P < 0.05$; **$P < 0.01$.

density (Fig. 2) after 4 weeks of NAC treatment. The reduction in femur length was correlated with the amount of weight gain at 4 weeks of treatment, independent of strain and treatment ($P < 0.001$, $R^2 = 0.235$). Mice treated with NAC had a tendency to have a smaller periosteal circumference at the midshaft and a thinner cortical shell at the midshaft (Table I), but the affect

TABLE 1   Femoral Morphology Measurements on NAC-Treated Mice and Controls After 4 Weeks of Treatment

Strain	Treatment	Femoral Length (mm)	Periosteal Circumference (mm)	Cortical Thickness (mm)
C57BL/6JBm	Control	14.8 ± 0.10	4.67 ± 0.069	0.246 ± 0.004
	NAC	14.1 ± 0.07**	4.56 ± 0.066	0.223 ± 0.006*
C3H/HeJ	Control	14.0 ± 0.16	4.13 ± 0.065	0.337 ± 0.005
	NAC	13.6 ± 0.14*	3.99 ± 0.064*	0.327 ± 0.005
129/SvJ	Control	14.8 ± 0.12	4.81 ± 0.055	0.341 ± 0.005
	NAC	13.7 ± 0.10**	4.36 ± 0.054**	0.289 ± 0.005**

Note: Comparisons for statistical purposes were made between NAC-treated mice and controls with a given strain. There were no statistically significant differences within strains at baseline. $*P < 0.05$; $**P < 0.01$.

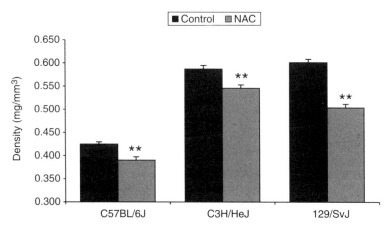

FIGURE 2   Bone mineral density in NAC-treated mice and controls after 4 weeks of treatment. $**P < 0.01$.

of NAC on these two measures of bone size was highly influenced by strain background. These two observations suggest that the femurs of the NAC-treated animals were weaker than the control femurs, but these femurs have not yet been tested for resistance to fracture.

SERUM IGF-I

Baseline serums measurements differed by strain but were consistent across the same strain. Treatment with NAC consistently resulted in

TABLE II   IGF-I in Control and NAC-Treated Mice at Baseline and After 4 Weeks
of Treatment

Strain	Treatment	IGF-I at Baseline	IGF-I at 4 Weeks of Treatment
C57BL/6JBm	Control	449.4 ± 7.9	387.8 ± 16.0
	NAC	492.4 ± 29.9	$312.2 \pm 6.3**$
C3H/HeJ	Control	464.8 ± 25.0	527.9 ± 25.6
	NAC	469.8 ± 18.9	$372.0 \pm 15.4**$
129/SvJ	Control	536.5 ± 17.4	456.5 ± 15.8
	NAC	479.6 ± 26.4	$229.0 \pm 14.6**$

Note: Comparisons for statistical purposes were made between NAC-treated mice and controls
with a given strain. There were no statistically significant differences within strains at
baseline. $**P < 0.01$.

reduction of serum IGF-I from baseline as compared to the control animals
for all strains (Table II).

DISCUSSION

Serum IGF-I levels, bone mineral density, and response to various drugs are
all highly influenced by genetics [5,14,15]. The three inbred strains of
mice used in this study have been well characterized for many aspects of
normal physiology. Both serum IGF-I and BMD are polygenic traits [16,17];
therefore, the genes and genetics controlling each of these phenotypes
depend on the strains being studied [16–20]. We have shown that NAC
supplementation in mice greatly reduces serum IGF-I levels in each of the
three strains used in this study, suggesting that the mode of action of NAC
on serum IGF-I is at a basic physiological level.

Mice treated with NAC had smaller femorae with lower bone mineral
density (Fig. 2, Table I), and, again, this effect appeared to be independent
of the genetics of the mouse studied. Reductions in serum IGF-1 have
been associated with certain dwarf phenotypes in mice [3], and serum IGF-I
levels have been correlated with BMD in healthy children [21]. In this study,
a moderate correlation between femur BMD and serum IGF-1 at the conclusion of the experiment was seen ($P < 0.001$, $R^2 = 0.274$; Fig. 3). A similar
correlation is seen between IGF-I and femur length at the conclusion of the
experiment (data not shown). It is likely that the reduction seen in the
serum IGF-I is responsible for the reduction in bone size and bone mineral
density seen in the NAC-treated mice.

In conclusion, treatment with NAC of the growing young mouse results
in a lower serum IGF-I level. This reduction in serum IGF-I may, in part,

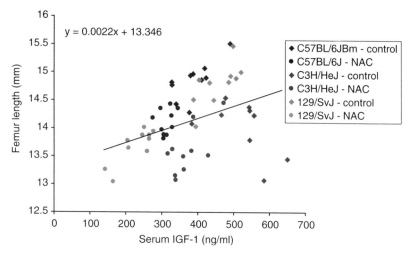

FIGURE 3   The relationship between femur bone mineral density and serum IGF-I levels for all mice after 4 weeks of placebo or NAC treatment. Trend-line and equation are for all data combined.

be responsible for the reduction in femoral length and femoral BMD seen in NAC-treated mice. The effect of NAC on growth of healthy children has not been documented, but the effect of NAC on growth seen in this study suggest that extreme caution should be used when treating children with NAC for long periods of time.

REFERENCES

1. Javaid, M. and Cooper, C. (2002). Prenatal and childhood influences on osteoporosis. *Best Pract. Res. Clin. Endocrinol. Metab.* 16(2): 349–367.
2. Le Roith, D. *et al.* (2001). The somatomedin hypothesis: 2001. *Endocrine Rev.* 22(1): 53–74.
3. Yakar, S. *et al.* (2002). Circulating levels of IGF-1 directly regulate bone growth and density. *J. Clin. Invest.* 10(6): 771–781.
4. Bouxsein, M. *et al.* (2002). Generation of a new congenic mouse strain to test the relationships among serum insulin-like growth factor I, bone mineral density, and skeletal morphology in vivo. *J. Bone Mineral Res.* 17(4): 570–579.
5. Rosen, C. *et al.* (1997). Circulating and skeletal insulin-like growth factor-I (IGF-I) concentrations in two inbred strains of mice with different bone mineral densities. *Bone* 21(3): 217–223.
6. Mohan, S. and Baylink, D. (1991). Bone growth factors. *Clin. Orthop.* 263: 30–48.
7. Lupu, F. *et al.* (2001). Roles of growth hormone and insulin-like growth factor 1 in mouse postnatal growth. *Dev. Biol.* 229(1): 141–162.
8. Levasseur, R. *et al.* (2003). Reversible skeletal abnormalities in γ-glutamyl transpeptidase-deficient mice. *Endocrinology* 144(7): 2761–2764.

9. Anon. (2001). N-Acetylcysteine. *Altern. Med. Rev.* 5(5): 467–471.

10. Zafarullah, M. *et al.* (2003). Molecular mechanisms of N-acetylcysteine actions. *Cell. Mol. Life Sci.* 60: 6–20.

11. Kelly, G. (1998). Clinical applications of N-acetylcysteine. *Altern. Med. Rev.* 3(2): 114–127.

12. Lieberman, M. *et al.* (1996). Growth retardation and cysteine deficiency in γ-glutamyl transpeptidase-deficient mice. *Proc. Natl. Acad. Sci. USA*, 93: 7923–7926.

13. Kinscherf, R. *et al.* (1996). Low plasma glutamine in combination with high glutamate levels indicate risk for loss of body cell mass in healthy individuals: the effect of N-acetylcysteine. *J. Mol. Med.* 74: 393–400.

14. Beamer, W., Donahue, L. and Baylink, D. (1996). Genetic variability in adult bone mineral density among inbred strains of mice. *Bone* 18(5): 397–403.

15. Nebert, D. (1999). Phamacogenetics and pharmacogenomics: why is this relevant to the clinical geneticist. *Clin. Genet.* 56(4): 247–258.

16. Beamer, W. *et al.* (2001). Quantitative trait loci for femoral and lumbar vertebral bone mineral density in C57BL/6J and C3H/HeJ inbred strains of mice. *J. Bone Mineral Res.* 16(7): 1195–1206.

17. Rosen, C. *et al.* (2000). Mapping quantitative trait loci for serum insulin-like growth factor-1 levels in mice. *Bone* 27(4): 521–528.

18. Masinde, G. *et al.* (2002). Quantitative trait loci for bone density in mice: the genes determining total skeletal density and femur density show little overlap in F2 mice. *Calcif. Tissue Int.* 71(5): 421–428.

19. Beamer, W. *et al.* (1999). Quantitative trait loci for bone density in C57BL/6J and CAST/EiJ inbred mice. *Mamm. Genome* 10(11): 1043–1049.

20. Klein, R. *et al.* (1998). Quantitative trait loci affecting peak bone mineral density in mice. *J. Bone Mineral Res.* 13(11): 1648–1656.

21. Moreira-Andres, M. *et al.* (1995). Correlations between bone mineral density, insulin-like growth factor I and auxological variables. *Eur. J. Endocrinol.* 132(5): 573–579.

CHAPTER 28

Dietary Protein Intakes and Bone Strength

René Rizzoli, Patrick Ammann, Thierry Chevalley, and Jean-Philippe Bonjour

Division of Bone Diseases, WHO Collaborating Center for Osteoporosis Prevention, Department of Rehabilitation and Geriatrics, University Hospital, Geneva, Switzerland

INTRODUCTION

Undernutrition is often observed in the elderly. It appears to be more severe in patients with hip fracture than in the general aging population [1–3]. Indeed, a state of undernutrition at hospital admission is consistently documented in elderly patients with hip fracture [3,4]. Close to 40% of hip fractures occur in nursing homes [5,6], where undernutrition is known to be particularly prevalent. In addition to an inadequate food intake during a hospital stay, the state of undernutrition before admission can adversely influence the clinical outcome [1,2,4,7]. A low protein intake could be particularly detrimental for both the acquisition of bone mass and the conservation of bone integrity with aging [8–11]. Bone strength is determined by various components (Table I), all of which could be influenced by changes in dietary protein intakes. Furthermore, protein undernutrition can favor the occurrence of hip fracture by increasing the propensity to fall as a result of muscle weakness and of impaired movement coordination by

Nutritional Aspects of Osteoporosis, Second Edition

TABLE I   Determinants of Bone Strength

Bone mass
Bone size
Microarchitecture
Bone remodeling rate
Intrinsic bone tissue properties

affecting protective mechanisms, such as reaction time or muscle strength [1] and/or by decreasing bone mass [10,12,13].

DIETARY PROTEIN AND BONE MASS GAIN

Peak bone mass is defined as the amount of bony tissue present at the end of skeletal maturation (for review, see [13–15]). In healthy Caucasian females with apparently adequate intakes of energy, protein, and calcium, bone mass accumulation can virtually be completed before the end of the second decade at both the lumbar spine and the femoral neck [16,17]. During puberty, the accumulation rate in areal bone mineral density (BMD) at both the lumbar spine and femoral neck levels increases 4- to 6-fold over a 3- and 4-year period in females and males, respectively [16,17]. Puberty affects bone size much more than volumetric mineral density. In a prospective survey carried out in a cohort of female and male subjects 9 to 19 years old, food intake was assessed twice, at a 1-year interval, using a 5-day dietary diary method requiring the weighing of all consumed foods [18]. In this adolescent cohort, we found a positive correlation between yearly lumbar and femoral bone mass gain and calcium or protein intake. The association remained statistically significant after adjustment for the alternate nutrient intake and appeared to be significant mainly in prepubertal children but not in those having reached a peri- or postpubertal stage (Fig. 1).

Impairment of bone mass gain can be observed in states of severe undernutrition, such as anorexia nervosa, which is frequently observed in young women. Bone mineral density is reduced at several skeletal sites in most women with anorexia nervosa. Young women with anorexia nervosa are at increased risk of fracture later in life [19]. Besides estrogen and calcium deficiency, low protein intake very likely contributes to the impaired bone acquisition or accelerated bone loss observed in anorexia nervosa patients. Experimental evidence obtained in adult female rats indicates that a normal calorie supply obtained by consuming carbohydrates cannot compensate for the detrimental effect on bone mass exerted by a low protein intake [20].

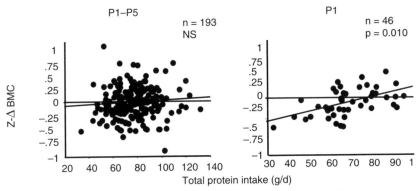

FIGURE 1   Relationship between age-adjusted increase in lumbar spine bone mineral content and dietary protein in infants and adolescents. (Adapted from Theintz *et al.* [16].)

In athletes or ballet dancers, intensive exercise can lead to hypothalamic dysfunction with delayed menarche and disturbances in menstrual cycles and to bone loss [21–25]. Nutritional restriction can play an important role in the disturbance of the female reproductive system resulting from intense physical activity. Insufficient energy intake with respect to energy expenditure is supposed to impair the secretion of gonadotropin-releasing hormone (GnRH) and thereby lead to a state of hypoestrogenism; however, the relative contribution of insufficient protein intake frequently associated with the low energy intake remains to be assessed. Indeed, experimental studies indicate that bone loss induced by isocaloric protein restriction in adult female rats is mediated by both sex-hormone deficiency-dependent and -independent mechanisms [20,26,27].

DIETARY PROTEIN AND BONE MINERAL MASS

In numerous studies, a positive association between bone mass at various skeletal sites and spontaneous protein intake has been detected in pre- or postmenopausal women as well as in men (Table II) [12,28–51]. In a survey carried out in hospitalized elderly, low protein intake was associated with decreased proximal femur BMD and with poor physical performance [12]. Undernutrition can concern all kinds of nutrients, and the specific role of a low protein intake besides low calorie consumption can be difficult to appraise in the elderly [12]. Protein supplements are associated with a favorable outcome [2], as one of the key nutrients responsible for a beneficial effect on fracture outcome seems to be proteins [52]. Unadjusted

TABLE II   Bone Mineral Density and Protein Intake

Refs.	Subjects (Duration)	Skeletal Site
	Cross-Sectional Studies	
Positive Association (BMD Proportional to Dietary Protein)		
[28]	5900 men and women	Proximal femur
[29]	258 postmenopausal women	Lumbar spine
[30]	72 premenopausal women	Distal radius, proximal femur
[12]	74 men and women	Femoral neck
[31]	161 premenopausal women	Forearm
[32]	1822 postmenopausal women	Proximal femur
[33]	178 pre- and postmenopausal women	Midradius
[34]	76 postmenopausal women	Hip
[35]	175 pre- and postmenopausal women	Total, lumbar spine, proximal femur
[36]	92 men	Midradius, lumbar spine
[37]	215 premenopausal women	Midradius, lumbar spine
[38]	375 postmenopausal women	Mid- and distal radius
No Association		
[39]	115 premenopausal women	Lumbar spine, proximal femur, forearm
[40]	200–300 premenopausal women	Lumbar spine, forearm
[41]	994 premenopausal women	Lumbar spine, proximal femur
[42]	139 premenopausal women	Lumbar spine, forearm
[43]	125 postmenopausal women	Lumbar spine, proximal femur
Negative Association (BMD Inversely Proportional to Dietary Protein)		
[44]	220 premenopausal women	Distal radius
[45]	38 premenopausal women	Distal radius
	Longitudinal Studies	
Inverse Relationship (Higher Intake → Lower Rate of Bone Loss)		
[46]	345 men and women (3 yr)	Femoral neck[a]
[47]	67 postmenopausal women (4 yr)	Forearm
[48]	615 men and women, 75 yr (4 yr)	Spine, femoral neck
No Association		
[49]	156 premenopausal women (3.4 yr)	Spine
[50]	122 postmenopausal women (2 yr)	Spine, hip
Positive Relationship (Higher Intake → Higher Rate of Bone Loss)		
[51]	1035 postmenopausal women, >65 yr	Femoral neck[b]

[a]In the group supplemented in calcium.
[b]Animal/vegetable ratio, adjusted for energy, calcium, protein, body weight.

bone mineral density (BMD) was found to be greater in the group with the higher protein intake in a large series of data collected by the Study of Osteoporotic Fracture [51]. There was a positive correlation between radial bone mineral content and protein intake in Japanese or American women [31]. Besides numerous cross-sectional studies showing a positive association between bone mass and protein intake, a longitudinal follow-up of the

Framingham study has demonstrated that the rate of bone mineral loss is inversely correlated to dietary protein intake (Table II) [48]. Recently, spontaneous higher protein intake was associated with an increase in BMD in a group of patients receiving calcium supplements who were followed longitudinally (Table II) [46]. In contrast, very few are the surveys in which high protein intake was accompanied with lower bone mass. In a cross-sectional study, a protein intake close to 2 g/kg body weight was associated with reduced bone mineral density only at one out of the two forearm sites measured in young college women [44]. With various adjustments, BMD was found to be lower in the group with the higher animal-to-vegetable protein ratio [51].

It has been claimed that high protein intake could be harmful for bone, based on the positive association between urinary calcium excretion and protein intake. This association between urinary calcium excretion and dietary protein suggested that high protein intake would induce a negative calcium balance and, consequently, would favor bone loss [53]. However, further studies indicated that a reduction in dietary protein led to a decline in calcium absorption and to secondary hyperparathyroidism [54]. An increase in parathyroid hormone (PTH) can be detected with dietary protein lower than 0.8 g/kg body weight [54]. There is some evidence that the favorable effect of increasing the protein intake on bone mineral mass as repeatedly observed in both genders [12,28,29,33–36,38,48] is better expressed with an adequate supply of both calcium and vitamin D [46,55–58].

The source of proteins, animal versus vegetable, has been claimed to influence calcium metabolism [56]. The hypothesis implies that animal proteins would generate more sulfuric acid from sulfur-containing amino acids than a vegetarian diet. Consequently, the nutrition-generated acid load would lead in healthy individuals to an increased bone dissolution, this by analogy to the classical physicochemical *in vitro* observation indicating that lowering pH favors the dissolution of calcium phosphate crystals, including those of hydroxyapatite. The theory suggesting that animal protein in contrast to vegetable protein would be more detrimental for bone health is not supported by convincing experimental evidence. Indeed, a vegetarian diet with protein derived from grains and vegetables appears to deliver as many millimoles of sulfur per gram proteins as would a purely meat-based diet [56]. Several recent human studies do not suggest that the protective effect of protein on either bone loss or osteoporotic fracture is due to vegetable rather than animal protein [46,48,59–61]. In contrast with these consistent results, a longitudinal follow-up study reported that individuals consuming diets with high ratios of animal to vegetable protein lost bone more rapidly than did those with lower ratios and had a greater risk of hip fracture [51]. The physiological meaning, particularly in terms of the impact on calcium-phosphate and bone metabolism of the animal-to-vegetable protein ratio remains mechanistically difficult to interprete, as a similar ratio can be achieved with a large variety of protein contents and thus of sulfur supply, if the acid load theory was valid. Indeed, a similar ratio can be obtained with markedly different absolute intakes of either animal or vegetable protein. More importantly, however, in this study [51] the statistically negative relationship between the animal-to-vegetable protein ratio and bone loss was obtained only after multiple adjustments, not only for age but also for energy intake, total calcium intake (dietary plus supplements), total protein intake, weight, current estrogen use, physical activity, smoking status, and alcohol use [51]. In sharp contrast, a positive relationship between the animal-to-vegetable protein ratio and baseline BMD was found when the statistical model was adjusted only for age [51]. An inconsistency according to the way the data were analyzed makes it difficult to generalize these finding in terms of nutritional recommendation for bone health and osteoporosis prevention [56].

Taken together, these results indicate that, whereas a gradual decline in calory intakes with age can be considered as an adequate adjustment to the progressive reduction in energy expenditure, the parallel reduction in protein intakes may be detrimental for maintaining the integrity and function of several organs or systems, including skeletal muscles and bone.

DIETARY PROTEIN AND BONE HOMEOSTASIS

Insulin-like growth factor I (IGF-I) is an essential factor for longitudinal bone growth [62]. IGF-I can also exert anabolic effects on bone mass during adulthood [63–66]. Furthermore, by its renal action on tubular reabsorption of phosphate and on the synthesis of calcitriol, through a direct action on renal cells [67,68], IGF-I can be considered as an important controller of the intestinal absorption and of the extracellular concentration of both calcium and phosphate, the main elements of bone mineral (Fig. 2). On the other hand, IGF-I can selectively stimulate the transport of inorganic phosphate across the plasma membrane in osteoblastic cell lines [69,70].

Experimental and clinical studies suggest that dietary protein, by influencing both the production and action of IGF-I, particularly the growth hormone (GH)–IGF system, could control bone anabolism [63,71]. The hepatic production and plasma levels of IGF-I are under the influence of dietary proteins [72–74]. Protein restriction has been shown to reduce IGF-I plasma levels by inducing a resistance to the action of GH at the hepatic level [75,76] and by an increase of IGF-I metabolic clearance rate [77]. Decreased levels of IGF-I have been found in states of undernutrition

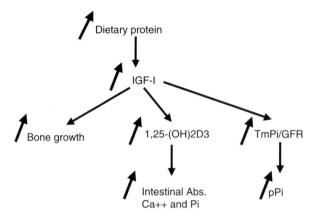

FIGURE 2   Role of dietary protein and IGF-I in calcium–phosphate metabolism.

such as marasmus, anorexia nervosa, celiac disease, or human immunodeficiency virus (HIV) [72,73,78,79]. Elevated protein intake is able to prevent the decrease in IGF-I usually observed in hypocaloric states [3,80]. Protein restriction appears to render target organs less sensitive to IGF-I. When IGF-I was given to growing rats maintained under a low-protein diet at doses normalizing the plasma levels, it failed to restore skeletal longitudinal growth [81]. When pharmacological doses of IGF-I were administered to produce a fivefold increase in IGF-I circulating levels in adult rats in an attempt to correct the negative influence of protein deficiency, no effects on bone were observed if the protein intake was insufficient [82].

Because undernutrition can concern all kinds of nutrients in the elderly [2], not only protein, we developed an experimental model in adult female rats of selective protein deprivation with isocaloric low-protein diets supplemented with identical amounts of minerals in order to study the specific influence of protein deficiency in the pathogenesis of osteoporosis [20]. This model enables the study of bone mineral mass, bone strength, and bone remodeling. A decrease of BMD is observed at the level of skeletal sites formed by trabecular or cortical bone in animals fed 2.5% casein but receiving the same amount of energy. This decrease is associated with a marked and early decrease in plasma IGF-I by 40%. In this model, the decrease in bone mass and bone strength is related to an early inhibition of bone formation and a later acceleration of bone resorption [20]. Whereas a rapid decrease in circulating IGF-I could account for the former, the latter might be related to estrogen deficiency caused by protein undernutrition. Indeed, under a low-protein diet, the normal cycling in female rats disappeared, and was recovered upon protein replenishment (Ammann et al., unpublished results). An isocaloric low protein (2.5% casein) diet decreased BMD and altered mechanical properties in male rats as well; the protein deficiency induced cortical and trabecular thinning in relation with a remodeling imbalance with impaired bone formation. This led to a decrease in bone mineral mass and bone strength [82]. At an early time point (1 month), histomorphometry analysis showed that the bone loss process was mainly related to a depressed bone formation [82]. Also in males, some state of hypogonadism was associated with long-term, isocaloric, low-protein diets. Adult male and female rats differed by the kinetics of the response to the isocaloric low-protein diet, with changes occurring more slowly in males than in females.

Because there was an alteration of the growth hormone–IGF-I bone axis in protein undernutrition with altered production of both hormones, decreased bone formation, increased bone resorption, and a marked increase in bone fragility, we investigated whether the administration of growth hormone or IGF-I could reverse this process. Under an isocaloric, low-protein diet, the IGF-I response to GH appeared to be blunted, but the most striking finding was that growth hormone was rather catabolic on bone, instead of anabolic, because there was a dose-dependent decrease of bone strength after 4 weeks of growth hormone treatment in animals fed the isocaloric, low-protein diet [83]. We then tested the effects of protein replenishment by administering essential amino acid supplements in the same relative proportion as in casein. These supplements caused an increase of IGF-I up to a level higher than in rats fed the control diet, increased biochemical bone formation, decreased markers of bone resorption, and improved bone strength more than bone mineral mass, probably due to an increase in cortical thickness, as demonstrated by micro-quantitative computerized tomography (Fig. 3) [83].

In addition to alterations in the control and action of the growth hormone–IGF-I system, protein undernutrition can be associated with alterations of cytokines secretion, such as interferon gamma (IFN-γ), tumor necrosis factor alpha (TNF-α), or transforming growth factor beta (TGF-β) [84,85]. Levels of TNF-α and interleukin-6 (IL-6) generally increase with age [86]. In a situation of cachexia, such as in chronic heart failure, an inverse correlation between bone mineral density and TNF-α levels has been found [87,88], further implicating a possible role of uncontrolled cytokines production in bone loss. Increased TNF-α can be a crucial factor in bone loss induced by a sex-hormone deficiency [89], but it also plays a role in the target organ resistance to insulin and possibly to IGF-I [90]. Along the same line, certain amino acids given to rats fed a low-protein diet can increase the liver protein synthesis response to TNF-α [91] ; however, an increase in bone resorption under a low-protein diet was also detected in ovariectomized

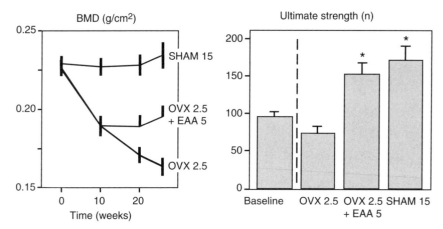

FIGURE 3   Effects of essential amino acids supplements on vertebral bone mineral density (A) and strength (B) in ovariectomized rats fed a low protein diet. (Adapted from Ammann et al. [83].)

animals, indicating the presence of a component that is low protein diet-dependent and sex hormone-independent [20]. Histomorphometry analysis and biochemical markers of bone remodeling results indicate that the low protein intake-induced decrease in bone mineral mass and bone strength is related to an uncoupling between bone formation and resorption [20]. The prevalence of bone resorption over formation could be partially explained by the altered sex hormone status; however, other mechanisms, including the effects of circulating or locally released cytokines, are likely [89,92]. The production and action of TNF-α play a central role in the accelerated bone loss caused by sex-hormone deficiency, as indicated by experiments carried out in transgenic mice overexpressing TNF-α receptor 1 protein, which blocks the effects of this factor. Indeed, in these animals, the influence of ovariectomy [89] or orchidectomy [92] is prevented in transgenic animals overexpressing the receptor. To address the issue of accelerated bone loss occurring under a low-protein diet, we used the model of transgenic mice that overexpresses the soluble TNF-α receptor. Blocking TNF-α activity prevented the component of increased bone resorption induced by the isocaloric, low-protein diet, without modifying the alterations in bone formation [93,94]. Similarly, we also assessed whether interleukin-1 (IL-1) could be involved in this process. The effects of an isocaloric, low-protein diet were studied in transgenic mice overexpressing an IL-1 receptor antagonist, a situation in which IL-1 cannot exert its biological action. In this model, bone loss in the mice overexpressing the IL-1 receptor antagonist and their negative littermates was identical [93,94]. In humans, too, the amino acid oxidation rate has been found to be lower in children with kwashiorkor who are treated with milk as compared with egg white, and protein breakdown and synthesis are inversely correlated to TNF-α levels [95].

EFFECTS OF CORRECTING PROTEIN INSUFFICIENCY

Taking into account these experimental and clinical observations, IGF-I could play a prominent role in the pathophysiology of osteoporosis, of osteoporotic fracture, and of its complications. Under these conditions, a restoration of the altered growth hormone–IGF-I system in the elderly by protein replenishment is likely to favorably influence not only bone mineral density but also muscle mass and strength, as these two variables are important determinants of the risk of falling [96,97]. The modulation of cytokine production and action by nutritional intake [98] and the strong implication of various cytokines in the regulation of bone remodeling [99] suggest a possible role of certain cytokines in the nutrition–bone link.

Intervention studies using a simple oral dietary preparation that normalizes protein intake [2] can improve the clinical outcome after hip fracture. It should be noted that a 20-g protein supplement has been shown to bring protein intake from a low level to a level that is still below the recommended daily allowance (0.8 g/kg body weight), thus avoiding the risk of an excess of dietary protein [2]. Follow-up showed a significant difference in the clinical course in the rehabilitation hospitals, with the supplemented patients doing better. The significantly lower rate of complications (bedsores, severe anemia, intercurrent lung or renal infections and deaths [44% versus 87%] was still observed at 6 months [40% versus 74%]) [2]. In this study [2], the total length of stay in the orthopedic ward and convalescent hospital was significantly shorter in supplemented patients than in controls (median: 24 versus 40 days). It was then shown that normalization of protein intake, independently of that of energy, calcium, and vitamin D, was in fact responsible for this more favorable outcome [52], as shown in a randomized controlled trial, in which protein intake was the primary variable accounting for the better outcome that was recorded. In undernourished elderly with a recent hip fracture, an increase in protein intake, from low to normal, can also be beneficial for bone integrity [59]. Indeed, in a double-blind, placebo-controlled study, protein repletion with 20 g of protein supplement daily for 6 months as compared to an isocaloric placebo produced greater gains in serum prealbumin, IGF-I, and immunoglobulin (IgM), as well as an attenuated proximal femur BMD decrease [59].

In this trial, all 82 patients (80.7 ± 1.2 years) were given 200,000 IU vitamin D once at baseline and 550 mg/day of calcium, starting within 1 week after an osteoporotic hip fracture. In a multiple regression analysis, baseline IGF-I concentrations, biceps muscle strength, and protein supplementation accounted for more than 30% of the variance of the length of stay in rehabilitation hopitals ($R^2 = 0.312$, $P < 0.0005$), which was reduced by 25% in the protein-supplemented group. Thus, the lower incidence of medical complications observed after a protein supplement [2,52] is also compatible with the hypothesis of IGF-I improving the immune status, as this growth factor can stimulate the proliferation of immunocompetent cells and modulate immunoglobulin secretion [100].

We recently completed short-term studies on the kinetics and determinants of the IGF-I response to protein supplements in a situation associated with low baseline IGF-I levels. In the elderly with a recent hip fracture, we found that a 20 g/day protein supplement increased serum IGF-I and IGF-binding protein-3 already by one week. The increase in bone turnover, as assessed by biochemical markers, was slightly delayed (Chevalley et al., unpublished results).

DIETARY PROTEIN AND FRACTURE RISK

Various studies, assessing the relationship between protein intake and bone metabolism [13,44,45,101–105] came to the conclusion that either a deficient or an excessive protein supply could negatively affect the balance of calcium. An indirect argument in favor of a deleterious effect of high protein intake on bone is that hip fracture appeared to be more frequent in countries with high protein intake of animal origin (Table III) [106,107]. But, as expected, the countries with the highest incidence are those with longest life expectancy, accounting for an elevated fracture incidence. In the large Nurse Health Study, a trend for a hip fracture incidence inversely related to protein intake has been reported [108]. Similarly, hip fracture was higher with low energy intake, low serum albumin levels, and low muscle strength in the NHANES I study [109]. In a prospective study carried out on more than 40,000 women in Iowa, higher protein intake was associated with a reduced risk of hip fracture [60]. The protective effect was observed with dietary protein of animal origin. In another survey, no association between hip fracture and non-dairy-animal protein intake could be detected [110]; however, in this study, fracture risk was increased when a high protein diet was accompanied by a low calcium intake, in agreement with the finding that the intake of calcium had to be sufficient to detect a favorable influence of dietary protein on bone.

TABLE III   Osteoporotic Fracture and Protein Intake

Refs.	Study Subjects (Duration)	Site of Fracture (Source of Protein)
Positive Association (Higher Intake → Higher Risk)		
[106]	Cross-cultural study	Hip (animal)
[108]	85,900 women (12 yr)	Forearm 1.2 × (animal)
[107]	Cross-cultural study	Hip
[110]	39,787 men and women	Hip (if low calcium intake in women)
[51]	1035 women (7 yr)	Hip (animal/vegetable ratio)
Inverse Relationship (Higher Intake → Lower Risk)		
[109]	2565 women (16 yr)	Hip
[60]	32,050 women (3 yr)	Hip (animal > vegetable)
[51]	1035 women (7 yr)	Hip (vegetable)
[111]	2501 men and women (5 yr)	Hip
No Association		
[108]	85,900 women, 12 yr	Hip (animal)

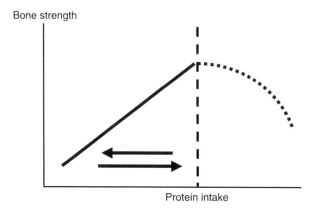

FIGURE 4   Bone strength and dietary protein.

In a longitudinal study, hip fracture incidence was positively related to a higher ratio of animal to vegetable protein intake [51], whereas protein of vegetable origin was rather protective.

CONCLUSIONS

There is a large body of evidence linking nutritional intakes, particularly protein undernutrition, to bone homeostasis, bone strength, and osteoporotic fractures. Sufficient dietary proteins are necessary for bone homeostasis and strength, during growth as well as in advanced years (Fig. 4). Several mechanisms, among them the growth hormone–IGF-I–target organ axis and various cytokines, are likely to be implicated.

ACKNOWLEDGMENTS

We thank Mrs. M. Perez for her secretarial assistance. The work quoted here by our group was supported by the Swiss National Science Research Foundation (32-32415.91, 32-49757.96, 32-58880.99, and 3200B0-100714) and by Novartis-Nutrition, Berne, Switzerland.

REFERENCES

1. Bastow, M.D., Rawlings, J., and Allison, S.P. (1983). Undernutrition, hypothermia, and injury in elderly women with fractured femur: an injury response to altered metabolism? *Lancet* 1: 143–146.
2. Delmi, M., Rapin, C.H., Bengoa, J.M., Delmas, P.D., Vasey, H., and Bonjour, J.P. (1990). Dietary supplementation in elderly patients with fractured neck of the femur. *Lancet* 335: 1013–1016.
3. Jensen, J.E., Jensen, T.G., Smith, T.K., Johnston, D.A., and Dudrick, S.J. (1982). Nutrition in orthopaedic surgery. *J. Bone Joint Surg.* (*Am.*) 64: 1263–1272.
4. Bastow, M.D., Rawlings, J., and Allison, S.P. (1983). Benefits of supplementary tube feeding after fractured neck of femur: a randomised controlled trial. *Br. Med. J.* 287: 1589–1592.
5. Schurch, M.A., Rizzoli, R., Mermillod, B., Vasey, H., Michel, J.P., and Bonjour, J.P. (1996). A prospective study on socioeconomic aspects of fracture of the proximal femur. *J. Bone Mineral Res.* 11: 1935–1942.
6. Nydegger, V., Rizzoli, R., Rapin, C.H., Vasey, H., and Bonjour, J.P. (1991). Epidemiology of fractures of the proximal femur in Geneva: incidence, clinical and social aspects. *Osteoporos Int.* 2: 42–47.
7. Patterson, B.M., Cornell, C.N., Carbone, B., Levine, B., and Chapman, D. (1992). Protein depletion and metabolic stress in elderly patients who have a fracture of the hip. *J. Bone Joint Surg.* (*Am.*) 74: 251–260.
8. Garn, S.M., Guzman, M.A., and Wagner, B. (1969). Subperiosteal gain and endosteal loss in protein-calorie malnutrition. *Am. J. Phys. Anthropol.* 30: 153–155.
9. Parfitt, A.M. (1983). Dietary risk factors for age-related bone loss and fractures. *Lancet* 2: 1181–1185.
10. Rizzoli, R., Ammann, P., Chevalley, T., and Bonjour, J.P. (2001). Protein intake and bone disorders in the elderly. *Joint Bone Spine* 68: 383–392.
11. Schaafsma, G., van Beresteyn, E.C., Raymakers, J.A., and Duursma, S.A. (1987). Nutritional aspects of osteoporosis. *World Rev. Nutr. Diet* 49: 121–159.
12. Geinoz, G., Rapin, C.H., Rizzoli, R., Kraemer, R., Buchs, B., Slosman, D., Michel, J.P., and Bonjour, J.P. (1993). Relationship between bone mineral density and dietary intakes in the elderly. *Osteoporos Int.* 3: 242–248.
13. Rizzoli, R. and Bonjour, J.P. (1999). Nutritional approaches to healing fractures in the elderly, in *The Aging Skeleton*, Rosen, C.J., Glowacki, J., and Bilezikian, J.P., Eds., Academic Press, San Diego, CA, pp. 399–409.

14. Bonjour, J.P., Chevalley, T., Ammann, P., Slosman, D., and Rizzoli, R. (2001). Gain in bone mineral mass in prepubertal girls 3.5 years after discontinuation of calcium supplementation: a follow-up study. *Lancet* 358: 1208–1212.
15. Bonjour, J.P., Theintz, G., Law, F., Slosman, D., and Rizzoli, R. (1994). Peak bone mass. *Osteoporos Int.* 4: 7–13.
16. Theintz, G., Buchs, B., Rizzoli, R., Slosman, D., Clavien, H., Sizonenko, P.C., and Bonjour, J.P. (1992). Longitudinal monitoring of bone mass accumulation in healthy adolescents: evidence for a marked reduction after 16 years of age at the levels of lumbar spine and femoral neck in female subjects. *J. Clin. Endocrinol. Metab.* 75: 1060–1065.
17. Bonjour, J.P., Theintz, G., Buchs, B., Slosman, D., and Rizzoli, R. (1991). Critical years and stages of puberty for spinal and femoral bone mass accumulation during adolescence. *J. Clin. Endocrinol. Metab.* 73: 555–563.
18. Clavien, H., Theintz, G., Rizzoli, R., and Bonjour, J.P. (1996). Does puberty alter dietary habits in adolescents living in a western society? *J. Adolesc. Health* 19: 68–75.
19. Lucas, A.R., Melton, III, L.J., Crowson, C.S., and O'Fallon, W.M. (1999). Long-term fracture risk among women with anorexia nervosa: a population-based cohort study. *Mayo Clin. Proc.* 74: 972–977.
20. Ammann, P., Bourrin, S., Bonjour, J.P., Meyer, J.M., and Rizzoli, R. (2000). Protein undernutrition-induced bone loss is associated with decreased IGF-I levels and estrogen deficiency. *J. Bone Mineral Res.* 15: 683–690.
21. Drinkwater, B.L., Nilson, K., Chesnut, III, C.H., Bremner, W.J., Shainholtz, S., and Southworth, M.B. (1984). Bone mineral content of amenorrheic and eumenorrheic athletes. *New Engl. J. Med.* 311: 277–281.
22. Marcus, R., Cann, C., Madvig, P., Minkoff, J., Goddard, M., Bayer, M., Martin, M., Gaudiani, L., Haskell, W., and Genant, H. (1985). Menstrual function and bone mass in elite women distance runners: endocrine and metabolic features. *Ann. Intern. Med.* 102: 158–163.
23. Warren, M.P. and Perlroth, N.E. (2001). The effects of intense exercise on the female reproductive system. *J. Endocrinol.* 170: 3–11.
24. Gremion, G., Rizzoli, R., Slosman, D., Theintz, G., and Bonjour, J.P. (2001). Oligo-amenorrheic long-distance runners may lose more bone in spine than in femur. *Med. Sci. Sports Exerc.* 33: 15–21.
25. Beck, B.R., Shaw, J., and Snow, C.M. (2001). Physical activity and osteoporosis, in *Osteoporosis*, 2nd ed., Marcus, R., Feldman, D., and Kelsey, J., Eds., Academic Press, San Diego, CA, pp. 701–720.
26. Ammann, P., Rizzoli, R., and Bonjour, J.P. (1998). Protein malnutrition-induced bone loss is associated with alteration of growth hormone–IGF-I axis and with estrogen deficiency in adult rats. *Osteoporos Int.* 8(suppl. 3), 10.
27. Ammann, P., Garcia, I., Bonjour, J.P., and Rizzoli, R. (1999). High expression of soluble tumor necrosis factor receptor-1 fusion protein prevents bone loss caused by testosterone deficiency. *Calcif. Tissue Int.* 64: S26.
28. Calvo, M.S., Barton, C.N., and Park, Y.K. (1998). Bone mass and high dietary intake of meat and protein: analyses of data from the Third National Health and Nutrition Examination Survey (NHANES III, 1988–94). *Bone* 23(suppl.): S290.
29. Chiu, J.F., Lan, S.J., Yang, C.Y., Wang, P.W., Yao, W.J., Su, L.H., and Hsieh, C.C. (1997). Long-term vegetarian diet and bone mineral density in postmenopausal Taiwanese women. *Calcif. Tissue Int.* 60: 245–249.
30. Cooper, C., Atkinson, E.J., Hensrud, D.D., Wahner, H.W., O'Fallon, W.M., Riggs, B.L., and Melton III, L.J. (1996). Dietary protein intake and bone mass in women. *Calcif. Tissue Int.* 58: 320–325.

31. Hirota, T., Nara, M., Ohguri, M., Manago, E., and Hirota, K. (1992). Effect of diet and lifestyle on bone mass in Asian young women. *Am. J. Clin. Nutr.* 55: 1168–1173.
32. Kerstetter, J.E., Looker, A.C., and Insogna, K.L. (2000). Low dietary protein and low bone density. *Calcif. Tissue Int.* 66: 313.
33. Lacey, J.M., Anderson, J.J., Fujita, T., Yoshimoto, Y., Fukase, M., Tsuchie, S., and Koch, G.G. (1991). Correlates of cortical bone mass among premenopausal and postmenopausal Japanese women. *J. Bone Mineral Res.* 6: 651–659.
34. Lau, E.M., Kwok, T., Woo, J., and Ho, S.C. (1998). Bone mineral density in Chinese elderly female vegetarians, vegans, lacto-vegetarians and omnivores. *Eur. J. Clin. Nutr.* 52: 60–64.
35. Michaelsson, K., Holmberg, L., Mallmin, H., Wolk, A., Bergstrom, R., and Ljunghall, S. (1995). Diet, bone mass, and osteocalcin: a cross-sectional study. *Calcif. Tissue Int.* 57: 86–93.
36. Orwoll, E.S., Weigel, R.M., Oviatt, S.K., Meier, D.E., and McClung, M.R. (1987). Serum protein concentrations and bone mineral content in aging normal men. *Am. J. Clin. Nutr.* 46: 614–621.
37. Teegarden, D., Lyle, R.M., McCabe, G. P., McCabe, L.D., Proulx, W.R., Michon, K., Knight, A.P., Johnston, C.C., and Weaver, C.M. (1998). Dietary calcium, protein, and phosphorus are related to bone mineral density and content in young women. *Am. J. Clin. Nutr.* 68: 749–754.
38. Tylavsky, F.A. and Anderson, J.J. (1988). Dietary factors in bone health of elderly lactoovovegetarian and omnivorous women. *Am. J. Clin. Nutr.* 48: 842–849.
39. Henderson, N.K., Price, R.I., Cole, J.H., Gutteridge, D.H., and Bhagat, C.I. (1995). Bone density in young women is associated with body weight and muscle strength but not dietary intakes. *J. Bone Mineral Res.* 10: 384–393.
40. Mazess, R.B. and Barden, H.S. (1991). Bone density in premenopausal women: effects of age, dietary intake, physical activity, smoking, and birth-control pills. *Am. J. Clin. Nutr.* 53: 132–142.
41. New, S.A., Bolton-Smith, C., Grubb, D.A., and Reid, D.M. (1997). Nutritional influences on bone mineral density: a cross-sectional study in premenopausal women. *Am. J. Clin. Nutr.* 65: 1831–1839.
42. Nieves, J.W., Golden, A.L., Siris, E., Kelsey, J.L., and Lindsay, R. (1995). Teenage and current calcium intake are related to bone mineral density of the hip and forearm in women aged 30–39 years. *Am. J. Epidemiol.* 141: 342–351.
43. Wang, M.C., Luz Villa, M., Marcus, R., and Kelsey, J.L. (1997). Associations of vitamin C, calcium and protein with bone mass in postmenopausal Mexican American women. *Osteoporos Int.* 7: 533–538.
44. Anderson, J.J. and Metz, J.A. (1995). Adverse association of high protein intake to bone density. *Challenges Modern Med.* 7: 407–412.
45. Metz, J.A., Anderson, J.J., and Gallagher, Jr., P.N. (1993). Intakes of calcium, phosphorus, and protein, and physical-activity level are related to radial bone mass in young adult women. *Am. J. Clin. Nutr.* 58: 537–542.
46. Dawson-Hughes, B. and Harris, S.S. (2002). Calcium intake influences the association of protein intake with rates of bone loss in elderly men and women. *Am. J. Clin. Nutr.* 75: 773–779.
47. Freudenheim, J.L., Johnson, N.E., and Smith, E.L. (1986). Relationships between usual nutrient intake and bone mineral content of women 35–65 years of age: longitudinal and cross-sectional analysis. *Am. J. Clin. Nutr.* 44: 863–876.
48. Hannan, M.T., Tucker, K.L., Dawson-Hughes, B., Cupples, L.A., Felson, D.T., and Kiel, D.P. (2000). Effect of dietary protein on bone loss in elderly men and women: the Framingham Osteoporosis Study. *J. Bone Mineral Res.* 15: 2504–2512.
49. Recker, R.R., Davies, K.M., Hinders, S.M., Heaney, R.P., Stegman, M.R., and Kimmel, D.B. (1992). Bone gain in young adult women. *JAMA* 268: 2403–2408.

50. Reid, I.R., Ames, R.W., Evans, M.C., Sharpe, S.J., and Gamble, G.D. (1994). Determinants of the rate of bone loss in normal postmenopausal women. *J. Clin. Endocrinol. Metab.* 79: 950–954.

51. Sellmeyer, D.E., Stone, K.L., Sebastian, A., and Cummings, S.R. (2001). A high ratio of dietary animal to vegetable protein increases the rate of bone loss and the risk of fracture in postmenopausal women. Study of Osteoporotic Fractures Research Group. *Am. J. Clin. Nutr.* 73: 118–122.

52. Tkatch, L., Rapin, C.H., Rizzoli, R., Slosman, D., Nydegger, V., Vasey, H., and Bonjour, J.P. (1992). Benefits of oral protein supplementation in elderly patients with fracture of the proximal femur. *J. Am. Coll. Nutr.* 11: 519–525.

53. Heaney, R.P. and Recker, R.R. (1982). Effects of nitrogen, phosphorus, and caffeine on calcium balance in women. *J. Lab. Clin. Med.* 99: 46–55.

54. Kerstetter, J.E., O'Brien, K., and Insogna, K.L. (2002). Dietary protein and intestinal calcium absorption. *Am. J. Clin. Nutr.* 73: 990–992.

55. Heaney, R.P. (2000). Calcium, dairy products and osteoporosis. *J. Am. Coll. Nutr.* 19: 83S–99S.

56. Heaney, R.P. (2001). Protein intake and bone health: the influence of belief systems on the conduct of nutritional science. *Am. J. Clin. Nutr.* 73: 5–6.

57. Heaney, R.P. (2002). Protein and calcium: antagonists or synergists? *Am. J. Clin. Nutr.* 75: 609–610.

58. Bell, J. and Whiting, S.J. (2002). Elderly women need dietary protein to maintain bone mass. *Nutr. Rev.* 60: 337–341.

59. Schurch, M.A., Rizzoli, R., Slosman, D., Vadas, L., Vergnaud, P., and Bonjour, J.P. (1998). Protein supplements increase serum insulin-like growth factor-I levels and attenuate proximal femur bone loss in patients with recent hip fracture. A randomized, double-blind, placebo-controlled trial. *Ann. Intern. Med.* 128: 801–809.

60. Munger, R.G., Cerhan, J.R., and Chiu, B.C. (1999). Prospective study of dietary protein intake and risk of hip fracture in postmenopausal women. *Am. J. Clin. Nutr.* 69: 147–152.

61. Promislow, J.H., Goodman-Gruen, D., Slymen, D.J., and Barrett-Connor, E. (2002). Protein consumption and bone mineral density in the elderly: the Rancho Bernardo Study. *Am. J. Epidemiol.* 155: 636–644.

62. Froesch, E.R., Schmid, C., Schwander, J., and Zapf, J. (1985). Actions of insulin-like growth factors. *Annu. Rev. Physiol.* 47: 443–467.

63. Rosen, C.J. and Donahue, L.R. (1995). Insulin-like growth-factor: potential therapeutic options for osteoporosis. *Trends Endocrinol. Metab.* 6: 235–241.

64. Ammann, P., Rizzoli, R., Meyer, J.M., and Bonjour, J.P. (1996). Bone density and shape as determinants of bone strength in IGF-1 and/or pamidronate-treated ovariectomized rats. *Osteoporos Int.* 6: 219–227.

65. Bagi, C., van der Meulen, M., Brommage, R., Rosen, D., and Sommer, A. (1995). The effect of systemically administered rhIGF-I/IGFBP-3 complex on cortical bone strength and structure in ovariectomized rats. *Bone* 16: 559–565.

66. Bagi, C.M., DeLeon, E., Brommage, R., Rosen, D., and Sommer, A. (1995). Treatment of ovariectomized rats with the complex of rhIGF-I/IGFBP-3 increases cortical and cancellous bone mass and improves structure in the femoral neck. *Calcif. Tissue Int.* 57: 40–46.

67. Caverzasio, J. and Bonjour, J.P. (1989). Insulin-like growth factor I stimulates Na-dependent Pi transport in cultured kidney cells. *Am. J. Physiol.* 257: F712–717.

68. Caverzasio, J., Montessuit, C., and Bonjour, J.P. (1990). Stimulatory effect of insulin-like growth factor-1 on renal Pi transport and plasma 1,25-dihydroxyvitamin D_3. *Endocrinology* 127: 453–459.

69. Palmer, G., Bonjour, J.P., and Caverzasio, J. (1996). Stimulation of inorganic phosphate transport by insulin-like growth factor I and vanadate in opossum kidney cells is mediated by distinct protein tyrosine phosphorylation processes. *Endocrinology* 137: 4699–4705.

70. Palmer, G., Bonjour, J.P., and Caverzasio, J. (1997). Expression of a newly identified phosphate transporter/retrovirus receptor in human SaOS-2 osteoblast-like cells and its regulation by insulin-like growth factor I. *Endocrinology* 138: 5202–5209.

71. Canalis, E. and Agnusdei, D. (1996). Insulin-like growth factors and their role in osteoporosis [editorial]. *Calcif. Tissue Int.* 58: 133–134.

72. Thissen, J.P., Ketelslegers, J.M., and Underwood, L.E. (1994). Nutritional regulation of the insulin-like growth factors. *Endocr. Rev.* 15: 80–101.

73. Thissen, J.P., Pucilowska, J.B., and Underwood, L.E. (1994). Differential regulation of insulin-like growth factor I (IGF-I) and IGF binding protein-1 messenger ribonucleic acids by amino acid availability and growth hormone in rat hepatocyte primary culture. *Endocrinology* 134: 1570–1576.

74. Isley, W.L., Underwood, L.E., and Clemmons, D.R. (1983). Dietary components that regulate serum somatomedin-C concentrations in humans. *J. Clin. Invest.* 71: 175–182.

75. Thissen, J.P., Triest, S., Maes, M., Underwood, L.E., and Ketelslegers, J.M. (1990). The decreased plasma concentration of insulin-like growth factor-I in protein-restricted rats is not due to decreased numbers of growth hormone receptors on isolated hepatocytes. *J. Endocrinol.* 124: 159–165.

76. VandeHaar, M.J., Moats-Staats, B.M., Davenport, M.L., Walker, J.L., Ketelslegers, J.M., Sharma, B.K., and Underwood, L.E. (1991). Reduced serum concentrations of insulin-like growth factor-I (IGF-I) in protein-restricted growing rats are accompanied by reduced IGF-I mRNA levels in liver and skeletal muscle. *J. Endocrinol.* 130: 305–312.

77. Thissen, J.P., and Underwood, L.E. (1992). Translational status of the insulin-like growth factor-I mRNAs in liver of protein-restricted rats. *J. Endocrinol.* 132: 141–147.

78. Sullivan, D.H. and Carter, W.J. (1994). Insulin-like growth factor I as an indicator of protein-energy undernutrition among metabolically stable hospitalized elderly. *J. Am. Coll. Nutr.* 13: 184–191.

79. Pucilowska, J.B., Davenport, M.L., Kabir, I., Clemmons, D.R., Thissen, J.P., Butler, T., and Underwood, L.E. (1993). The effect of dietary protein supplementation on insulin-like growth factors (IGFs) and IGF-binding proteins in children with shigellosis. *J. Clin. Endocrinol. Metab.* 77: 1516–1521.

80. Musey, V.C., Goldstein, S., Farmer, P.K., Moore, P.B., and Phillips, L.S. (1993). Differential regulation of IGF-1 and IGF-binding protein-1 by dietary composition in humans. *Am. J. Med. Sci.* 305: 131–138.

81. Thissen, J.P., Triest, S., Moats-Staats, B.M., Underwood, L.E., Mauerhoff, T., Maiter, D., and Ketelslegers, J.M. (1991). Evidence that pretranslational and translational defects decrease serum insulin-like growth factor-I concentrations during dietary protein restriction. *Endocrinology* 129: 429–435.

82. Bourrin, S., Ammann, P., Bonjour, J.P., and Rizzoli, R. (2000). Dietary protein restriction lowers plasma insulin-like growth factor I (IGF-I), impairs cortical bone formation, and induces osteoblastic resistance to IGF-I in adult female rats. *Endocrinology* 141: 3149–3155.

83. Ammann, P., Laib, A., Bonjour, J.P., Meyer, J.M., Ruegsegger, P., and Rizzoli, R. (2002). Dietary essential amino acid supplements increase bone strength by influencing bone mass and bone microarchitecture in ovariectomized adult rats fed an isocaloric low-protein diet. *J. Bone Mineral Res.* 17: 1264–1272.

84. Chan, J., Tian, Y., Tanaka, K.E., Tsang, M.S., Yu, K., Salgame, P., Carroll, D., Kress, Y., Teitelbaum, R., and Bloom, B.R. (1996). Effects of protein calorie malnutrition on tuberculosis in mice. *Proc. Natl. Acad. Sci. USA* 93: 14857–14861.

85. Dai, G. and McMurray, D.N. (1998). Altered cytokine production and impaired antimycobacterial immunity in protein-malnourished guinea pigs. *Infect. Immun.* 66: 3562–3568.

86. Spaulding, C.C., Walford, R.L., and Effros, R.B. (1997). Calorie restriction inhibits the Age-related dysregulation of the cytokines TNF-alpha and IL-6 in C3B10RF1 mice. *Mech. Ageing Dev.* 93: 87–94.

87. Anker, S.D., Clark, A.L., Teixeira, M.M., Hellewell, P.G., and Coats, A.J. (1999). Loss of bone mineral in patients with cachexia due to chronic heart failure. *Am. J. Cardiol.* 83: 612–615.

88. Anker, S.D. and Coats, A.J. (1999). Cardiac cachexia: a syndrome with impaired survival and immune and neuroendocrine activation. *Chest* 115: 836–847.

89. Ammann, P., Rizzoli, R., Bonjour, J.P., Bourrin, S., Meyer, J.M., Vassalli, P., and Garcia, I. (1997). Transgenic mice expressing soluble tumor necrosis factor-receptor are protected against bone loss caused by estrogen deficiency. *J. Clin. Invest.* 99: 1699–1703.

90. Hotamisligil, G.S. (1999). Mechanisms of TNF-alpha-induced insulin resistance. *Exp. Clin. Endocrinol. Diabetes* 107: 119–125.

91. Grimble, R.F., Jackson, A.A., Persaud, C., Wride, M.J., Delers, F., and Engler, R. (1992). Cysteine and glycine supplementation modulate the metabolic response to tumor necrosis factor alpha in rats fed a low protein diet. *J. Nutr.* 122: 2066–2073.

92. Ammann, P., Bourrin, S., Bonjour, J.P., Brunner, F., Meyer, J.M., and Rizzoli, R. (1999). The new selective estrogen receptor modulator MDL 103:323 increases bone mineral density and bone strength in adult ovariectomized rats. *Osteoporos Int.* 10: 369–376.

93. Ammann, P., Gabay, C., Palmer, G., Garcia, I., and Rizzoli, R. (2002). Tumor necrosis factor alpha but not interleukine-1 is involved in protein undernutrition-induced bone resorption. *J. Bone Mineral Res.* 17(suppl. 1), S205.

94. Ammann, P., Aubert, M.L., Meyer, J.M., and Rizzoli, R. (2002). Protein undernutrition-induced bone resorption is dependent on tumor necrosis factor alpha (TNF). *Osteoporos Int.* 13(suppl. 1), S5.

95. Manary, M.J., Brewster, D.R., Broadhead, R.L., Graham, S.M., Hart, C.A., Crowley, J.R., Fjeld, C.R., and Yarasheski, K.E. (1997). Whole-body protein kinetics in children with kwashiorkor and infection: a comparison of egg white and milk as dietary sources of protein. *Am. J. Clin. Nutr.* 66: 643–648.

96. Aniansson, A., Zetterberg, C., Hedberg, M., and Henriksson, K.G. (1984). Impaired muscle function with aging. A background factor in the incidence of fractures of the proximal end of the femur. *Clin. Orthop.* 193–201.

97. Castaneda, C., Gordon, P.L., Fielding, R.A., Evans, W.J., and Crim, M.C. (2000). Marginal protein intake results in reduced plasma IGF-I levels and skeletal muscle fiber atrophy in elderly women. *J. Nutr. Health Aging* 4: 85–90.

98. Grimble, R.F. (1998). Nutritional modulation of cytokine biology. *Nutrition* 14: 634–640.

99. Jilka, R.L. (1998). Cytokines, bone remodeling, and estrogen deficiency: a 1998 update. *Bone* 23: 75–81.

100. Auernhammer, C.J. and Strasburger, C.J. (1995). Effects of growth hormone and insulin-like growth factor I on the immune system. *Eur. J. Endocrinol.* 133: 635–645.

101. Bonjour, J.P., Schurch, M.A., and Rizzoli, R. (1996). Nutritional aspects of hip fractures. *Bone* 18: 139S–144S.

102. Orwoll, E.S., Ware, M., Stribrska, L., Bikle, D., Sanchez, T., Andon, M., and Li, H. (1992). Effects of dietary protein deficiency on mineral metabolism and bone mineral density. *Am. J. Clin. Nutr.* 56: 314–319.

103. Orwoll, E.S. (1992). The effects of dietary protein insufficiency and excess on skeletal health. *Bone* 13: 343–350.

104. Rizzoli, R. and Bonjour, J.P. (1999). Determinants of peak bone mass and mechanisms of bone loss. *Osteoporos Int.* 9: S17–S23.

105. Rizzoli, R., Schürch, M.A., Chevalley, T., and Bonjour, J.P. (1998). Protein intake and osteoporosis, in *Nutritional Aspects of Osteoporosis*, Burckhardt, P., Dawson-Hughes, B., and Heaney, R.P. Eds., Springer-Verlag, New York, pp. 141–154.
106. Abelow, B.J., Holford, T.R., and Insogna, K.L. (1992). Cross-cultural association between dietary animal protein and hip fracture: a hypothesis. *Calcif. Tissue Int.* 50: 14–18.
107. Frassetto, L.A., Todd, K.M., Morris, R.C., Jr., and Sebastian, A. (2000). Worldwide incidence of hip fracture in elderly women: relation to consumption of animal and vegetable foods. *J. Gerontol. A Biol. Sci. Med. Sci.* 55: M585–592.
108. Feskanich, D., Willett, W.C., Stampfer, M.J., and Colditz, G.A. (1996). Protein consumption and bone fractures in women. *Am. J. Epidemiol.* 143: 472–479.
109. Huang, Z., Himes, J.H., and McGovern, P.G. (1996). Nutrition and subsequent hip fracture risk among a national cohort of white women. *Am. J. Epidemiol.* 144: 124–134.
110. Meyer, H.E., Pedersen, J.I., Loken, E.B., and Tverdal, A. (1997). Dietary factors and the incidence of hip fracture in middle-aged Norwegians: a prospective study. *Am. J. Epidemiol.* 145: 117–123.
111. Wengreen, H.J., Munger, R.G., West, N.A., Cutler, D.R., Corcoran, C.O., Zhang, J., and Sassano, N.E. (2004). Dietary protein intake and risk of osteoporotic hip fracture in elderly residents of Utah. *J. Bone Miner. Res.* 19: 537–545.

CHAPTER 29

Dietary Protein and the Skeleton*

BESS DAWSON-HUGHES

Bone Metabolism Laboratory, Jean Mayer U.S.D.A. Human Nutrition Research Center on Aging at Tufts University, Boston, Massachusetts

ABSTRACT

Currently, there is no consensus on the impact of dietary protein on calcium and bone metabolism. Increasing protein intake increases the circulating level of insulin-like growth factor-1 (IGF-1), a compound that promotes bone formation. Increasing protein intake also increases urinary calcium excretion, although this finding is less consistent when protein from food sources (as opposed to purified protein) is used, presumably because many protein-rich foods are rich in phosphorus, which mitigates calciuria. There is some evidence that the net effect of dietary protein on bone mass is dependent upon the level of calcium intake. This chapter addresses the evidence that protein influences bone health, and it considers the dietary setting in which protein may have its optimal effect.

*This material is based on work supported by the U.S. Department of Agriculture, under agreement no. 58-1950-9001. Any opinions, findings, conclusions, or recommendations expressed in this publication are those of the authors, and do not necessarily reflect the view of the U.S. Department of Agriculture.

Dietary protein has several effects on calcium handling, and its net impact on the skeleton may depend upon the acid–base balance of the diet, the calcium intake, the length of time on the diet, and other factors. The purpose of this paper is to consider:

- The impact of dietary protein on IGF-1 and the impact of IGF-1 on bone remodeling
- The effect of dietary protein on calcium excretion, calcium absorption, and bone remodeling
- Whether the level of calcium intake influences any effect of protein on bone

DIETARY PROTEIN AND SERUM IGF-1

Insulin-like growth factor-1 is a small polypeptide that is synthesized in liver, bone (by osteoblasts), and other tissues. It binds to IGF-1 receptors in many tissues to stimulate cell responses related to growth. IGF-1 synthesis in tissues requires adequate energy and protein and, as such, serves as an intermediate signaling system to target cells that adequate substrate is available to support anabolic activity. In classical experiments, Isley et al. [1] found that fasting for 5 days lowered serum IGF-1 levels by about 65% in healthy young subjects. Refeeding normal calories and graded amounts of protein resulted in progressive recovery of IGF-1 levels with increasing protein intake up to an intake of 1.0 g/kg/day. Clemmons et al. [2] found that IGF-1 recovery after a 5-day fast was better with refeeding of essential rather than non-essential amino acids. Serum IGF-1 levels were correlated with nitrogen balance in this study [2]. With aging, serum IGF-1 levels decline in men and women [3,4]. There is some evidence that chronic metabolic acidosis decreases serum IGF-1 levels in humans [5,6]; however, Maurer et al. [7] found no significant change in serum IGF-1 levels after administering bicarbonate to young volunteers for one week.

There is some evidence that increasing intake of protein alters IGF-1 levels in elderly populations. In one study, adult men and women who consumed three extra servings of milk per day (containing a total of 27 g of protein, and other nutrients) for 12 weeks had significant (14%) increases in serum IGF-1, whereas the control group did not change [8]. Schurch et al. [9] administered 20 g of protein to elderly acute hip fracture patients. These patients had a usual protein intake of 45 g/day (or 0.75 g/kg/day). Both the protein intervention and control patients received daily calcium and vitamin D supplements. After 6 months of supplementation, serum IGF-1 levels had increased 80% in the protein group and were unchanged in the controls.

We have recently found that supplementation of older men and women with basal protein intakes no higher than 0.7 g/kg/day with meats providing an additional 0.75 g/kg/day of protein significantly increased their IGF-1 levels by about 25%. The RDA for dietary protein is currently 0.8 g/kg/day [10]. According to the third National Health and Examination Survey (NHANES III) survey, women in the United States ages 50 and older had a median protein intake of 58 g/day and 25% consumed less than 44 g/day [11].

Nutrient intake can also influence the circulating levels of IGF-1 binding proteins. The most abundant binding protein, IGF BP-3, is a large glycoprotein that associates with IGF-1 in the circulation and prevents its rapid extravasation from blood. Serum IGF BP-3 levels decline after a prolonged fast [12] but remain stable throughout the day in subjects on normal diets [13]. IGF binding proteins are also located in extracellular spaces, where they may modulate the action of IGF-1 at the surface of target cells [14].

The clearest evidence that IGF-1 affects bone remodeling comes from experiments in which biochemical markers of bone turnover are measured after administration of IGF-1. Ebeling et al. [15] treated postmenopausal women for 6 days with IGF-1 and noted a significant increase in type 1 procollagen but not in osteocalcin levels, both markers of bone formation. The women had a significant increase in urinary pyridinoline, a marker of bone resorption. Serum PTH, calcium, and phosphorus were unchanged. Johansson et al. [16] administered IGF-1 to osteoporotic men daily for one week and observed that markers of bone formation and resorption increased by about 20%, but levels of serum IGF-BP3, parathyroid hormone (PTH), and 1,25-dihydroxyvitamin D and urine calcium did not change significantly. These studies indicate that the effect of IGF-1 on bone is anabolic and that it is probably not mediated by PTH.

PROTEIN AND ACID–BASE BALANCE

Protein of both animal and plant origin produces endogenous acid as it is metabolized. There is a strong relationship between the amount of acid–ash consumed in the diet and the amount of acid produced [17,18]. On a daily basis, adults on normal Western diets generate approximately 1 mEq of acid [19]. As individuals age, their renal function and the ability to excrete acid decline [20], and they become more acidic. An acid environment affects bone in several ways. First, it increases osteoclastic activity. In an in vitro study in rats [21], a reduction in medium pH from 7.4 to 6.8 was associated with a 14-fold increase in mean area resorbed per bone slice ($P < 0.01$). In a similar *in vitro* study [22], changes in resorption rate were detectable within the physiologic range of pH. The number of resorption pits was 6-fold higher at pH 7.15 than at pH 7.25. Second, acidosis inhibits osteoblastic activity. In isolated cultured osteoblasts, acidosis reduced collagen synthesis and reduced formation of nodules of apatitic bone [23–27]. Third, acid appears to have a direct physicochemical effect on bone. In a synthetic bone mineral model in which there was no cell-mediated resorption [28], Bushinsky has shown that H^+ ions cause efflux of calcium from the apatite surface. Thus, bone serves as a buffer, and, in the process of neutralizing acidity arising from Western diets, calcium is lost from bone.

PROTEIN AND URINE CALCIUM EXCRETION

It has long been recognized that dietary protein induces calciuria [20–32]. Evidence that hypercalciuria results from losses of bone calcium in humans is found in several studies. Sebastian and Morris [33] reported that in postmenopausal women neutralization of endogenous acid production leads to inhibition of bone resorption and positive calcium balance. More recently, Maurer *et al.* [7] documented significant declines in biochemical markers of bone resorption within one week of administering bicarbonate and reversal of these changes within a week of discontinuing the bicarbonate in healthy young volunteers studied on metabolic diets. In an earlier study, ingestion of acid dramatically increased urinary calcium and hydroxyproline excretion without altering PTH levels in healthy men [34]. There has been some suggestion from studies employing potassium bicarbonate ingestion that it is the potassium rather than the bicarbonate that reduces calciuria in humans [35]. A similar conclusion was drawn in a potassium citrate supplement study [36]. This conclusion, however, has been refuted in the recent study of Maurer *et al.* [7], in which sodium bicarbonate and potassium bicarbonate had similar effects on calciuria and markers of bone resorption.

PROTEIN AND CALCIUM ABSORPTION

Dietary protein may affect intestinal calcium absorption, but the evidence for this is mixed. Rats on high-protein diets appear to compensate for increased urinary calcium losses by increasing net calcium absorption [37]. Lutz and Linkswiler [38] found that increased protein intake significantly increased net calcium absorption and urinary calcium excretion in postmenopausal women [38]. In young women with a mean calcium intake of 800 mg/day, decreasing protein intake from 158 to 52 g/day lowered calcium absorption over the following 4 days, consistent with at least a transient effect of dietary protein on absorption [39]. Longer-term balance studies in humans, however, have found little to no effect of dietary protein on calcium absorption [29,40,41].

DIETARY PROTEIN AND BONE TURNOVER

Several early studies reported increases in hydroxyproline in response to increases in protein intake [42,43], but one must be cautious in concluding that the hydroxyproline reflects bone resorption, as meat in the diet increases urine excretion of hydroxyproline. Recent protein intervention studies have addressed this question. Kerstetter *et al.* [32] observed higher levels of urine N-telopeptide in subjects on high-protein diets compared with low-protein diets. This study in young subjects had short diet intervention periods of only 4 days. In a careful metabolic study with 8-week diet periods, Roughead *et al.* [44] found no change in markers of bone formation or resorption after increasing dietary protein from 12 to 20% of energy. Serum IGF-1 levels did not change in this study either. The authors concluded that protein did not have a negative impact on bone turnover. In a relatively malnourished group of very elderly patients with recent hip fractures, treatment with 20 g/day of protein for 6 months resulted in no changes in bone turnover, although there were trends toward higher serum osteocalcin and lower urine pyridinoline levels [9]. As noted earlier, serum IGF-1 levels rose by 80% but serum PTH levels were unchanged. We have recently found that increasing meat intake for 2 months resulted in a significant reduction in urinary excretion of N-telopeptide. Serum osteocalcin and PTH levels did not change significantly in this study. From these studies, it is clear that changes in bone turnover induced by protein and by IGF-1 administration (described earlier) are not precisely matched. This indicates that dietary protein affects bone turnover not only through its effect on IGF-1 but also by other mechanisms, including the acid load that accompanies protein and perhaps other components of protein-rich foods such as vitamin B_{12}.

PROTEIN, BONE LOSS, AND FRACTURES

In the original Framingham cohort, elderly subjects with lower total and animal protein intakes had greater rates of bone loss from the femoral neck and spine than subjects consuming more protein [45]. In a controlled, 6-month intervention study, 20 g/day of supplemental protein improved hip bone mineral density in elderly patients with recent hip fractures (Fig. 1) [9]. All of the patients received supplemental calcium and vitamin D.

Munger *et al.* [46] reported that higher total (and animal) protein intakes were associated with a reduced incidence of hip fractures in postmenopausal women. In contrast, a high ratio of animal to plant protein intake has been associated with greater bone loss from the femoral neck and a greater risk of hip fracture in women age 65 years and older [47]. Higher total and higher animal protein intakes have also been associated with increased risk of forearm fracture in younger postmenopausal women [48]. Thus, evidence for the effects of dietary proteins of both animal and plant origin on the skeleton is conflicting.

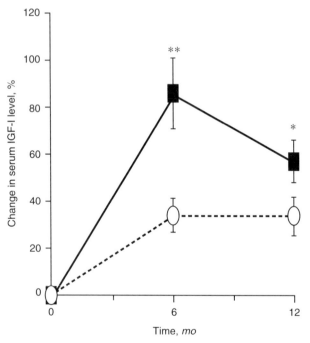

FIGURE 1   Protein supplementation for 6 months and change in hip bone mineral density in elderly patients with recent hip fractures. (From Schurch, M.A. *et al.*, *Ann. Intern. Med.* 128, 801–809, 1998. With permission.)

POTENTIAL IMPACT OF CALCIUM INTAKE ON LINK BETWEEN PROTEIN AND BONE

A higher calcium intake might be expected to offset the negative effect of protein on urine calcium losses and induce a more positive net effect of protein on bone. Little evidence is available to address this hypothesis. Meyer *et al.* [49] noted no association between protein intake and risk of hip fracture in most women, but among those with very low calcium intakes (<400 mg/day), a higher protein intake was associated with increased risk of hip fracture. In a recent analysis of men and women who had participated in our 3-year calcium and vitamin D supplementation trial [50], higher protein intakes (both animal and total) were associated with beneficial changes in bone mineral density of the total body and femoral neck in the supplemented group but *not* in the placebo group (Fig. 2) [51].

The men and women in the lowest protein tertile consumed < 0.86 g/kg/day of protein (mean 0.7g/kg/day) and those in the highest

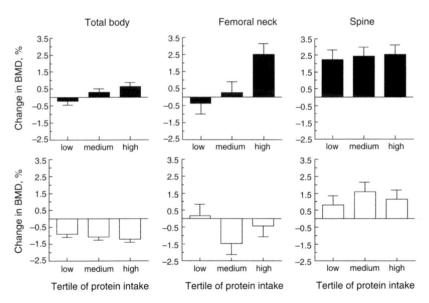

FIGURE 2   The association of protein intake with rates of bone loss in elderly men and women treated for 3 years with 500 mg calcium as citrate malate plus 700 IU of vitamin D (solid bars) and with placebo (open bars). For the total body, there was a significant interaction of treatment group with protein tertile ($P = 0.44$). (From Dawson-Hughes, B., and Harris, S.S., *Am. J. Clin. Nutr.* 75, 773–779, 2002. With permission.)

tertile consumed >1.2 g/kg/day (mean, 1.57 g/kg/day). Total calcium and vitamin D intakes were 1300 mg and 900 IU, respectively, in the supplemented group and 800 mg and 200 IU, respectively, in the placebo group. There were no significant differences across the protein tertiles in intake of calcium, potassium, or magnesium in 24-hour urinary sodium or potassium excretion or in citrate intake from the calcium supplements. These findings suggest that a higher calcium intake may promote a favorable impact of dietary protein on the skeleton. A protein intervention study is needed to confirm these associations.

In summary, dietary protein has multiple effects on calcium and bone metabolism—some positive, like its trophic effect on IGF-1, and others that are negative, such as calciuria. Predicting the net effect of dietary protein on rates of bone loss is difficult and will require long-term protein intervention studies. These studies should take into account potential interactions with other aspects of the diet, such as acid–base balance and calcium intake.

REFERENCES

1. Isley, W.L., Underwood, L.E., and Clemmons, D.R. (1983). Dietary components that regulate serum somatomedin-C concentrations in humans. *J. Clin. Invest.* 71: 175–182.
2. Clemmons, D.R., Seek, M.M., and Underwood, L.E. (1985). Supplemental essential amino acids augment the somatomedin-C/insulin-like growth factor I response to refeeding after fasting. *Metabolism* 34: 391–395.
3. Harris, T.B., Kiel, D., Roubenoff, R., Langlois, J., Hannan, M., Havlik, R., and Wilson, P. (1997). Association of insulin-like growth factor-I with body composition, weight history, and past health behaviors in the very old: the Framingham Heart Study. *J. Am. Geriatr. Soc.* 45: 133–139.
4. Landin-Wilhelmsen, K., Wilhelmsen, L., Lappas, G., Rosen, T., Lindstedt, G., Lundberg, P.A., and Bengtsson, B.A. (1994). Serum insulin-like growth factor I in a random population sample of men and women: relation to age, sex, smoking habits, coffee consumption and physical activity, blood pressure and concentrations of plasma lipids, fibrinogen, parathyroid hormone and osteocalcin. *Clin. Endocrinol.* 41: 351–357.
5. Brungger, M., Hulter, H.N., and Krapf, R. (1997). Effect of chronic metabolic acidosis on thyroid hormone homeostasis in humans. *Am. J. Physiol.* 272: F648–F653.
6. Challa, A., Chan, W., Krieg, Jr., R.J., Thabet, M.A., Liu, F., Hintz, R.L., and Chan, J.C. (1993). Effect of metabolic acidosis on the expression of insulin-like growth factor and growth hormone receptor. *Kidney Int.* 44: 1224–1227.
7. Maurer, M., Riesen, W., Muser, J., Hulter, H.N., and Krapf, R. (2003). Neutralization of Western diet inhibits bone resorption independently of K intake and reduces cortisol secretion in humans. *Am. J. Physiol. Renal* 284: F32–F40.
8. Heaney, R.P., McCarron, D.A., Dawson-Hughes, B., Oparil, S., Berga, S.L., Stern, J.S., Barr, S.I., and Rosen, C.J. (1999). Dietary changes favorably affect bone remodeling in older adults. *J. Am. Diet. Assoc.* 99: 1228–1233.

9. Schurch, M.A., Rizzoli, R., Slosman, D., Vadas, L., Vergnaud, P., and Bonjour, J.P. (1998). Protein supplements increase serum insulin-like growth factor-I levels and attenuate proximal femur bone loss in patients with recent hip fracture. A randomized, double-blind, placebo-controlled trial. *Ann. Intern. Med.* 128: 801–809.

10. Subcommittee on the Tenth Edition of the RDAs Food and Nutrition Board Commission on Life Sciences National Research Council. (1989). *Recommended Dietary Allowances*, National Academy Press, Washington, D.C.

11. Kerstetter, J.E., Looker, A.C., and Insogna, K.L. (2000). Low dietary protein and low bone density. *Calcif. Tissue Int.* 66: 313.

12. Clemmons, D.R., Thissen, J.P., Maes, M., Ketelslegers, J.M., and Underwood, L.E. (1989). Insulin-like growth factor-I (IGF-I) infusion into hypophysectomized or protein-deprived rats induces specific IGF-binding proteins in serum. *Endocrinology* 125: 2967–2972.

13. Baxter, R.C., and Martin, J.L. (1989). Binding proteins for the insulin-like growth factors: structure, regulation and function. *Prog. Growth Factor Res.* 1: 49–68.

14. De Mellow, J.S., and Baxter, R.C. (1988). Growth hormone-dependent insulin-like growth factor (IGF) binding protein both inhibits and potentiates IGF-I-stimulated DNA synthesis in human skin fibroblasts. *Biochem. Biophys. Res. Commun.* 156: 199–204.

15. Ebeling, P.R., Jones, J.D., O'Fallon, W.M., Janes, C.H., and Riggs, B.L. (1993). Short-term effects of recombinant human insulin-like growth factor I on bone turnover in normal women. *J. Clin. Endocrinol. Metab.* 77: 1384–1387.

16. Johansson, A.G., Lindh, E., Blum, W.F., Kollerup, G., Sorensen, O.H., and Ljunghall, S. (1996). Effects of growth hormone and insulin-like growth factor I in men with idiopathic osteoporosis. *J. Clin. Endocrinol. Metab.* 81: 44–48.

17. Remer, T. and Manz, F. (1994). Estimation of the renal net acid excretion by adults consuming diets containing variable amounts of protein. *Am. J. Clin. Nutr.* 59: 1356–1361.

18. Bushinsky, D.A. (1997). Acid–base imbalance and the skeleton, in *Nutritional Aspects of Osteoporosis 1997: Proceedings of the 3rd International Symposium on Nutritional Aspects of Osteoporosis*, Burckhardt, P., Dawson-Hughes, B., Heaney, R.P., Eds., Ares-Serono Symposia Publications, Italy, pp. 208–217.

19. Kurtz, I., Maher, T., Hulter, H.N., Schambelan, M., and Sebastian, A. (1983). Effect of diet on plasma acid–base composition in normal humans. *Kidney Int.* 24: 670–680.

20. Frassetto, L.A., Todd, K.M., Morris, Jr., R.C., and Sebastian, A. (1998). Estimation of net endogenous noncarbonic acid production in humans from diet potassium and protein contents. *Am. J. Clin. Nutr.* 68: 576–583.

21. Arnett, T.R. and Dempster, D.W. (1986). Effect of pH on bone resorption by rat osteoclasts *in vitro*. *Endocrinology* 119: 119–124.

22. Arnett, T.R. and Spowage, M. (1996). Modulation of the resorptive activity of rat osteoclasts by small changes in extracellular pH near the physiological range. *Bone* 18: 277–279.

23. Sprague, S.M., Krieger, N.S., and Bushinsky, D.A. (1994). Greater inhibition of *in vitro* bone mineralization with metabolic than respiratory acidosis. *Kidney Int.* 46: 1199–1206.

24. Bhargava, U., Bar-Lev, M., Bellows, C.G., and Aubin, J.E. (1988). Ultrastructural analysis of bone nodules formed in vitro by isolated fetal rat calvaria cells. *Bone* 9: 155–163.

25. Ecarot-Charrier, B., Glorieux, F.H., van der, R.M., and Pereira, G. (1983). Osteoblasts isolated from mouse calvaria initiate matrix mineralization in culture. *J. Cell Biol.* 96: 639–643.

26. Sudo, H., Kodama, H.A., Amagai, Y., Yamamoto, S., and Kasai, S. (1983). *In vitro* differentiation and calcification in a new clonal osteogenic cell line derived from newborn mouse calvaria. *J. Cell Biol.* 96: 191–198.

27. Sprague, S.M., Krieger, N.S., and Bushinsky, D.A. (1993). Aluminum inhibits bone nodule formation and calcification *in vitro*. *Am. J. Physiol.* 264: F882–F890.

28. Bushinsky, D.A. (1996). Metabolic alkalosis decreases bone calcium efflux by suppressing osteoclasts and stimulating osteoblasts. *Am. J. Physiol.* 271: F216–F222.
29. Hegsted, M. and Linkswiler, H.M. (1981). Long-term effects of level of protein intake on calcium metabolism in young adult women. *J. Nutr.* 111: 244–251.
30. Pannemans, D.L., Schaafsma, G., and Westerterp, K.R. (1997). Calcium excretion, apparent calcium absorption and calcium balance in young and elderly subjects: influence of protein intake. *Br. J. Nutr.* 77: 721–729.
31. Linkswiler, H.M., Joyce, C.L., and Anand, C.R. (1974). Calcium retention of young adult males as affected by level of protein and of calcium intake. *Trans. N.Y. Acad. Sci.* 36: 333–340.
32. Kerstetter, J.E., Mitnick, M.E., Gundberg, C.M., Caseria, D.M., Ellison, A.F., Carpenter, T.O., and Insogna, K.L. (1999). Changes in bone turnover in young women consuming different levels of dietary protein. *J. Clin. Endocrinol. Metab.* 84: 1052–1055.
33. Sebastian, A., and Morris, Jr., R.C. (1994). Improved mineral balance and skeletal metabolism in postmenopausal women treated with potassium bicarbonate. *New Engl. J. Med.* 331: 279.
34. Lemann, Jr., J., Gray, R.W., Maierhofer, W.J., and Cheung, H.S. (1986). The importance of renal net acid excretion as a determinant of fasting urinary calcium excretion. *Kidney Int.* 29: 743–746.
35. Lemann, Jr., J., Gray, R.W., and Pleuss, J.A. (1989). Potassium bicarbonate, but not sodium bicarbonate, reduces urinary calcium excretion and improves calcium balance in healthy men. *Kidney Int.* 35: 688–695.
36. Sellmeyer, D.E., Schloetter, M., and Sebastian, A. (2002). Potassium citrate prevents increased urine calcium excretion and bone resorption induced by a high sodium chloride diet. *J. Clin. Endocrinol. Metab.* 87: 2008–2012.
37. Whiting, S.J. and Draper, H.H. (1981). Effect of chronic high protein feeding on bone composition in the adult rat. *J. Nutr.* 111: 178–183.
38. Lutz, J. and Linkswiler, H.M. (1981). Calcium metabolism in postmenopausal and osteoporotic women consuming two levels of dietary protein. *Am. J. Clin. Nutr.* 34: 2178–2186.
39. Kerstetter, J.E., O'Brien, K.O., and Insogna, K.L. (1998). Dietary protein affects intestinal calcium absorption. *Am. J. Clin. Nutr.* 68: 859–865.
40. Heaney, R.P. and Recker, R.R. (1982). Effects of nitrogen, phosphorus, and caffeine on calcium balance in women. *J. Lab. Clin. Med.* 99: 46–55.
41. Spencer, H., Kramer, L., Osis, D., and Norris, C. (1978). Effect of a high protein (meat) intake on calcium metabolism in man. *Am. J. Clin. Nutr.* 31: 2167–2180.
42. Schuette, S.A., Hegsted, M., Zemel, M.B., and Linkswiler, H.M. (1981). Renal acid, urinary cyclic AMP, and hydroxyproline excretion as affected by level of protein, sulfur amino acid, and phosphorus intake. *J. Nutr.* 111: 2106–2116.
43. Chan, E.L. and Swaminathan, R. (1994). The effect of high protein and high salt intake for 4 months on calcium and hydroxyproline excretion in normal and oophorectomized rats. *J. Lab. Clin. Med.* 124: 37–41.
44. Roughead, Z.K., Johnson, L.K., Lykken, G.I., and Hunt, J.R. (2003). Controlled high meat diets do not affect calcium retention or indices of bone status in healthy postmenopausal women. *J. Nutr.* 133: 1020–1026.
45. Hannan, M.T., Tucker, K.L., Dawson-Hughes, B., Cupples, L.A., Felson, D.T., and Kiel, D.P. (2000). Effect of dietary protein on bone loss in elderly men and women: the Framingham Osteoporosis Study. *J. Bone Mineral Res.* 15: 2504–2512.
46. Munger, R.G., Cerhan, J.R., and Chiu, B.C. (1999). Prospective study of dietary protein intake and risk of hip fracture in postmenopausal women. *Am. J. Clin. Nutr.* 69: 147–152.

47. Sellmeyer, D.E., Stone, K.L., Sebastian, A., and Cummings, S.R. (2001). A high ratio of dietary animal to vegetable protein increases the rate of bone loss and the risk of fracture in postmenopausal women. Study of Osteoporotic Fractures Research Group. *Am. J. Clin. Nutr.* 73: 118–122.
48. Feskanich, D., Willett, W.C., Stampfer, M.J., and Colditz, G.A. (1996). Protein consumption and bone fractures in women. *Am. J. Epidemiol.* 143: 472–479.
49. Meyer, H.E., Pedersen, J.I., Loken, E.B., and Tverdal, A. (1997). Dietary factors and the incidence of hip fracture in middle-aged Norwegians: a prospective study. *Am. J. Epidemiol.* 145: 117–123.
50. Dawson-Hughes, B., Harris, S.S., Krall, E.A., and Dallal, G.E. (1997). Effect of calcium and vitamin D supplementation on bone density in men and women 65 years of age or older. *New Engl. J. Med.* 337: 670–676.
51. Dawson-Hughes, B. and Harris, S.S. (2002). Calcium intake influences the association of protein intake with rates of bone loss in elderly men and women. *Am. J. Clin. Nutr.* 75: 773–779.

PART X

Protein—Mineral Water

Milk Basic Protein Increases Bone Mineral Density and Improves Bone Metabolism in Humans

YUKIHIRO TAKADA,[1] SEIICHIRO AOE,[2] YASUHIRO TOBA,[1]
KAZUHIRO UENISHI,[3] AKIRA TAKEUCHI,[4] and AKIRA ITABASHI[5]

[1]Technology & Research Institute, Snow Brand Milk Products Co., Ltd., Saitama, Japan;
[2]Department of Home Economics, Otsuma Women's University, Chiyoda-ku,
Tokyo, Japan; [3]Laboratory of Physiological Nutrition, Kagawa Nutrition University, Tokyo, Japan;
[4]Luke Hospital, Nakano, Tokyo, Japan; [5]Department of Clinical Laboratory Medicine,
Saitama Medical School, Saitama, Japan

ABSTRACT

Milk contains not only a bioavailable calcium source but also other components effective for bone health. Earlier we found that milk basic protein (MBP) strongly stimulated both bone formation and bone resorption. In the study discussed here, we examined the effect of daily intake of MBP on bone mineral density (BMD) and bone metabolism in two human studies. Human Study 1: The gain of calcaneus BMD in the MBP group was significantly higher than that in the placebo group, and the radial BMD value in the MBP group was also increased significantly at both the 1/6 and 1/10 portions from the distal end of the radius. Human Study 2: The serum osteocalcin (BGP) concentration, as a marker for bone formation, increased significantly, and the serum propeptide of human type I procollagen (PICP), another marker of bone formation, slightly increased, after the intake of MBP. On the other hand, the urinary level of cross-linked N-teleopeptides of type I collagen (NTX), a bone resorption marker, was lower in the MBP group. These results suggest that MBP promoted bone formation and

Nutritional Aspects of Osteoporosis, Second Edition

413

suppressed bone resorption in humans, that MBP increased BMD by promoting bone formation and suppressing bone resorption, and that it affected bone metabolism while maintaining a balance of bone remodeling. Thus, MBP might become a novel, natural, and desirable nutritional supplement for bone health.

INTRODUCTION

In bone tissue, the bone formation and bone resorption are always occurring, so that the integrity of the bone tissue is maintained. This continual bone remodeling or bone turnover is presumably important for maintaining the structural integrity and strength of bones. Bone tissue consists of a wide variety of cells of bone-forming and bone-resorbing cell lineages. Especially, both osteoblasts and osteoclasts are important for bone remodeling (Fig. 1). This remodeling begins with a phase of osteoclastic bone resorption that is relatively short lived. Osteoclasts are formed from precursor cells in the hematopoietic bone marrow that are common not only to osteoclasts but also to the formed elements of the blood. Under the direction of local signals, osteoclasts form and then attach to bone and start to resorb it. The phase of osteoclastic bone resorption lasts about 10 days and is followed by reversal phase, in which the osteoclasts are replaced by mononuclear cells that line the lacunae formed by the osteoclasts.

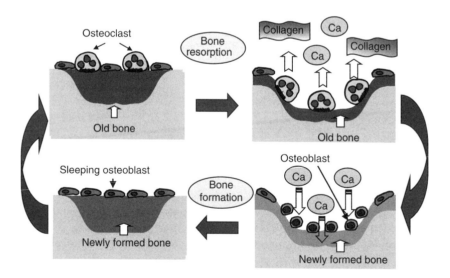

FIGURE 1   Bone remodeling by osteoclasts and osteoblasts.

These mononuclear cells are soon replaced by osteoblast precursors that are attracted to the site of the defect made by the osteoclasts, and these precursors are stimulated to replicate and differentiate into mature osteoblasts. These cells are capable of forming new bone that, over a period of several months, replaces the defect made by the osteoclasts. The activities of bone cells are regulated by many hormones and factors. For bone health, it is important to maintain the proper balance of bone formation and resorption. While this balance of the bone formation and bone resorption is maintained properly in the young, in older individuals the bone resorption becomes predominant. This alteration in the balance between bone resorption and formation occurs for various reasons, such as menopause or aging. With the population of the aged increasing, the incidence of bone metabolic diseases such as osteoporosis and bone fracture has also been increasing; therefore, it is particularly important to develop food stuffs capable of increasing bone formation or suppressing bone resorption for the improvement of the unbalanced bone metabolism that occurs in later life.

Milk is a safe food taken over long decades of life and is beneficial for human health. It is also a good source of calcium that is easily absorbed and bioavailable [1–3]. Additionally, milk contains several components useful for calcium absorption in the intestines, such as lactose and phosphopeptides formed by the proteolytic digestion of milk casein [3,5]. Milk plays functional roles in the growth of newborn animals. Thus, we speculated earlier that milk contains proteins that affect bone metabolism [6]. A previous report of ours showed that milk whey protein (WP) stimulated the proliferation and differentiation of osteoblastic MC3T3-E1 cells [7]. WP also suppressed osteoclast cell formation and bone resorption [8]. The administration of WP was effective for increasing bone strength and the contents of collagen-typical amino acids such as hydroxyproline in young ovariectomized (OVX) rats [9,10].

We attempted to concentrate the active components from WP and estimate their biological activity. We found that a milk protein fraction with a basic isoelectric point, termed milk basic protein (MBP), strongly stimulated bone formation and suppressed bone resorption [11]. Milk proteins generally constitute approximately 3.5% of milk. They are composed of a number of fractions of which the casein constitutes approximately 2.9% and whey proteins 0.6%. The main whey protein fractions are acidic and contain α-lactoglobulin, β-lactoalbumin, and serum albumin. MBP in milk is a small fraction of whey. Proteins in MBP have basic isoelectric points approximately from 7.0 to 10.5 as judged from isoelectric focusing disc gel electrophoresis. In terms of the amino acid composition, MBP has much higher amounts of lysine and arginine (basic amino acids) of MBP than casein. Almost all of the growth factors in milk possess basic isoelectric points [12].

In earlier studies, we investigated the effect of MBP on bone metabolism *in vitro* and *in vivo*. MBP increased the [³H] thymidine incorporation and PICP contents dose dependently in osteoblastic cells and suppressed both the area of pits formed by preexisting osteoclasts and newly formed osteoclasts [13] and isolated osteoclasts [11].These results show that MBP contains components that are active in the promotion of bone formation and the suppression of bone resorption. In 5-week-old OVX rats, the bone strength of the MBP-fed group was significantly higher than that in the control group [14]. In 55-week-old OVX rats, both BMD and bone strength in the group fed 0.1% MBP were significantly higher than those in the control group at weeks 12 and 16. Urinary deoxypyridinoline (D-Pyr) excretion of the group fed 0.01% MBP was significantly lower than that of the control group [15]. These results show that MBP is also effective for bone formation and bone resorption *in vivo*. In the remainder of this review, we describe the effects of MBP on bone metabolism as found by human studies.

HUMAN STUDY 1

SUBJECTS AND PROTOCOL

Thirty-three healthy women were recruited, and written informed consent was obtained from each subject. The level of physical activity of all subjects was moderate, and women were excluded from the study if they had used estrogen, glucocorticoids, or other medications known to affect bone metabolism for the last 3 years. In this 6-month, double-blind, placebo-controlled trial, the volunteers were randomly assigned to either the placebo or the MBP group. The baseline characteristics of the women are shown in Table I [16]. Overall, there was no significant difference between the MBP and placebo groups in any of the parameters indicated in the Table I.

Seventeen women received the experimental beverage containing 40 mg of MBP, and the other 16 received the matching placebo beverage. Each beverage contained lactic acid, a sweetener, and flavoring agent as masking ingredients in 50 mL of water. Women in each group were instructed to drink 1 bottle (50 mL) of the beverage daily at any time. They were advised to maintain their usual diets and to avoid taking supplemental minerals and vitamins on their own throughout the 6-month study. Prior to the experiment and at the end of 3 and 6 months, urine and blood measurements were taken for each subject. At the baseline and 6-month evaluation, they were also measured for BMD. During the study period (0 to 6 months), a prospective standardized 3-day food record was completed by each subject at 3 and

TABLE I Characteristics of the Subjects (Human Study 1)

	Placebo	MBP
No. of subjects	16	17
Age (yr)	27 ± 8	30 ± 9
Weight (kg)	50 ± 4	51 ± 6
Height (m)	1.58 ± 0.04	1.58 ± 0.05
Body mass index	20.0 ± 2.0	20.5 ± 2.4

Note: Each value is the mean ± SD.

6 months. Nutrient content of the diets was quantified by using a computer program based on the *Standard Tables of Food Composition* [17].

The calcaneus BMD was measured by dual-energy x-ray absorptiometry (DEXA) with the use of a DX2000 scanner (Kyoto Daiichi Kagaku, Japan); the coefficient of variation for the measurements was 2.0%. The radial BMD was measured by DEXA with a DX600 EX scanner (Aloka, Japan). The validation of the machine was less than 1.0%, and the coefficient of variation for the measurements was 0.86%.

Blood was drawn between 9:00 a.m. and 11:00 a.m. after the subjects had fasted for at least 8 hours. Second spontaneous urine was collected between 9:00 and 10:00 a.m. before breakfast. Aliquots of samples were frozen at −20°C until analysis could be performed. Assays for the following items were conducted: serum bone-specific alkaline phosphatase (B-ALP), measured by an immunoselective enzyme assay (Alkphase-B, Metra Biosystems, Palo Alto, CA); osteocalcin (BGP), by an immunoradiometric assay (BGP IRMA; Mitsubishi Kagaku, Tokyo, Japan); NTX, by enzyme-linked immunosorbent assay (ELISA; Osteomark, Ostex International, Seattle, WA); and D-Pyr, by an ELISA (Pyrlinks-D, Metra Biosystems, Palo Alto, CA). The coefficients of variation for these assays ranged from 5.0 to 8.0%. All biochemical markers of bone metabolism were analyzed by Mitsubishi Bio-Clinical Laboratories (Tokyo, Japan). Other blood and urine assays were analyzed by use of Clinical Analyzers (Models 7450 and 7070, respectively; Hitachi, Tokyo).

During the 6-month study period, no bloating, diarrhea, or allergy was observed in either group, and no one withdrew from the study. All volunteers completed the study according to the protocol based on the Helsinki Declaration.

CHANGE IN BMD

The initial mean values for BMD of the calcaneus were similar for the two groups. The increase in calcaneus BMD was significantly greater in the

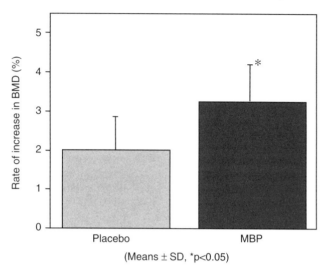

(Means ± SD, *p<0.05)

FIGURE 2   Rates of increase in BMD (calcaneus).

TABLE II   Change of the Radial BMD in the Placebo and MBP Group

	Before	After 6 Months	Paired t-Test/P Value
Radius distal 1/10			
Placebo group	0.450 ± 0.044	0.446 ± 0.044	0.1506/< 0.0001*
MBP group	0.440 ± 0.057	0.457 ± 0.056	
Radius distal 1/6			
Placebo group	0.553 ± 0.047	0.546 ± 0.0440	0395[#]/< 0.0001*
MBP group	0.532 ± 0.067	0.548 ± 0.068	

Note: Each value is the mean ± SD. Differences are considered significant if P< 0.05 (*, + change; #, – change).

MBP group than in the placebo group. The mean (± SD) gain in calcaneus BMD was significantly higher in the MBP group (3.42 ± 2.05%) than in the placebo group (Fig. 2) [16]. As shown in Table II and Fig. 3, the mean of the individual BMD at the 1/6 and 1/10 portions from the distal end of the radial bone was significantly higher in the MBP group than in the placebo group [18]. There was no significant difference in calcium, phosphorus, magnesium, and vitamin D, K, or C level between the groups by the Mann-Whitney U test. Correlation coefficients between gain of BMD and dietary intake of minerals and vitamins are shown in Table III. There was no significant correlation between gain of BMD and intake of any dietary

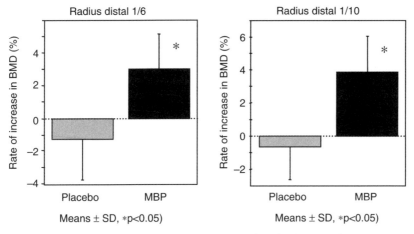

FIGURE 3   Rates of increase in BMD (radius distal 1/6, 1/10).

TABLE III   Change of the Radial BMD in the Placebo and MBP Group

| | BMD Gain Versus | | |
	Before	After 6 Months	Paired t-Test/P Value
1 month – 3 months			
Placebo group	−0.259 −0.195	−0.169 −0.161	−0.492/−0.229
MBP group	−0.259 −0.334	−0.26 −0.263	−0.259/−0.388
4 month – 6 months			
Placebo group	−0.012 −0.123	0.145 0.298	−0.250/−0.332
MBP group	−0.038 −0.072	−0.196 0.218	−0.328/−0.402

Note: No significant correlation coefficient was observed.

minerals or vitamins in the placebo and MBP groups. These data suggest that the significant increase in BMD in the MBP group was independent of the dietary intake of minerals (calcium, phosphorus, and magnesium) and vitamins (vitamins D, K, and C) [16]. We found that MBP could be one of the nutritional components to increase peak bone mass and reduce the future risk of osteoporosis for premenopausal women.

BIOCHEMICAL MARKERS OF BONE METABOLISM

Biochemical parameters in serum and urine are being used clinically to assess the rate of bone formation and resorption. A biochemical marker of

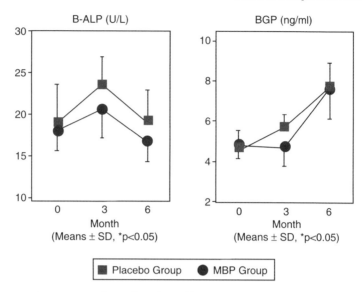

FIGURE 4   Biochemical markers of bone metabolism (bone formation).

bone turnover that reflects bone changes faster than BMD is available for measuring serum or urine. It was reported that serum B-ALP, BGP, and urinary D-Pyr, as indicators of skeletal health, are more sensitive than BMD [19]. Biochemical indexes of bone metabolism in the two groups were similar at the baseline. B-ALP and BGP concentrations (bone formation markers) showed no difference between the groups (Fig. 4). On the other hand, the mean urinary values for NTX and D-Pyr (bone resorption markers) were lower in the MBP group than in the placebo group at both 3 and 6 months (Fig. 5). These results indicate that MBP supplementation led to a reduction in the rate of bone resorption. Previously, we reported that MBP clearly reduced the urinary excretion level of D-Pyr by directly suppressing osteoclast-mediated bone resorption in aged ovariectomized rats [15]. That result is consistent with the findings in our human study. Also, the values of B-ALP/NTX and BGP/NTX for the MBP group were significantly higher than those for the placebo group at 6 months (Fig. 6) [20], suggesting that MBP could also promote bone formation. Other biochemical parameters were normal and did not change in the two groups throughout the study period.

Bones are continuously undergoing a remodeling process through repeated cycles of destruction and rebuilding. In healthy young adults, the amount of new bone formation approximately balances the amount of bone resorption. As we age, however, the balance shifts to favor bone

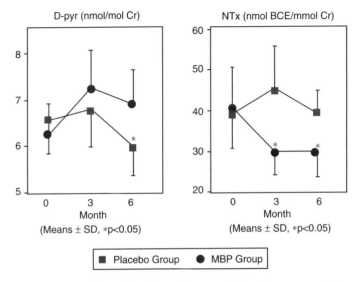

FIGURE 5   Biochemical markers of bone metabolism (bone resorption).

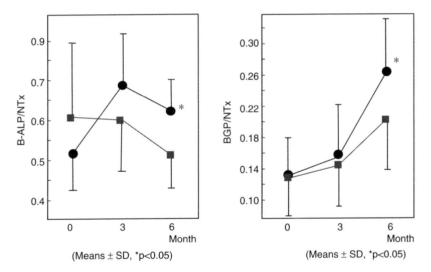

FIGURE 6   Values of B-ALP/NTX and BGP/NTX.

resorption, which can result in debilitating diseases such as osteoporosis. Efforts to treat bone diseases have been primarily concentrated on the development of drugs to block bone resorption (*i.e.*, to decrease the formation or activity of osteoclasts) [21].To prevent bone diseases, it might be questionable to strongly block bone resorption because this will unbalance bone remodeling [22]. It is important to investigate whether MBP actually causes a loss in the balance of bone remodeling, because it has a suppressive effect on bone resorption. In the present study, the NTX excretion (a biochemical marker of bone resorption) was not found to be related to the serum BGP concentration (a biochemical marker of bone formation) before the ingestion of MBP but was found to be related to it after 6 months of ingestion (Fig. 7) [20]. These results indicate that the subjects who had a higher activity of bone formation also had a higher activity of bone resorption after 6 months of ingestion. This phenomenon suggests that, while MBP suppressed bone resorption, it did not block bone resorption by bone remodeling. Thus, the results of this study suggest that MBP promoted bone formation and suppressed bone resorption while maintaining the balance of bone remodeling.

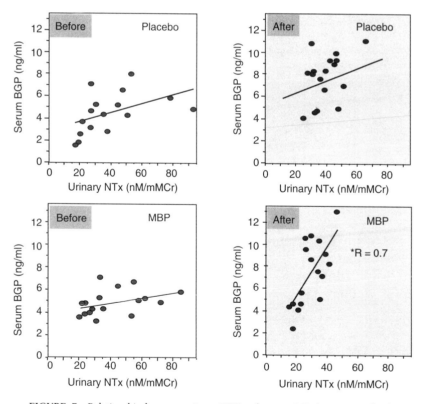

FIGURE 7   Relationship between urinary NTX and serum BGP (Human Study 1).

HUMAN STUDY 2

SUBJECTS AND PROTOCOL

Thirty healthy men were recruited, and written informed consent was obtained from each subject. The study complied with the code of ethics of the World Medical Association (Helsinki Declaration of 1964 as revised in 1989). Thirty men received an experimental beverage containing MBP (300 mg of MBP). The beverage also contained an acidifier, sweetener, and flavor agent to provide a pleasant taste for the volunteers. The subjects were instructed to drink the beverage daily within any 2-hour period for 16 days and were advised to maintain their usual diets. Each subject received a physical checkup every day and was measured for urine and blood parameters before and after the 16 days of ingestion. Blood and urine samples were collected as described in Human Study 1. The BGP and NTX were also measured as described as Human Study 1. Serum PICP was measured by radioimmunoassay (Orion Diagnostica, Oulunsalo, Finland). Calcium in the serum and urine was analyzed by clinical analyzer models 7450 and 7070, respectively (Hitachi, Tokyo). Table IV presents the subjects' characteristics. There was no significant difference in the parameters before and after 16 days of ingestion of MBP [23].

BIOCHEMICAL MARKERS OF BONE METABOLISM

The serum calcium level and urinary calcium excretion were unchanged after 16 days of ingesting the experimental beverage containing MBP (Table V). We measured serum BGP and PICP as markers of bone formation. The products of collagen breakdown, including collagen cross-links, can be used to assess bone resorption. We measured NTX as the biochemical marker of bone resorption, because NTX is reportedly more

TABLE IV Characteristics of the Subjects (Human Study 2)

	Before	After 16 Days
No. of subjects	30	30
Age (yr)	36 ± 9	36 ± 9
Weight (kg)	67 ± 9	
Height (m)	1.71 ± 0.04	1.71 ± 0.04
Body mass index	22.9 ± 2.5	23.0 ± 2.6

Note: Each value is the mean $\pm$ SD.

424

Nutritional Aspects of Osteoporosis

TABLE V   Biochemical Markers of the Subjects Before and After 16 Days

	Before	After 16 Days	Paired t-Test, P Value
Serum			
Calcium (mmol/L)	2.3 ± 0.1	2.3 ± 0.1	0.4820
BGP (ng/mL)	3.7 ± 1.8	5.4 ± 1.8	<0.0001
PICP (ng/mL)	122.3 ± 37.0	130.0 ± 44.1	0.0872
Urine			
Calcium (mmol/mmol Cr)	0.21 ± 0.11	0.23 ± 0.10	0.3535
NTx (nmol/mmol Cr)	31.5 ± 10.2	26.8 ± 9.6	<0.0001

Note: Each value is the mean ± SD ($n = 30$). Differences are considered significant if $P < 0.05$.

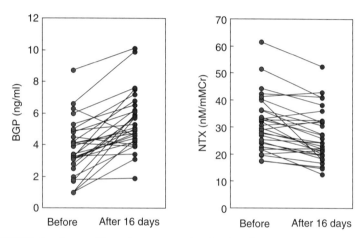

FIGURE 8   Change of bone formation marker (BGP) and resorption marker (NTX).

sensitive to a change in bone metabolism than is D-Pyr [24]. In this study, we found that MBP supplementation increased the serum BGP and PICP and decreased the NTX excretion, suggesting that MBP promoted bone formation and suppressed bone resorption. The serum osteocalcin concentration increased significantly after 16 days of ingestion (Table V), and the serum PICP level tended to increase, too, although the difference was not significant (Table V, $P = 0.0872$). The decrease in urinary NTX excretion after 16 days of ingestion was highly significant (Table V). Individual changes in the serum BGP concentration and urinary NTX excretion after 16 days of ingestion are shown in Fig. 8. An increase in the serum concentration of BGP was found in 28 (93%) of the 30 subjects, and a decrease in urinary NTX excretion was observed in 24 (80%) of them [23].

We demonstrated in previous *in vitro* and animal studies that MBP promoted bone formation by activating osteoblasts and suppressed bone resorption by its direct and/or indirect effects on osteoclasts [7,8,11,14,15]. Our results from the present human study are consistent with those from such *in vitro* and animal studies. In Human Study 1, we found that MBP supplementation (40 mg of MBP a day) increased BMD and suppressed the urinary level of NTX. Our results regarding the effect of MBP on bone resorption from the present human study are consistent with those from a previous human study [16]; however, we failed to find a clear effect of MBP on the serum BGP concentration. When slightly more MBP (300 mg of MBP a day) was ingested in the present human study, we observed an increase in the BGP. The present human study indicates that the increased levels of BMD might have been caused by the promoting effect of MBP on bone formation and by its suppressing effect on bone resorption.

Bones are continuously undergoing a remodeling process through repeated cycles of destruction and rebuilding, as mentioned earlier. It is important to investigate whether MBP actually causes a loss in the balance of bone remodeling, because it has a suppressive effect on bone resorption. In Human Study 1, NTX was found to be related to BGP after 6 months of MBP ingestion. Figure 9 presents the correlation between the NTX and the BGP concentration in Human Study 2. The NTX level was not related to the serum BGP concentration before the ingestion of MBP but was 16 days after it, with a correlation coefficient of 0.6457 ($P < 0.0001$) [23]. These results indicate that the subjects who had a higher activity of bone formation also had a higher activity of bone resorption after 16 days of ingestion.

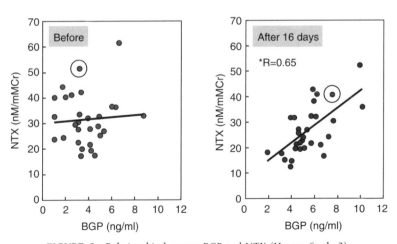

FIGURE 9   Relationship between BGP and NTX (Human Study 2).

These results also suggest that MBP promoted bone formation and suppressed bone resorption while maintaining the balance of bone remodeling as demonstrated by Human Study 1.

CONCLUSION

Milk basic protein, which has basic isoelectric points, is believed to contain an array of the profitable factors in milk. Since the ancient Egyptians first domesticated the dairy cow in 4000 B.C., milk has made a major contribution to human health. We propose that the active components in the MBP play an important role in bone metabolism (Fig. 10). The yield of the MBP from whey protein showed that approximately 400 to 800 mL of milk is equivalent to a 40-mg dose of the MBP. Although many long-term studies demonstrated that calcium supplementation is effective to prevent bone loss [25–27], our study, for the first time, provided evidence of a direct effect of MBP from milk on bone metabolism in humans. We also demonstrated that the active components responsible for the promotion of bone formation and suppression of bone resorption maintained their biological activity after gastrointestinal digestion and, by the everted gut-sac method, showed that they could be absorbed through the intestines [7,8,28]. Thus, the active components in the MBP or partially digested MBP might be absorbed through the intestine and promote bone formation and inhibit bone resorption directly by physiological processes.

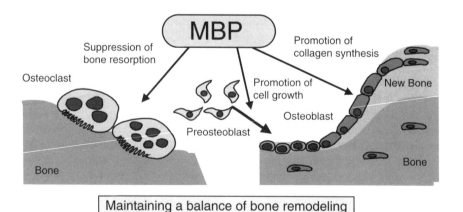

FIGURE 10 Milk basic protein effects: MBP promotes bone formation, suppresses bone resorption, and increases BMD.

We previously demonstrated by means of a bioassay using osteoblastic MC3T3-E1 cells that the active components in MBP related to bone formation were a high mobility group including, for example, protein and kininogen fragment 1·2 [29,30]. Also, we found that milk cystatin purified from milk suppressed osteoclast-mediated bone resorption. It is known that cathepsin, a protease secreted by osteoclasts, is responsible for bone resorption. It has been reported that cystatin C inhibited cathepsin as a protease inhibitor [31,32].We thus consider that milk cystatin in the MBP fraction is one of the possible components that prevents bone resorption. MBP is itself complex; it is a polyvalent fraction containing many profitable factors. Its effect on bone health is likely to be more than can be accounted for by any single constituent, and the totality of the effect of MBP may be more than the sum of the parts. MBP might maintain the balance of bone remodeling because it contains several effective components for both bone formation and resorption.

In conclusion, our results suggest that MBP promotes bone formation and suppresses bone resorption in humans and that it affects bone metabolism while maintaining a balance of bone remodeling. We believe that MBP might become a novel, natural, and desirable nutritional supplement for bone health.

REFERENCES

1. Kansal, V.K. and Chaudhary, S. (1982). Biological availability of calcium, phosphorus and magnesium from dairy products. *Milchwissenschaft* 37: 261–263.
2. Toba, Y., Kato, K., Takada, Tanaka, Y., Nakano, T., Aoki, T., and Aoe, S. (1999). Bioavailability of milk micellar calcium phosphate–phosphopeptide complex in rats. *J. Nutr. Sci. Vitaminol.* 45: 311–323.
3. Wong, N.P. and LaCroix, D.E. (1980). Biological availability of calcium in dairy products. *Nutr. Rep. Intern.* 21: 673–680.
4. Wasserman, R.H. (1964). Lactose-stimulated intestinal absorption of calcium: a theory. *Nature* 201: 997–999.
5. Toba, Y., Takada, Y., Tanaka, M., and Aoe, S. (1999). Comparison of the effects of milk components and calcium source on calcium bioavailability in growing male rats. *Nutr. Res.* 19: 449–459.
6. Takada, Y., Yahiro, M., and Nakajima, I. (1993). Effect of milk components on calcium absorption and bone metabolism, in *Characterization of Milk Components and Health*, Yamauchi, K., Imamura, T., and Morita, T., Eds., Kouseikan, Tokyo, 1993, pp. 171–185.
7. Takada, Y., Aoe, S., and Kumegawa, M. (1996). Whey protein stimulates the proliferation and differentiation of osteoblastic MC3T3-E1 cells. *Biochem. Biophys. Res. Commun.* 223: 445–449.
8. Takada, Y., Kobayashi, N., Matsuyama, H., Kato, K., Yamamura, J., Yahiro, M., and Aoe, S. (1997). Whey protein suppresses the osteoclast-mediated bone resorption and osteoclast cell formation. *Int. Dairy J.* 7: 821–825.

9. Takada, Y., Kobayashi, N., Kato, K., Matsuyama, H., Yahiro, M., and Aoe, S. (1997). Effect of whey protein on calcium and bone metabolism in ovariectomized rats. *J. Nutr. Sci. Vitaminol.* 43: 199–210.

10. Takada, Y., Matsuyama, H., Kato, K., Kobayashi, N., Yamamura, J., Yahiro, M., and Aoe, S., (1997). Milk whey protein enhances the bone breaking force in ovariectomized rats. *Nutr. Res.* 17: 1709–1720.

11. Takada, Y., Yoba, Y., Aoe, S., Kumegawa, M., and Itabashi, A. (2001). Milk basic protein (MBP) promotes bone formation and suppresses bone resorption. *Nutritional Aspects of Osteoporosis*, pp. 141–153.

12. Francis, G.L., Regester, H.A., Webb, H.A., and Ballard, F.J. (1995). Extraction from cheese whey by cation-exchange chromatography of factors that stimulate the growth of mammalian cells. *J. Dairy Sci.* 78: 1209–1218.

13. Takada, Y., Kusuda, M., Hiura, K., Sato, T., Mochizuki, H., Nagao, Y., Tomura, M., Yahiro, M., Hakeda, Y., Kawashima, H., and Kumegawa, M. (1992). A simple method to assess osteoclast-mediated bone resorption using unfractionated bone cells. *Bone and Miner.* 17: 347–359.

14. Kato, K., Toba, Y., Matsuyama, H., Yamamura, J., Matsuoka, Y., Kawakami, H., Itabashi, A., Kumegawa, M., Aoe, S., and Takada, Y. (2000). Milk basic protein enhances the bone strength in ovariectomized rats. *J. Food Biochem.* 24: 467–478.

15. Toba, Y., Takada, Y., Yamamura, J., Tanaka, M., Matsuoka, Y., Kawakami, H., Itabashi, A., Aoe, S., and Kumegawa M., (2000). Milk basic protein: a novel protective function of milk against osteoporosis. *Bone* 27: 403–408.

16. Aoe, S., Toba, Y., Yamamura, J., Kawakami, H., Yahiro, Kumegawa, M., Itabashi, A., and Takada, Y. (2001). A controlled trial of the effect of milk basic protein (MBP) supplementation on bone metabolism in healthy adult women. *Biosci. Biotechnol. Biochem.* 65: 913–918.

17. Resources Council, Science and Technology Agency. (1982). *Standard Tables of Food Composition In Japan*, 4th ed., Ministry of Finance, Printing Bureau, Tokyo.

18. Yamamura, J., Aoe, S., Toba, Y., Kawakami, H., Kumegawa, M., Itabashi, A., and Takada, Y. (2002). Milk basic protein (MBP) increases radial bone mineral density in healthy adult women. *Biosci. Biotechnol. Biochem.* 66: 702–714.

19. Blumsohn, A., Hannon, R.A., Wrate, R., Barton, J., Al-Dehaimi, A.W., Colwell, A., and Eastell, R. (1994). Biochemical markers of bone turnover in girls during puberty. *Clin. Endocrinol.* 40: 663–670.

20. Takada Y., Aoe, S., Ohta, H., and Itabashi, A. (2003). Milk basic protein (MBP) increases BMD and improves bone metabolism in human study. *J. Jpn. Menopause Soc.* 11: 19–26.

21. Ott, S.M. (1996). Theoretical and methodological approach, in *Principles of Bone Biology*, Bilezikian, J.P., Raisz, L.G., and Rodan, G.A., Eds., Academic Press, San Diego, CA, pp. 231–241.

22. Rodan, G.A. and Martin, T.J. (2000). Therapeutic approaches to bone diseases. *Science* 289: 1508–1514.

23. Toba, Y., Takada, Y., Matsuoka, Y., Morita, Y., Motouri, M., Hirai, T., Suguri, T., Aoe, S., Kawakami, H., Kumegawa, M., Takeuchi, A., and Itabashi. A. (2001). Milk basic protein promotes bone formation and suppresses bone resorption in healthy adult men. *Biosci. Biotechnol. Biochem.* 65: 1353–1357.

24. Hanson, D.A., Weis, M.A., Bollen, A.M., Maslan, S.L., Singer, F.R., and Eyre, D.R. (1992). A specific immunoassay for monitoring human bone resorption: quantitation of type I collagen cross-linked N-telopeptides in urine. *J. Bone Mineral Res.* 7: 1251–1258.

25. Prince, R.L., Smith, M., Dick, I.M., Prince, R.I., Webb, P.G., Henderson, N.K., and Harris, M.M. (1991). Prevention of postmenopausal osteoporosis: a comparative study of

exercise, calcium supplementation, and hormone-replacement therapy. *New Engl. J. Med.* 325: 1189–1195.

26. Recker, R.R., Saville, P.D., and Heaney, R.P. (1977). Effect of estrogens and calcium carbonate on bone loss in postmenopausal women. *Ann. Intern. Med.* 87: 649–655.

27. Smith, E.L., Gilligan, C., Smith, P.E., and Sempos, C.T. (1989). Calcium supplementation and bone loss in middle-aged women. *Am. J. Clin. Nutr.* 50: 833–842.

28. Martin D.L. and Deluca H.F. (1969). Influence of sodium on calcium transport by the rat small intestine. *Am. J. Physiol.* 216: 1351–1359.

29. Yamamura, J., Takada, Y., Goto, M., Kumegawa, M., and Aoe, S. (1999). High mobility group-like protein in bovine milk stimulates the proliferation of osteoblastic MC3T3-E1 cells. *Biochem. Biophys. Res. Commun.* 261: 113–117.

30. Yamamura, J., Takada, Y., Goto, M., Kumegawa, M., and Aoe, S. (2000). Bovine milk kininogen fragment 1·2 promotes the proliferation of osteoblastic MC3T3-E1 cells. *Biochem. Biophys. Res. Commun.* 269: 628–632.

31. Lerner, U.H. and Grubb, A. (1992). Human cystatin C, a cysteine proteinase inhibitor, inhibits bone resorption *in vitro* stimulated by parathyroid hormone and parathyroid hormone-related peptide of malignancy. *J. Bone Mineral Res.* 7: 433–440.

32. Matsuoka, Y., Serizawa, A., Yoshioka, T., Yamamura, J., Morita, Y., Kawakami, H., Toba, H., Takada, Y., and Kumegawa. M. (2002). Cystatin C in milk basic protein (MBP) and its inhibitory effect on bone resorption *in vitro*. *Biosci. Biotechnol. Biochem.* 66: 2531–2536.

CHAPTER 31

Dietary Balance in Physically Active and Inactive Girls

JAANA A. NURMI-LAWTON,[1] ADAM BAXTER-JONES,[2] PAT TAYLOR,[3]
CYRUS COOPER,[3] JACKI BISHOP,[1] and SUSAN NEW[1]

[1]Centre for Nutrition and Food Safety, School of Biomedical and Life Sciences, University of Surrey, Guildford, Surrey, United Kingdom; [2]College of Kinesiology, University of Saskatchewan, Saskatoon, Canada; [3]MRC Environmental Epidemiology Unit, Southampton General Hospital, Southampton, United Kingdom

ABSTRACT

The effect of dietary protein on skeletal health is controversial. It remains to be determined whether variations in protein intake, within normal range, can influence peak bone mass (PBM) development, especially in combination with a physically active or non-active lifestyle. As part of a 3-year longitudinal investigation we examined potential dietary influences on skeletal growth in physically active and sedentary adolescent girls. At baseline, 45 female competitive gymnasts (G) and 52 controls (C), ages 8 to 17, were recruited. Data on anthropometry, maturity status, dietary intake, bone mass, and several other aspects were collected. A multilevel regression model was fitted and the independent effects of body size, maturity, physical activity, and diet were identified over time.

The gymnasts were significantly shorter and lighter compared with controls and had higher bone mineral density (BMD), bone mineral content (BMC), and ultrasound values. Weight-adjusted protein intake was greater among the gymnasts. Longitudinal analysis of the predictor

Nutritional Aspects of Osteoporosis, Second Edition
Copyright © 2004 by Elsevier Science (USA)
All rights of reproduction in any form reserved.

variables on total body (TB) BMC showed that, after adjusting for body size, maturity, and exercise, protein intake (g/day) had a small but significant independent positive effect on TB BMC. Energy intake had a small, significant, independent, negative effect. When the G group alone was analyzed, no significant dietary effects were found, whereas in the C group the protein and energy effects still existed.

The positive protein effects may possibly be explained by the requirements of growth, indicating good nutritional status and hence contribution to BMC; however, these data would lend support to the theory that high-impact physical training may have an overriding influence on the nutritional factors affecting PBM development and is an area for further research.

INTRODUCTION

Peak bone mass (PBM), the maximum amount of bone achieved by the end of skeletal maturation, is generally achieved before the end of third decade, depending on skeletal site [1]. The main determinant of PBM is genetics, leaving still plenty of influential role for modifiable factors such as diet, physical activity, and hormonal status. Skeleton is believed to be particularly responsive to the influence of these factors during and/or just before longitudinal bone growth and pubertal maturation [2,3]. It is however difficult to determine the role of external factors due to strong simultaneous confounding events of normal development [4]. Of dietary determinants, calcium has received most research interest over the years. The effect of calcium in a form of supplement and dairy produce has demonstrated short-term skeletal benefits in the younger population [5], but longitudinal effects still need to be proven. Less is known about the role of dietary protein, although its importance for bone mass is acknowledged. Optimal range for protein intake is unclear, although both extremes of high and low intakes can have negative effects when examined as part of normal diet [6,7]. It has been suggested that low protein intake *per se* could be particularly detrimental for the acquisition of bone mass [8], but whether variations in normal protein intake range affect skeletal growth requires further study. In addition to dietary factors, exercise is one of the modifiable determinants of PBM. There is plenty of evidence for skeletal benefits resulting from physically active lifestyle during growth. Most exercise benefits overall health, but the most effective bone response is achieved through weight-bearing activities [9]. In girls, benefits have been shown to be particularly clear and significantly stronger when exercise was started before the end of pubertal maturation (*i.e.*, menarche) rather than after [10]; however, the optimal timing, duration, and type of exercise providing most benefit for the skeleton are not yet known. Exercise and dietary factors are both important for achieving optimal PBM, and they are believed to interact, although evidence is not conclusive.

AIMS

This research is part of a 3-year longitudinal investigation on the effects of diet and physical activity on PBM development in young females. The aims were (1) to examine the potential dietary influences on skeletal growth, and (2) to investigate differences in determinants of bone mass between physically active and sedentary adolescent girls.

SUBJECTS AND METHODS

A total of 45 competitive female gymnasts (G) and 52 sedentary controls (C), ages 8 to 17 years, were recruited at baseline. Measurements on anthropometry, physical activity levels, diet, and other important factors were repeated over 3 years. Dietary intake was measured using 7-day (at baseline) or 3-day (at 6, 9, 12, and 24 months) estimated food records and analyzed using Diet-5 computer software. Maturity status was assessed using secondary sex characteristics and by estimation of age from peak height velocity (PHV) [11]. Bone mass was measured by dual-energy x-ray absorptiometry (DEXA) scans at baseline and at 12 and 24 months (total body and lumbar spine; Lunar DPX). Mean differences were compared using t-test or ANCOVA. For longitudinal statistical analysis, a multilevel regression model (MLRM) [12] was fitted, and the independent effects of body size, maturity, physical activity, and diet were identified over time.

RESULTS

Descriptive data are shown in Table I. The gymnasts were significantly shorter and lighter compared with controls. There were no differences in dietary intakes of energy and most nutrients when absolute values were compared, but weight-adjusted protein intake was greater in gymnasts. The gymnasts also had higher BMC and BMD after controlling for body size and maturity. At baseline, the median for stage of breast development was I for gymnasts and II for controls. The estimated age at PHV was significantly later in gymnasts than controls (13.0 ± 0.7 versus 12.0 ± 0.5 years; $P < 0.001$). Longitudinal MLRM analysis of the predictor variables on TB BMC showed

TABLE I   Descriptive Data at Baseline[a]

Variable	Gymnasts ($n = 45$)	Controls ($n = 52$)
Age (yr)	11.3 ± 2.3	11.3 ± 1.9
Height (m)	$1.36 \pm 0.1^*$	1.48 ± 0.1
Weight (kg)	$31.7 \pm 8.4^*$	41.0 ± 11.1
Energy (MJ/day)	7.1 ± 1.5	7.7 ± 1.1
Calcium (mg/day)	728 ± 211	764 ± 190
Protein (g/day)	55.6 ± 11.9	58.0 ± 9.9
Protein (g/kg/day)	$1.9 \pm 0.5^*$	1.5 ± 0.4
TB BMC (g)[b]	$1603 \pm 22^*$	1373 ± 20
TB BMD (g/cm^2)[b]	$0.981 \pm 0.010^*$	0.914 ± 0.009

[a]Values are mean $\pm$ SD.
[b]Values are mean $\pm$ SE (adjusted for height, weight, maturity).
*Significantly different from the control group ($P < 0.05$)

TABLE II   Percentage (%) Contribution of Predictors of Total Body Bone Mineral Content at Peak Height Velocity

Variable	All Subjects(%)	Controls Only(%)	Gymnasts Only(%)
Height	55.4	64.8	49.5
Weight	31.4	26.0	50.5
Protein	3.5	4.6	—
Energy	3.6	4.6	—
Exercise group	6.0	Not applicable	Not applicable

Note: At PHV (peak height velocity) maturity age $= 0$ and therefore makes no contribution to the predicted BMC value. Height, weight, energy, and protein values were taken from the average group values at PHV.

that protein intake (g/day) had a small but significant independent positive effect on TB BMC (after adjusting for body size, maturity, and exercise). The percentage contribution of each predictor variable (controlled for maturity) is shown in Table II. In the analysis of the whole study group, height and weight were the strongest independent determinants of TB BMC. The exercise factor had a 6% influence. Protein intake had a 3.5% positive effect (in quantity, this was around 100 g bone mineral), and energy intake had a similar size negative effect in explaining the variation in TB BMC. When the groups were analyzed separately, the significant protein and energy effects were maintained in the control group, with both factors having a 4.6% influence on TB BMC. Within the gymnast group, only height and weight had a significant influence, with no effect determined by dietary factors.

DISCUSSION

The importance of nutrition or physical activity on skeletal growth has separately been shown in a number of studies. The two factors are also believed to interact, although the mechanisms are not yet known. Restricted amounts of either can have detrimental effects on bone health, as extreme cases of anorexia nervosa and bed rest have shown. The combined effect of physical activity and nutrients has not been studied conclusively, although a number of studies have addressed the issue [13–18]. A recent experimental study on 3- to 5-year old children, however, found that calcium intake modified bone response to activity, with significant interaction between calcium supplement and activity groups [19]. Strongest evidence for a single nutrient has been gathered for calcium, with several supplementation studies demonstrating a positive effect on bone. As part of dairy foods, nutrients including calcium, phosphate, vitamin D, and protein have been associated with increased bone mass during growth [20,21].

It has previously been shown that dietary protein intake is positively associated with bone mass in children and adolescents [3], and our results clearly support this data. It is difficult, however, to determine the true role of protein effect during development; while bone mass increases, both protein and total energy intakes increase to meet the requirements of normal growth. Our results from this longitudinal study provide evidence of an independent positive protein effect on bone mass in sedentary (normally active) girls, when influence of normal growth and energy intake was accounted for. One possible explanation for this is protein providing a marker for good nutritional status and an overall healthy diet. It is also likely that dietary protein contributes to bone mass via insulin-like growth factor I (IGF-I) [21]. IGF-I is an essential factor for bone formation and also for longitudinal bone growth, because it stimulates proliferation and differentiation of chondrocytes in the epiphyseal plate. It also has an important role in calcium-phosphate metabolism during normal growth. Nutrition is a primary regulator of IGF-I [3,22]. In what way is not yet clear, however, and prospective studies are required to find out whether varying levels of normal protein intake can influence bone growth or IGF-I levels and hence modulate the genetic potential in PBM attainment in well-nourished children and adolescents [8].

Our results also demonstrated an independent negative influence for total energy intake, which was an unexpected finding. In theory, greater energy intake and body size could be assumed to be beneficial for the skeleton. Larger body size has a protective influence on bone health, partly due to greater load-bearing impact and supportive padding in the event of trauma. Potential explanation for our finding is that protein and energy may act as surrogate markers for dietary quality. Hence, a larger proportion of energy from protein sources (high nutrient density foods: positive protein effect) and a smaller proportion of energy from sources high in sugars and fats (low nutrient density foods: negative energy effect) could well provide the most favorable environment for optimal skeletal growth. Animal studies suggest that an increase in the consumption of simple sugars and saturated fatty acids may affect bone mass in the long term by, for example, disturbing calcium metabolism and bone mineralization, immature bones being more vulnerable than mature bones (as reviewed by Sarazin et al. [23]).

Habitual exercise, especially during childhood and adolescence, is associated with long-term benefits for overall bone health. Exercise intervention studies with high-impact weight-bearing training regime have resulted in increased bone mineral acquisition in children [24], although lifelong benefits are yet to be proven. Excessive training, especially in sports where aesthetic appearance is highly valued, is sometimes associated with having a negative influence on bone mass. This is likely to result from the combined effects of continuous vigorous exercise with low body weight, restricted dietary intake, and disturbed hormonal function.

Artistic gymnastics seem to have a positive influence on bone mass, with participants having low body fat but relatively high lean mass. A study on collegiate gymnasts suggested that IGF-I may mediate the relationship between bone and lean mass, but that diet was unlikely to be a major contributor to the higher IGF-I levels found in gymnasts than in controls as no differences were found in dietary intake [25]. In general, dietary intake seems to be adequate for requirements in the youngest gymnasts but lacking after adolescence [26,27]. It has been suggested that gymnastic training, rather than differences in diet, is a reason for higher bone mass in gymnasts than in controls [28]. Maneuvers associated with gymnastics may provide such a strong osteogenic stimulus for bone that single nutrient effects cannot be detected (providing that diet is not deficient). As stated by Heaney, the more one exercises, the more bone one will have, nutrition permitting [29].

In conclusion, dietary protein and energy were shown to have an independent influence on bone mass in young sedentary females, thus highlighting the importance of dietary determinants of PBM. These effects were not found in girls involved in gymnastic training, hence suggesting that in physically active individuals, due to the strong independent effect of exercise, single nutrients may not express such an important role in achieving optimal PBM. Further research is needed to understand the role of dietary balance, including the important contribution from protein intake, in both normal and exercise-induced bone gain during growth.

REFERENCES

1. Matkovic, V., Jelic, T., Wardlaw, G.M., Ilich, J.Z., Goel, P.K., Wright, J.K., Andon, M.B., Smith, K.T., Heaney, R.P. (1994). Timing of peak bone mass in Caucasian females and its implication for the prevention of osteoporosis. Inference from a cross-sectional model. *J. Clin. Invest.* 93: 799–808.
2. Bass, S.L. (2000). The prepubertal years: a uniquely opportune stage of growth when the skeleton is most responsive to exercise? *Sports Med.* 30: 73–78.
3. Bonjour, J.P., Ammann, P., Chevalley, T., and Rizzoli, R. (2001). Protein intake and bone growth. *Can. J. Appl. Physiol.* 26(suppl.): S153–S166.
4. Rogol, A.D., Clark, P.A., and Roemmich, J.N. (2000). Growth and pubertal development in children and adolescents: effects of diet and physical activity. *Am. J. Clin. Nutr.* 72(suppl.): 521S–528S.
5. Kerstetter, J.E. (1995). Do dairy products improve bone density in adolescent girls? *Nutr. Rev.* 53: 328–332.
6. Kerstetter, J.E., Mitnick, M.E., Gundberg, C.M., Caseria, D.M., Ellison, A.F., Carpenter, T.O., and Insogna, K.L. (1999). Changes in bone turnover in young women consuming different levels of dietary protein. *J. Clin. Endocrinol. Metab.* 84: 1052–1055.
7. Kerstetter, J.E., O'Brien, K.O., and Insogna, K.L. (2003). Low protein intake: the impact on calcium and bone homeostasis in humans. *J. Nutr.* 133(suppl.): 855S–861S.
8. Bonjour, J.P., Schurch, M.A., Chevalley, T., Ammann, P., and Rizzoli, R. (1997). Protein intake, IGF-1 and osteoporosis. *Osteoporosis Int.* 7(suppl.): S36–S42.
9. Courteix, D., Lespessailles, E., Peres, S. L., Obert, P., Germain, P., Benhamou, C. L. (1998). Effect of physical training on bone mineral density in prepubertal girls: a comparative study between impact-loading and non-impact-loading sports. *Osteoporosis Int.* 8: 152–158.
10. Kannus, P., Haapasalo, H., Sankelo, M., Sievanen, H., Pasanen, M., Heinonen, A., Oja, P., and Vuori, I. (1995). Effect of starting age of physical activity on bone mass in the dominant arm of tennis and squash players. *Ann. Intern. Med.* 123: 27–31.
11. Mirwald, R.L., Baxter-Jones, A.D., Bailey, D.A., and Beunen, G.P. (2002). An assessment of maturity from anthropometric measurements. *Med. Sci. Sports Exerc.* 34: 689–694.
12. Baxter-Jones, A., and Mirwald, R. (2004). Multilevel modelling. In *Methods in Human Growth Research*, Hauspie, R.C., Cameron, N., and Molinari, L., Eds., Cambridge University Press, Cambridge, UK, pp. 306–330.
13. Fehily, A.M., Coles, R.J., Evans, W.D., and Elwood, P.C. (1992). Factors affecting bone density in young adults. *Am. J. Clin. Nutr.* 56: 579–586.
14. Tylavsky, F.A., Anderson, J.J.B., Talmage, R.V., and Taft, T.N. (1992). Are calcium intakes and physical activity patterns during adolescence related to radial bone mass of white college-age females? *Osteoporosis Int.* 2: 232–240.
15. Welten, D.C., Kemper, H.C.G., Post, G.B., van Mechelen, W., Twisk, J., Lips, P., and Teule, G.J. (1994). Weight-bearing activity during youth is a more important factor for peak bone mass than calcium intake. *J. Bone Mineral Res.* 9: 1089–1096.
16. Ilich, J.Z., Skugor, M., Hangartner, T., Baoshe, A., and Matkovic, V. (1998). Relation of nutrition, body composition and physical activity to skeletal development: a cross-sectional study in preadolescent females. *J. Am. Coll. Nutr.* 17: 136–147.
17. Lloyd, T., Chinchilli, V. M., Johnson-Rollings, N., Kieselhorst, K., Eggli, D.F., and Marcus, R. (2000). Adult female hip bone density reflects teenage sports-exercise patterns but not teenage calcium intake. *Pediatrics* 106: 40–44.
18. Uusi-Rasi, K., Sievanen, H., Pasanen, M., Oja, P., and Vuori, I. (2002). Associations of calcium intake and physical activity with bone density and size in premenopausal and

postmenopausal women: a peripheral quantitative computed tomography study. *J. Bone Mineral Res.* 17: 544–552.

19. Specker, B. and Binkley, T. (2003). Randomized trial of physical activity and calcium supplementation on bone mineral content in 3- to 5-year-old children. *J. Bone Mineral Res.* 18: 885–892.

20. Chan, G.M., Hoffman, K., and McMurry, M. (1995). Effects of dairy products on bone and body composition in pubertal girls. *J. Pediatr.* 126: 551–556.

21. Cadogan, J., Eastell, R., Jones, N., and Barker, M.E. (1997). Milk intake and bone mineral acquisition in adolescent girls: randomised, controlled intervention trial. *Br. Med. J.* 315: 1255–1260.

22. Price, J.S., Oyajobi, B.O., and Russell, R.G. (1994). The cell biology of bone growth. *Eur. J. Clin. Nutr.* 48(suppl.): S131–S149.

23. Sarazin, M., Alexandre, C., and Thomas, T. (2000). Influence on bone metabolism of dietary trace elements, protein, fat, carbohydrates, and vitamins. *Joint Bone Spine* 67: 408–418.

24. Morris, F.L., Naughton, G.A., Gibbs, J.L., Carlson, J.S., and Wark, J.D. (1997). Prospective ten-month exercise intervention in premenarcheal girls: positive effects on bone and lean mass. *J. Bone Mineral Res.* 12: 1453–1462.

25. Snow, C.M., Rosen, C.J., and Robinson, T.L. (2000). Serum IGF-1 is higher in gymnasts than runners and predicts bone and lean mass. *Med. Sci. Sports Exerc.* 32: 1902–1907.

26. Nickols-Richardson, S.M., O'Connor, P.J., Shapses, S.A., and Lewis, R.D. (1999). Longitudinal bone mineral density changes in female child artistic gymnasts. *J. Bone Mineral Res.* 14: 994–1002.

27. Nova, E., Montero, A., Lopez-Varela, S., and Marcos, A. (2001). Are elite gymnasts really malnourished? Evaluation of diet, anthropometry and immunocompetence. *Nutr. Res.* 21: 15–29.

28. Dyson, K., Blimkie, C.J., Davison, K.S., Webber, C.E., and Adachi, J.D. (1997). Gymnastic training and bone density in pre-adolescent females. *Med. Sci. Sports Exerc.* 29: 443–450.

29. Heaney, R.P. (1996). Bone mass, nutrition, and other lifestyle factors. *Nutr. Rev.* 54(suppl.): S3–S10.

CHAPTER 32

Mineral Waters: Effects on Bone and Bone Metabolism

PETER BURCKHARDT
Department of Medicine, CHUV, Lausanne, Switzerland

INTRODUCTION

The term *mineral waters* includes spring water and processed tap water, both being sold as still or carbonated water. Because processed tap water usually has a mineral concentration of minor interest, this chapter deals with spring water that is sold as natural or as pumped spring water, both denominations being equal in this context. The water being artificially or naturally carbonated is of secondary interest in this context [1]. Because bottled water is increasingly used as drinking water in place of tap water (*e.g.*, in 20% of American households) and because several mineral waters claim to have specific health effects, the question arises as to whether or not mineral waters can have a positive effect on bone health. There are, indeed, mineral waters with surprisingly high contents of calcium, sodium, potassium, fluoride, bicarbonate, and fluoride. As examples, Contrexeville (France) contains about 550 mg calcium per liter; Vichy Célestins (France), 3486 mg bicarbonate per liter. If 1 liter of such a water is regularly consumed over several years, it might well influence bone metabolism and bone

Nutritional Aspects of Osteoporosis, Second Edition
Copyright © 2004 by Elsevier Science (USA)
All rights of reproduction in any form reserved.

439

TABLE I   Mineral Content: Geographical Differences

Water (n)	Na (mg/L) > 300 mg/L	Mg (mg/L) > 50 mg/L	Ca		Ref.
			> 200 mg/L	> 400 mg/L	
North American waters (28)	11%	27%	5%	0%	[2]
Swiss waters (23)	<1%	17%	43%	17%	[5]
European waters (20)	20%	30%	35%	15%	[2]
German waters (220)	—	—	28%	12%	[4]
European waters (72)	—	—	24%	11%	[3]

health. The mineral content depends partially on the geographic area. American waters very rarely contain more than 200 mg of calcium per liter, while this concentration of calcium is found in 28% of German waters and in 43% of Swiss mineral waters. In general, mineral waters very rich in calcium seem to be typical for alpine regions. More than 400 mg/L calcium can be found in 17% of Swiss mineral waters and in 12% of German mineral waters, but in none of the American waters mentioned in the literature (Table I) [2–5]. For this reason, the effects of mineral waters on bone might also be geographically variable.

CALCIUM

The effect of calcium in mineral water has been the subject of several studies. Calcium from mineral water is quickly absorbed [6–10], and the absorption fraction is independent of the concentration of calcium in the given water. It depends on the amount of calcium consumed, as shown by absorption studies—about 25% at a concentration of 250 mg calcium per liter and almost 50% at a low concentration of 100 mg per liter [11]. But, when the amount of calcium is kept unchanged and the quantity of water varies as a function of the calcium concentration, the fraction absorption is the same for all waters and does not depend on the chemical content of the mineral water [10]. On average, absorption from mineral water is faster than from milk [6] and occurs within the first hour after consumption. This has the consequence that parathyroid hormone (PTH) secretion drops significantly during the first hour after consumption of a mineral water with a high calcium content (344.7 mg/L), when compared with the consumption of a low calcium water (9.9 mg/L) [12]. In parallel, there is a marked decrease in bone resorption, as measured by serum CTX. In a more recent study over 6 months, a high-calcium mineral water (596 mg/L) was consumed by postmenopausal women with a low average calcium intake of less than

700 mg/day. After this period, a 15% decrease of osteocalcine and alkaline phosphatase, as well as of resorption markers and plasma PTH, could be measured, all these modifications being significant in comparison with a group of women drinking a low-calcium (9 mg/L) water.

More difficult to demonstrate than the effect on bone metabolism is that on bone density. A cross-sectional study showed that postmenopausal women regularly drinking a calcium-rich mineral water (318 mg/L) not only had a higher total calcium intake than the control group (1300 versus 1042 mg/day) but also had a significantly higher bone mineral density at the lumbar spine (1.044 versus 1.002 g/cm^2; $P = 0.003$) [13]. A similar effect could be shown in a follow-up study over ± 13 months in early postmenopausal women. The group consuming 1 liter of a calcium-rich water (408 mg/L) showed over 13 months a smaller and nonsignificant decrease in bone mineral density of distal radius (–1.5%) than the control group consuming a low-calcium water (–5.7%), the difference being significant ($P < 0.05$) [14]. This shows that the immediate effect of the quickly absorbed calcium from mineral water on PTH secretion and bone resorption markers is still present after a longer period, and that regular consumption of calcium-rich mineral water has a positive effect on bone mineral density. Therefore, high-calcium water can be used as a calcium supplement.

There is some concern if the regular consumption of a calcium-rich water increases the incidence of renal stones. The formation of urinary stones depends on the urinary concentration of the crystallizing minerals. Any high fluid intake lowers this concentration by dilution, also the high intake of mineral water, independently of its mineral content. A low-calcium water increases urinary excretion of oxalate; a high-calcium water decreases it and lowers the oxalate × calcium product, despite the increase of calcium excretion [15].

SODIUM

The fact that sodium increases renal calcium excretion and even increases bone resorption [16] raises the question of whether sodium contained in mineral water can have a negative impact on calcium balance. In fact, the concentration of sodium in mineral waters is usually very modest; more than 300 mg/L can be found in only 9% of Swiss mineral waters, 20% of U.S. mineral waters, and 17% of European mineral waters sold in the United States. High concentrations (*i.e.*, between 1 and 2 g/L) are rare and usually associated with high concentrations of calcium and bicarbonate. But, such a water, when regularly consumed, can add sodium to the diet corresponding to about 4 g of salt, which might be too little to influence bone health but too much in cases of heart or renal failure. The American Heart Association recommends water with not more than 20 mg/L Na for individuals on a severe sodium-restricted diet. Still, however, it has to be remembered that an increase in natriuresis will increase urinary calcium excretion [16]. Although it is unlikely that a high sodium content can counterbalance the positive effect of a given mineral water, there are no data to exclude it.

SULFATES

Sulfates in mineral waters are perceived negatively, but there is no justification for that. Sulfates given in high amounts (e.g., 4 g/kg dry food) increased urinary calcium excretion in animals [17–19] but there are no data proving such an effect in humans. Urinary sulfate is not correlated with calcium [8]. Also, the content of sulfate in 1 liter of mineral water is usually lower than that found by normal intake of food. Very rarely, mineral waters contain more than 1 g/L of sulfates (e.g., Sissacher-Switzerland, 1494 mg/L).

CARBONATED BEVERAGES

A large study in school girls reported that the regular consumption of carbonated beverages is associated with an increased incidence of bone fractures, with a significant odds ratio of 3.14 [20]. This negative effect of carbonated waters was thought to be caused by an eventual acid load and by increased calciuria. But, a comparative study on carbonated beverages showed that the caffeine-containing beverages exerted a mild and transient sodium diuretic effect, which showed the expected relation to calcium excretion and hardly could be responsible for a negative calcium balance. The increased risk fracture in girls consuming regularly carbonated beverages is rather the consequence of the absence of a more healthy drinks, including the consumption of milk [21].

FLUORIDE

Some mineral waters are rich in fluoride. Most waters contain less than 1 mg/L of fluoride, but more than 2 mg/L can be found in 16% of mineral waters consumed in the United States [1], in 9% of Swiss mineral waters [5], and in 4% of German mineral waters [4]. The exceptionally high content in fluoride of the Royal Source St. Yorre (Vichy, France), which can reach 9 mg/L, was associated with higher bone density. Subjects who consumed at least 0.75 L/day (which corresponds to 6.38 mg fluoride) for 5 years or more showed a significantly increased osteocalcin level and increased serum and urinary fluoride levels, compared to a normal control population. When the mineral water consumption of these subjects was quantified with a consumption index (liters/day consumed multiplied by the number of years), a significant correlation appeared between the consumption of this water and bone mineral density at the lumbar spine ($P = 0.002$) [22]. In this case, as well as with other mineral waters, exact identification of the source has to be taken into account, as another St-Yorre water from the same region contains only 2.2 mg fluoride per liter. It could be argued that this permanent low-dose fluoride intake could have a positive effect on bone health. The dose of fluoride taken in this form is much lower than that used in the therapeutic trials for the treatment of osteoporosis, which showed no decrease of fracture incidence. But, it is still not known if low-dose fluoride treatment has a positive effect on bone or not [23]. The range of bone fluoride concentration in rats with the highest mechanical strength was found to be close that of persons living in regions with fluoridated water [24], but studies relating the regular consumption of such a water to fracture incidence are missing.

ACID LOAD

Each nutrient, beverages included, can be characterized by its potential renal acid load [25]. This is calculated by the sum of the major anions minus the sum of cations contained in the nutrient: ($Cl + P + SO_4$ + organic acid) − ($Na + K + Ca + Mg$), expressed in mEq/100 g. This approach can by applied to mineral waters. Carbonated and sweetened beverages certainly represent an acid load. The acid load of phosphoric-acid-containing colas leads to increased acid excretion, which amounts to less than half of the ingested acid load [21].

The question could be asked if mineral waters can represent an acid load big enough to have a negative impact on bone health. An oral acid load in form of 2 mmol ammonium chloride per kg led to a significant increase of net urinary acid excretion as well as of calcium excretion [26]. The acid load of a mineral water can be calculated by subtracting anions from cations, each ion being included in the formula as the product of its concentration and its average absorption fraction and expressed in mEq/L; for calcium, the concentration (in milligrams) in the mineral water would be multiplied by 0.25 (25% absorbed) and 0.025. The potential renal acid load calculated in this way sums up to only 5 to 15 mEq/L, and if bicarbonate is included in the calculation between to 3 and 13 mEq/L. Compared to the acid load induced by food (50 to 150 mEq noncarbonic protons per day), this is a low figure that is not likely to interfere with bone metabolism.

ALKALINE LOAD

On the other hand, it is conceivable that some mineral waters represent a substantial nutritional alkaline load and might have a beneficial effect on bone metabolism. Bicarbonate given as an oral supplement is anticalciuric [27]; it decreases not only calciuria but also improves calcium balance and lowers bone resorption [28], in addition to decreasing renal acid excretion [29]. Such an effect can hardly be expected from most of the mineral waters, as their bicarbonate concentration varies from 50 mg to several grams per liter, the high concentrations being rather exceptional. But, some mineral waters contain to 2 to 5 g bicarbonate per liter (e.g., Vichy Célestins, France; Malavella, Spain; Radenska, Slovenia; St. Yorre, France), and it could be that this amount of bicarbonate has a measurable bone effect. Indeed, when 1 liter of such a water was given to normal volunteers in addition to a diet with a low acid load, urinary calcium excretion dropped by almost half and urinary markers of bone resorption by about 15%, although the intake of sodium, calcium, protein, and calories was equal in the treated and the control groups on a high acid load diet [30]. In another, 1-month trial, three mineral waters were given to healthy volunteers, who maintained a free diet. One water contained double the amount of calcium than the other two, the second water was rich in bicarbonate, and the third water served as a comparable control with neither a high calcium nor a high bicarbonate content. Although the large variation in nutritional intakes of these volunteers affected the significance of most of the results, urinary pH increased among those drinking the bicarbonate-rich mineral water, and the markers of bone resorption (telopeptides) decreased significantly by 30% over the month. Urinary calcium excretion did not increase among those who drank the bicarbonate-rich water, but it did increase among those who drank water of comparable calcium content. These two trials showed that mineral water rich in bicarbonate decreases bone resorption in healthy volunteers even on a free diet, independently of the calcium content. Obviously, we need more data to confirm this.

The alkalinity of a mineral water is also expressed as its content of $CaCO_3$ [1], where a water with more than 500 mg/L is considered alkaline. The above-mentioned effects can hardly be expected with such waters.

According to this definition, 15 of the 37 waters sold in the United States would be considered alkaline [1], but this limit corresponds to only 310 mg/L bicarbonate, a rather low value considering that some waters contain several grams.

POTASSIUM

It can be argued, that the above-mentioned effects of bicarbonate-rich mineral waters are due to the high potassium content, although potassium excretion did not increase. Indeed, the effects of potassium and of the alkaline load are difficult to separate. There is a highly significant relationship between calcium excretion and urinary net acid excretion as determined by dietary protein plus potassium [31], but only potassium bicarbonate and not sodium bicarbonate could reduce urinary calcium excretion and improve calcium balance in healthy men [32], while both forms of bicarbonate cause a similar increase of renal base excretion [33]. In addition, the thiazide-induced reduction of urinary calcium excretion is not enhanced when only potassium chloride is added, while it is almost doubled by the addition of potassium bicarbonate [34]. Although the mechanism by which potassium lowers urinary calcium excretion is unknown, it can at least be concluded that potassium and bicarbonate have additional effects on calciuria, potassium bicarbonate being stronger than potassium chloride [34]. This raises the question of whether mineral waters rich in both potassium and bicarbonate have an especially positive effect on bone metabolism. The above-mentioned studies seemed to suggest this [30,35].

CONCLUSIONS

Some mineral waters are so rich in minerals that their regular consumption can influence bone metabolism and bone mineral density. Calcium from mineral water is readily absorbed, lowers PTH and markers of bone resorption, and has a long-term effect on BMD. Bicarbonate and potassium lower urinary calcium excretion, and mineral waters rich in these electrolytes also inhibit bone resorption.

REFERENCES

1. Allen, H.E., Alley-Henderson, M.A., and Hass, C.N. (1989). Chemical composition of bottled mineral water. *Arch. Environ. Health* 44(2): 102–116.

2. Garzon, P. and Eisenberg, M.J. (1998). Variation in the mineral content of commercially available bottled waters: implications for health and disease. *Am. J. Med.* 105: 125–130.

3. Azoulay, A., Garzon, P., and Eisenberg, M.J. (2001). Comparison of the mineral content of tap water and bottled waters. *J. Gen. Intern. Med.* 16: 168–175.

4. Willershausen, B., Kroes, H., and Brandenbusch, M. (2000). Evaluation of the contents of mineral water, spring water, table water and spa water. *Eur. J. Med. Res.* 5: 251–262.

5. Mineralwassermarkt Schweiz. Ed. 2002.

6. Halpern, G.M., de Water, J.V., Delabroise, A.M., Keen C.L., and Gershwin, E. (1991). Comparative uptake of calcium from milk and a calcium-rich mineral water in lactose intolerant adults: implications for treatment of osteoporosis. *Am. J. Prev. Med.* 7(6): 379–383.

7. Heaney, R.P. and Dowell, M.S. (1994). Absorbability of the calcium in a high-calcium mineral water. *Osteoporosis Int.* 4: 323–324.

8. Couzy, F., Kastenmayer, P., Vigo, M., Clough, J., Munoz-Box, R., and Barclay, D.V. (1995). Calcium bioavailability from a calcium- and sulfate-rich mineral water, compared with milk, in young adult women. *Am. J. Clin. Nutr.* 62: 1239–1244.

9. Van Dokum, W., De La Guéronnière, V., Schaafsma, G., Bouley, C., Luten, J., and Latgé, C. (1996). Bioavailability of calcium of fresh cheeses, enteral food and mineral water. A study with stable calcium isotopes in young adult women. *Br. J. Nutr.* 75: 893–903.

10. Wynckel, A., Hanrotel, C., Wuillai, A., and Chanard, J. (1997). Intestinal calcium absorption from mineral water. *Mineral Electrol. Metab.* 23: 88–92.

11. Böhmer, H., Müller, H., and Resch, K.L. (2000). Calcium supplementation with calcium-rich mineral waters: a systematic review and meta-analysis of its bioavailability. *Osteoporos Int.* 11: 938–943.

12. Guillemant, J., Le, H.T., Accarie, C. *et al.* (2000). Mineral water as a source of dietary calcium: acute effects on parathyroid function and bone resorption in young men. *Am. J. Clin. Nutr.* 71: 999–1002.

13. Costi, D., Calcaterra, P.G., Iori, N., Vourna, S., Nappi, G., and Passeri, M. (1999). Importance of bioavailable calcium drinking water for the maintenance of bone mass in post-menopausal women. *J. Endocrinol. Invest.* 22: 852–856.

14. Cepollaro, C., Orlandi, G., Gonnelli, S., Ferrucci, G., Arditti, J.C., Borracelli, D., Toti, E., and Gennari, C. (1996). Effect of calcium supplementation as a high-calcium mineral water on bone loss in early postmenopausal women. *Calcif. Tissue Int.* 59: 238–239.

15. Jaeger, P., Portmann, L., Jacquet, A.F., and Burckhardt, P. (1984). Drinking water for stone formers: is the calcium content relevant? *Eur. Urol.* 10: 53–54.

16. Massey, L.K. and Whiting, S.J. (1996). Dietary salt, urinary calcium, and bone loss. *J. Bone Mineral Res.* 11: 731–736

17. Guéguen, L. and Besançon, P. (1972). Influence des sulfates sur le métabolisme phospho-calcique. *Ann. Biol. Anim. Bioch. Biophys.* 12: 589–598.

18. Walser, M. and Browder, AA. (1959). Ion association III. The effect of sulfate infusion on calcium excretion. *J. Clin. Invest.* 38: 1404–1411.

19. Whiting, S.J. and Draper, H.H. (1981). Effect of a chronic acid load as sulphate or sulphur amino acids on bone metabolism in adult rats. *J. Nutr.* 111: 1721–1726.

20. Wyshak, G. (2000). Teenaged girls, carbonated beverage consumption, and bone fractures. *Arch. Pediatr. Adolescent Med.* 154(6): 610–613.

21. Heaney, R.P. and Rafferty, K. (2001). Carbonated beverages and urinary calcium excretion. *Am. J. Clin. Nutr.* 74(3): 343–347.

22. Meunier, P.J., Femenias, M., Duboeuf, F., Chapuy, M.C., and Delmas, P.D. (1989). Increased vertebral bone density in heavy drinkers of mineral water rich in fluoride [letter to the editor]. *Lancet* i: 152.

23. Ringe, J.D., Dorst, A., Kipshoven, C., Rovati, L.C., and Setnikar, I. (1998). Avoidance of vertebral fractures in men with idiopathic osteoporosis by a three year therapy with calcium and low-dose intermittent monofluorophosphate. *Osteoporosis Int.* 8: 47–52.

24. Turner, C.H., Akhter, M.P., and Heaney, R.P. (1992). The effects of fluoridated water on bone strength. *J. Orthoped. Res.* 10: 581–587.

25. Remer, Th. and Manz, F. (1995). Potential renal acid load of foods and its influence on urine pH. *J. Am. Dietetic Assoc.* 95(7): 791–797.

26. Houillier, P., Normand, M., Froissart, M. *et al.* (1996). Calciuric response to an acute acid load in healthy subjects and hypercalciuric calcium stone formers. *Kidney Int.* 50: 987–997.

27. Lemann, J., Pleuss, J.A., Hornick, L., and Hoffman, R.G. (1995). Dietary NaCl restriction prevents the calciuria of KCl deprivation and blunts the calciuria of KHCO$_3$ deprivation in healthy adults. *Kidney Int.* 47: 899–906.

28. Sebastian, A., Harris, S.T., Ottaway, J.H., Todd, K.M., and Morris, R.C. (1994). Improved mineral balance and skeletal metabolism in postmenopausal women treated with potassium bicarbonate. *New Engl. J. Med.* 330(25): 1776–1781.

29. Frassetto, L., Morris, R.C., and Sebastian, A. (1997). Potassium bicarbonate reduces urinary nitrogen excretion in postmenopausal women. *J. Clin. Endocrinol. Metab.* 82(1): 254–259.

30. Buclin, T., Cosma, M., Appenzeller, M., Jacquet, A.F., Décosterd, L.A., Biollaz, J., and Burckhardt, P. (2001). Diet acids and alkalis influence calcium retention in bone. *Osteoporosis Int.* 12: 493–499.

31. Lemann, J. (1999). Relationship between urinary calcium and net acid excretion as determined by dietary protein and potassium: a review. *Nephron* 81(suppl. 1): 18–25.

32. Lemann, J., Gray, R.W., and Pleuss, J.A. (1989). Potassium bicarbonate, but not sodium bicarbonate, reduces urinary calcium excretion and improves calcium balance in healthy men. *Kidney Int.* 35: 688–695.

33. Lindinger, M.I., Franklin, T.W., Lands, L.C., Federsen, P.K., Welsh, D.G., and Heisenhauser, G.J.F. (2000). NaHCO$_3$ ingestion rapidly increases renal electrolyte excretion in humans. *J. Appl. Physiol.* 88: 540–550.

34. Frassetto, L.A., Nash, E., Morris, R.C., and Sebastian, A. (2000). Comparative effects of potassium chloride and bicarbonate on thiazide-induced reduction in urinary calcium excretion. *Kidney Int.* 58: 748–752.

35. Waldvogel-Abramowski, S., Burckhardt, P., Arnaud, M., and Aeschlimann, J.M. (2004). Bicarbonate in mineral water inhibits bone resorption, in *Nutritional Aspects of Osteoporosis*, Burckhardt, P., Dawson-Hughes, B., and Heaney, R.P., Eds., Elsevier, Amsterdam.

INDEX

A

Acid-base balance
  acid producing metabolic states, 290,
    317, 361
  chronic acidosis, 273–274, 278–281,
    316–317, 334–335, 360–362
  extracellular pH, 186, 274
  metabolic alkalosis, 288–290, 320–321
  metabolic setpoints, 274–279
  mobility of skeletal base, 283–288
  normal system pH, 281, 316
  ovine model, 331–335
  See also Diet acid load; Foodstuffs and
    beverages inhibiting bone resorption;
    Fruits and vegetables
Acid-base relationship to bone health, 360–361
Acid load
  effects of on bone health
    acid balance, 278–279
    chronic acidosis and bone wasting,
      279–281
    dietary setpoint, 275–276
    estimating diet net acid load, 277–278
    intervention studies manipulating diet
      composition, 282–283
    metabolic response to acidosis, 273–274
    renal function, 276–279
    respiratory setpoint, 274–275
    trade-offs of chronic adaptation, 274,
      281–282
    in vitro systems, 273–274, 280–281
    in vivo systems, 274, 281–282
  low-grade metabolic alkalosis (Stone Age
    diets for the 21st century), 349–362
    acid-base relationship to bone health,
      360–361

analysis applied to modern diet, 356–358
ancient dietary patterns vs. contemporary,
  350–351
estimation of ancestral diet net acid load,
  351–356
further research, 351, 361–362
NEAP of ancestral diet, 356
overview, 349–350, 361
potassium intake, 358–360
  of mineral water, 443–444
  ovine model for dietary acid base, estrogen
    depletion and bone health, 331–347
    dietary strong ions, 333–336
    effect of low DCAD diet on OVX ewes,
      339–345
    equations for estimating, 336–337
    overview, 331–332, 345
    postparturient hypocalcemia in dairy
      cattle, 336, 338
    preliminary studies, 338–339
    sheep as animal models, 331, 332–333
  Western diet generation per day, 317
Acid producing metabolic states, 290, 317, 361
Alkaline load of mineral water, 444–445
Alkali supplementation, 274, 319–320,
  324–325, 335–336
Alkalosis, 288–290
Alveolar bone, 153, 154
  See also Nutrition and teeth
Anabolic therapies, 69–70, 73
Ancient dietary patterns vs. contemporary,
  350–351
Anorexia nervosa, 166, 380
Anticoagulants, 81, 88–89
Antiresorptive therapies, 69, 73, 421–422
Atherosclerosis, 83

B

Beverages
  caffeinated, 111, 304–305, 442
  carbonated, 67, 305–306, 442
  effects on bone resorption, 304–306
  milk, 55, 63–64 (*see also* Milk basic protein)
  mineral water effects on bone metabolism, 439–447
    acid load, 443–444
    alkaline load, 444–445
    calcium, 440–441
    carbonated beverages, 442
    fluoride, 442–443
    mineral content by geographic area, 440
    potassium, 445
    sodium, 441–442
    sulfates, 442
  phosphorus levels, 67–68
Bicarbonate
  potential, 349–350
  supplementation, 400, 402
  potassium *vs.* sodium, 402, 445
Bicarbonate-to-chloride ratio in diet, 352
Bone development. *See* Skeletal development
Bone remodeling
  protein intake, 66, 403, 413, 416
  serum IGF-1 levels, 401
Bone resorption
  antiresorptive therapies, 69, 73, 421–422
  bone response to calcium deficiency, 184, 186
  cytokine promoted, 110
  foodstuffs and beverages inhibiting bone resorption, 297–313, 324
    beverages, 304–306
    carbohydrates, 304
    essential oils and monoterpenes, 307–309
    fruits, 303–304, 309
    methods, 299–302
    mushrooms, 304
    nuts, beans and seeds, 304
    overview, 297–299, 309–311
    pharmacologically active compound *vs.* base excess, 306–307, 309
    vegetables, salads and herbs, 302–303
  nutrient release, 66, 69
  pH drop response, 279–281, 286–287, 318
Bone size influences. *See* IGF-1 (insulin-like growth factor); Physical activity; Skeletal development

Bone strength
  effects of dietary protein, 379–397
    acid load, 383–384
    bone mass gain, 380–381
    bone mineral mass, 381–384
    bone strength determinants, 380
    cytokine secretion, 386–388
    fracture risk, 389–390
    GH-IGF-1 system, 384–386, 388
    overview, 379–380, 390–391
    protein supplementation, 388–389
  fragility expressed with age, 41, 120

C

Caffeinated beverages, 111, 304–305, 442
Calcification, non-inflammatory, 83
Calcification, vascular, 82–83
Calcium buffering
  capacity, 317
  mechanisms, 287, 334–335
  See also Calcium excretion, urinary
Calcium carbonate, 287, 444
Calcium carbonate in adolescent boys and girls and serum IGF-1 levels, 45–56, 400
Calcium citrate, 287
Calcium deficiency, insufficiency, 232
Calcium economy and vitamin D serum levels reference ranges, 227–228, 232
Calcium excretion, urinary
  and bone breakdown in low pH conditions, 287–288, 320, 334–335, 360–361
  caffeinated beverages increase, 305
  fruit and vegetable intake effects, 320–321, 360
  management of postparturient dairy cattle, 338
  potassium bicarbonate effects, 335, 349–350, 402
  protein effects, 65–66, 68, 383, 399, 402, 405–406
Calcium metabolism
  absorption, 94, 183, 184, 186, 228–231, 402–403
  acid-base homeostasis, 324
  calcium salts compared, 69, 73–74, 287
  chromium picolinate effects on bone and calcium metabolism, 141–152
  diet quality, 61–65
  effects on oral bone, 153, 157
  gender influences, 21–22

homeostasis, 184, 186
phosphorous interactions, 67–74
race influences, 19–21
Calcium phosphate, 383–384
    methods, 18–19
    overview, 17, 22
    threshold intake for African-American
        girls, 20
    threshold intake for Caucasian girls, 17, 18
    total body salt levels, 20–21
Cancers
    fruit and vegetable effects, 310, 316–317
    methylene tetrahydrofolate reductase link,
        130–131
    vitamin D deficiency, 189, 191–192
Carbohydrates, 304, 380, 435–436
    See also Grain products
Carbonated beverages, 67, 305–306, 442
Cardiovascular disease
    potential hesperidin effects, 111–112
    vitamin D role, 189, 190
    vitamin K role, 85–86
Childhood. See Peak bone mass; Skeletal
    development
Children, effects of Asian traditional diet and
    sitting style on bone mineral gain, 25–34
    Asian diet, 29–30
    Asian floor sitting, 25, 30, 31
    effects of education, 26, 30, 31, 32
    stiffness index values, 27–29
    dietary restraint, cortisol and bone density,
        165–177
    assessment scales, 167–168
    association between restraint and BMD,
        173–175
    bone loss, 167, 168
    menstrual cycle, 168–172
    girls, 174–175
Cholecalciferol (vitamin D₃). See Vitamin D
Chromium picolinate effects on bone and
    calcium metabolism, 141–152
    local production of 1,25(OH)₂D, 191, 193
    metabolic pathways, 183–186
    See also specific disease
Clinical attachment loss (CAL), 153
Cod liver oil, 215
Collagen
    acidic conditions in vitro, 402
    insulin modulator, 143
    linked with mineralization, 55

post-translational modification, 66
procollagen increases with protein,
    401, 413
vitamin D deficiency and, 187–188
Corticosteroids, 86, 142, 166, 167, 172–173
Co-twin calcium intervention trial, cortical
    bone effects by hip structural analysis,
    35–43
Coumarin, 88–89
Cytokines, 388
    associated with osteoclastic resorption, 110
    and protein undernutrition, 386–388
    retinoic acid role, 94

D
Daidzein, 298–299
Dairy products; See also Milk
    B-complex content, 133
    diet quality improved by, 62–65
    fortified with vitamin D, 195
    hypocalcemia management, 336, 338
    Japanese consumption vs. Western, 31
    Metabolic syndrome, 64
    milk, 55, 63–65 (see also Milk basic protein)
    reduction in nonskeletal disorders, 64–65
Dairy protein
    effect on plasma IGF-1 levels, 46, 55
    milk basic protein, 413–429
        bone remodeling, 414–415
        milk components, 415–416
        biochemical markers, 419–423
        BMD changes, 416–419, 423, 426
DASH (dietary approaches to stopping
    hypertension), 64, 315–316, 320–321
DCAD (dietary cation-anion difference),
    332–336, 339
    See also Ovine model for dietary acid base,
    estrogen depletion and bone health
Dental health. See Nutrition and teeth
Dental Longitudinal Study, Veterans
    Administration, 158
Diabetes, 142, 143, 189
Diet and lifestyle intervention in children,
    effects of Asian traditional diet and
    sitting style, 25–34
    effects of Asian diet, 29–30
    effects of education, 26, 30, 31, 32
    overview, 25–26, 31–32
    stiffness index values, 27–29
    traditional Asian floor sitting, 25, 30, 31

Dietary balance in active and inactive girls, 431–438
bone mineral content at peak height velocity, 433–434
factors effecting achievement of peak bone mass, 432–433
overview, 431–432, 435–436
subjects and methods, 433
Dietary restraint, cortisol and bone density, 165–177
assessment scales, 167–168
association between restraint and BMD, 173–175
cortisol, 166, 167, 172–173
menstrual cycle, 168–172
Dietary strong ions (DCAD). See Ovine model for dietary acid base, estrogen depletion and bone health
Docosahexaeanoic acid, 31

E
Elderly populations
cognitive decline, 130–131
fruit intake, 31
homocysteine levels, 130–131, 135
phosphorous insufficiency, 70
protein intake and plasma IGF-1, 46, 400–402
protein intake, 67, 379, 381, 385 (*see also* Dietary protein)
serum levels of 25(OH)D in the elderly, 203–209
tooth loss relationship to lower BMD, 155, 156 (*see also* Teeth, nutrition and)
vitamin A metabolism, 104
Ergocalciferol (vitamin D₂). See Vitamin D
Essential oils, 302, 307–309
Estrogen-depletion-associated osteoporosis
alternatives to classical HRT, 298–299
cytokine association, 110, 386–387
site sensitivities to estrogen deficiency, 120
Ethylene diamine tetraacetic acid (EDTA), 80

F
Falling
increased risk and low protein, 379–380
reduced risk and vitamin D, 266
Fish, whole, 31
Flavonoids, 298–299
flavanones, 111–112

See also Hesperidin, improved bone acquisition and prevention of skeletal impairment
Fluoride in mineral water, 442–443
Fruits and vegetables
antioxidant properties, 110–111, 119
blood pressure, 64
bone resorption, 303–304, 309
effects on bone status, 29, 31–32, 309–311, 320–321
effects on bone resorption, 303–304, 309
effects on disease, 316–317
osteoporosis prevention, 315–328
acid-base homeostasis, 316–318
alkaline supplements, 319–320
buffering role of calcium, 317, 324
intervention studies, 320–321
NEAP, 321, 323
pharmacologically active compound *vs.* base excess, 306–307, 309
phytochemical interaction, 123
potential renal acid loads, 318–319
role, 315–328
See also Foodstuffs and beverages inhibiting bone resorption; Hesperidin, improved bone acquisition and prevention of skeletal impairment

G
Gene-nutrient interaction, 26, 128.
See Vitamin B-complex, methylene tetrahydrofolate reductase polymorphism and bone
Genistein, 298–299
Gla proteins, 79–82, 84
Glucose tolerance factor (GTF), 147–148
Gonadotropin-releasing hormone (GnRH), 381
Grain products
acid load, 273, 318, 352, 359–360
sulfur per gram protein, 383
Growth hormone, 384, 386, 388

H
Hesperidin, improved bone acquisition and prevention of skeletal impairment, 109–126
body composition and uterine weight, 115–116
bone mineral density, 116–118

bone size and strength, 118
bone turnover and plasma hesperidin,
    118–119
    mechanism, 121–122
Hip fractures
    antioxidant actions of vitamin E, 122
    calcium intake, protein and risk,
        403–406
    Japanese vs. Western rates, 31, 85
    nursing home residents, 84, 379
    protein effects, 65, 67, 379, 388–390,
        403–404
    vitamin A association, 94–95, 106
    vitamin D supplementation in elderly after
        hip fracture, adherence
        methods, 254–255
        overview, 253–254, 258–259
        patient evaluation and risk assessment,
            256–258
        recommendations, 258–259
Hip structural analysis (HSA), 37, 38–39, 42
Homocysteine levels. See Vitamin B-complex,
    methylene tetrahydrofolate reductase
    polymorphism and bone
Homocystinuria, 127, 131
Hormone replacement therapy (HRT), 83,
    298–299; See Estrogens
HSA analysis, 37, 38–39, 42
Hydroxyapatite
    deposition and osteocalcin role, 81, 82
    phosphorous-calcium ratio, 288
    released in metabolic acidosis, 335
    of tooth enamel and bone, 154
    vitamin D effects, 187
Hydroxyproline
    alkali supplementation effects, 319–320,
        335–336
    chromium intake, 141, 143, 148
    excretion in metabolic acidosis, 280
    nonspecific marker of bone resorption,
        403
Hypercalciuria. See Calcium excretion
Hypertension, 64, 189
    DASH (dietary approaches to stopping
        hypertension), 64, 315–316, 320–321
Hypocalcemia in dairy cattle, 336, 338
Hypophosphatemia, 67–68
Hypothalamic-pituitary-adrenal (HPA) axis
    effects of dietary restraint, 165, 167–168,
        172–173, 175

I
Icosapentaenoic acid, 31
IGF-1 binding proteins, 46, 55, 401
IGF-1 (insulin-like growth factor)
    calcium carbonate supplementation, 45–56
        bone size and IGF-1 influence, 46–47, 55
        effects on girls and boys, 51–55
        methods, 47–51
    and chronic metabolic acidosis, 400
    N-acetyl cysteine supplementation, bone
        characteristics and serum IGF-1,
            369–377
        biological activity of NAC, 370–371
        bone density and morphology, 372–374,
            375
        materials and methods, 371–372
        reduced body weight gain, 372
        serum IGF-1 levels, 374–376
    and protein intake, 46, 66–67, 384–388,
        389, 400–401, 403
    threshold characteristics, 66–67
Insulin, 148
    chromium effects, 142
    dairy consumption, 64
Insulin-like growth factor 1. See IGF-1
    (insulin-like growth factor)
Interleukin-1 (IL-1), 387–388
Ischemic heart disease
    importance of fruits and vegetables,
        316–317

M
Matrix Gla protein (MGP), 79, 80, 82, 84
Meat intake, 352, 354, 355, 401
Menstrual cycle, 168–169
    dietary restraint effects, 170–172
    disturbances and bone loss, 172
    effects of protein restriction in athletes, 381
    effects of protein restriction in rats, 385
Metabolic syndrome and dairy consumption, 64
Methylation reactions, B_6 role, 129
Methylene tetrahydrofolate reductase
    polymorphism, vitamin B-complex and
    bone. See Vitamin B-complex
Milk (See also Dairy products) basic protein,
    increased bone mineral density and
    improved bone metabolism, 413–429
    bone remodeling, 414–415
    component nutrients, 415–416, 427
    overview, 413–414, 426–427

Milk basic protein (*Continued*)
  study one (female)
    biochemical markers, 419–426
    BMD changes, 417–419
    subjects and protocols, 416–417, 423
Minerals. *See specific mineral*
Mineral waters, effects on bone metabolism, 439–447
  acid load, 443–444
  alkaline load, 444–445
  calcium, 440–441
  carbonated beverages, 442
  fluoride, 442–443
  mineral content by geographic area, 440
  potassium, 445
  sodium, 441–442
  sulfates, 442
Monoterpenes, 298, 302, 307–309
Multiple sclerosis, 189
Mushrooms, 304

N
N-acetyl cysteine supplementation, bone characteristics and serum IGF-1, 369–377
  biological activity of NAC, 370–371
  bone density and morphology, 372–374, 375
  materials and methods, 371–372
  reduced body weight gain, 372
  serum IGF-1 levels, 374–376
NEAP (net endogenous noncarbonic acid production)
  of ancestral humans *vs.* modern, 350, 356–358
  estimation equations, 337
  food group values, 354, 357–358
  protein-to-potassium ratio, 321, 323, 324, 360, 361
  relationship to bone mineral density, 360–361
  relationship to RNAE and acidosis, 273, 277–279, 286
  setpoint determinants, 274–279
  See also Acid load
N-telopeptide excretion, 360, 403
Nutrients
  interactions and food sources, 61–79
    diet quality and calcium intake, 62–65
    phosphorus and calcium relationships, 67–74
    protein and calcium relationships, 65–67

  See also specific nutrient
Nuts, beans, and seeds, 304

O
Onions, 111, 298, 302, 306–307
Orange juice, 67, 111, 122, 195
Osteoblasts
  chromium effects, 144
  hesperidin effects, 122
  pH change response, 274
Osteocalcin
  alkali administration, 274, 319
  calcium supplementation, 54–55
  milk basic protein effects, 413
  vitamin K effects, 79, 80, 81, 85, 88 (*see also* Vitamin K)
Osteocalcin total antigen, 81
Osteoclasts, 186, 274, 414–415
Osteomalacia, 187–188, 203, 219, 232
  vitamin D optimal amount for osteoporosis, 211–223
    comparison of evidence, 214–215
    dosage determination, 215–217
    dosage recommendations, 219–220
    hormonal nature of 1,25(OH)$_2$D, 217–219
    overview, 211–212, 219–220

P
Parathyroid hormone (PTH)
  calcium effects, 186, 335
  chromium effects, 144, 148
  dietary protein effects, 383, 401
  metabolic acidosis relationship, 274, 335
  phosphorus effects, 73–74
  vitamin D relationship, 186, 187, 204, 206–207, 236
Peak bone mass, 26, 36, 46, 289
  age of achievement, 21, 25, 30, 432
  diet and exercise, 432–433 (*see also* Physical activity)
  peak bone mineral velocity and gender, 21
  See also IGF-1 (insulin-like growth factor); Skeletal development
Peanuts (Charles Schulz), 198
Phosphorus
  absorption efficiency, 68, 69, 70–72
  antiresorptive therapies, 69
  calcium effects, 67–74, 288
  effects on PTH secretion, 73–74

protein effects, 65–66, 68
reference values, 68–69
Physical activity
BMC at peak height velocity, 433–434
dietary balance in active and inactive girls, 431–438
mechanical stress on growing bones, 14, 29, 31, 432–433, 436
nutritional inadequacies, 381
peak bone mass, 432–433
serum IGF-1 levels, 54, 435
See also Skeletal development
Postmenopausal bone health
calcium and phosphorus supplementation, 73–74, 401
neutralizing diet net acid load, 287–288
protein, 66, 381–383, 402–403
protein and calcium absorption, 402–403
protein increases procollagen, 401
PTH, sensitivity to, 335
tooth loss and rates of total body bone loss, 156
vitamin D supplementation, 245–251
vitamin D therapy, 228–229
vitamin K therapy, 86
See also Estrogen-depletion-associated osteoporosis; Hesperidin, improved bone acquisition and prevention of skeletal impairment; Osteoporosis prevention; Ovine model for dietary acid base, estrogen depletion and bone health
Potassium
ancestral intake vs. modern, 349–350, 358–362
content in various foods, 354
metabolic acidosis induced by reduction, 337, 349
in mineral water, 445
Potassium bicarbonate, 349–350, 402
supplementation, 287–288, 335–336
vs. potassium chloride, 445
Potassium intake in ancestrial diet, 358–360
Potassium citrate, 349, 402
Potassium-to-protein ratio and net acid excretion, 321, 323, 324, 352, 360, 361
Potassium-to-sodium ratio, 352
Potential renal acid load (PRAL), 318–319, 443–444

Protein. See Dietary protein
acid-base balance, 401–402
ancestral vs. modern intake, 352
animal vs. plant sources, 383–384, 390, 404
calcium effects, 65–67, 402–403
effect on BMD, 381, 384, 413, 414
effects, 65–66, 68, 383, 389, 399, 402–403, 405–406
impact on the skeleton, 399–409
acid-base balance, 401–402
bone loss and fracture, 403–405
bone turnover, 403
calcium absorption, 402–403
IGF-1 levels, 400–401
insufficiency, 380–381, 388–389
intake and bone strength, 379–397
acid load, 383–384
bone mineral mass, 380–384
bone strength determinants, 380
cytokine secretion, 386–388
fracture risk, 389–390
GH-IGF-1 system, 384–386, 388
protein supplementation, 388–389
net acid load, 273, 352, 383–384
plant protein, 352–353
pubertal status, 4, 6, 80, 380
purified protein, 65, 66, 399
recommended daily allowance, 388
soy, 298–299
sulfur production, 355
vegetarian vs. omnivorous, 170–171, 318
Protein S, 82
Prunes, 303–304
Pubertal status
BMD responses to calcium, 31, 55
effects of calcium and protein on bone size, 380
growth spurts, 4, 6, 30, 380

R
Renal acid load, potential (PRAL), 318–319
of mineral water, 443–444
Renal function
age related decline, 219, 276–277, 335
effects of IGF-1, 384
phosphorus retention, 67
Renal net acid excretion (RNAE), 273–274, 276–279

Renal net acid excretion (RNAE) (*Continued*)
average excretion per day, 285–286
changes in after addition of single food
item, 353
equations for estimating DCAD, 336–337
predictive of calcium excretion, 321, 323,
360
relation to bone mineral density, 360–361
See also Calcium excretion, urinary; NEAP
(net endogenous noncarbonic acid
production)
Renal stones, 68, 282
Respiratory setpoints in acid-base balance,
274–275
Retinoic acid, serum, 93, 99, 105–106
See also Vitamin A
Retinoic acid nuclear receptors, 94, 186
Rheumatoid arthritis, 83, 189
Rickets, 186–187, 188, 219, 232, 237

S
Secondary hyperparathyroidism, 203
and reduction in dietary protein, 383
vitamin D deficiency, 187
Sheep, 331–333
Skeletal development
BMD of skull and lower extremities during
growth and calcium supplementation,
3–15
lower extremity mineralization, 7–10, 12,
13
mechanical stresses, 14
methods, 5–6
overview, 3–4, 10–14
skull mineralization, 6–7, 8, 11
whole-body scans, 4, 14
calcium carbonate supplementation in
adolescent boys and girls and serum
IGF-1 levels, 45–56, 400
bone size and IGF-1 influence, 46–47
effects on boys, 54–55
effects on girls, 51–53
methods, 47–51
overview, 45–47, 54–55
calcium retention in adolescence as a
function of calcium intake, influence of
race and gender, 17–23
gender influences, 21–22
methods, 18–19
overview, 17, 22

race influences, 19–21
threshold intake for African-American
girls, 20
threshold intake for Caucasian girls,
17, 18
total body salt levels, 20–21
co-twin calcium intervention trial, cortical
bone effects by hip structural analysis,
35–43
bone response to calcium intervention,
41–42
femoral bone assessment, 39–41
influences on bone geometry and
strength, 37–38
overview, 36, 41–42
participants and study design, 38–39
genetic variance *vs.* modifiable factors, 26, 36
protein relationship, 380–381
See also Diet and lifestyle intervention in
children, effects of Asian traditional
diet and sitting style; Dietary balance in
active and inactive girls; N-acetyl
cysteine supplementation
Sodium
ancestral intake *vs.* modern, 352
consumption per day, 352
in metabolic acidosis, 337
in mineral water, 441–442
Sodium bicarbonate, 402
Sodium-to-potassium ratio, 352
Soy isoflavones, 111
Soy protein, 298–299
Stone Age diets for the 21st century (low-grade
metabolic alkalosis), 349–362
Sulfates in mineral water, 442
Sulfur byproducts of protein metabolism, 306,
337, 355–356, 383–384
Sunscreen, 183, 187, 194

T
Tea beverages, 111
Teeth, nutrition and, 153–164
bacterial inflammation, 154, 155
key nutrients, 154, 158–162
oral bone loss and BMD, 154–156
periodontal disease and tooth loss,
156–158
Teriparatide, 73
Tumor necrosis factor alpha (TNF-∞),
386–387

U

UVB radiation and cutaneous production of D_3
 artificial sources, 183, 189–190
 natural sunlight, 182–186
 See also Vitamin D

V

Vascular elasticity
 vitamin K effects, 79, 87
VDRs, 186, 189, 191, 193
Vegetables, effect on bone, 302–303
 See also Fruits and vegetables
Vitamin A
 negative relationship to BMD in
  postmenopausal women, 93–108
 baseline evaluations, 98–99
 food sources, 104
 hypervitaminosis A, 94
 serum retinol, 93–94, 105
Vitamin B-complex, methylene
  tetrahydrofolate reductase polymorphism
  and bone, 127–138
 B complex and bone health, 132–133
 B complex and reduction homocysteine
  levels, 132
 dietary intake of B-complex vitamins,
  133–135
 folate, 133, 135
 gene-nutrient interaction evidence, 132,
  133
 MTHFR and bone health, 131–132
 MTHFR and chronic disease, 130–131
 MTHFR functions, 128–129
 MTHFR polymorphism, 129–130
Vitamin D
 breakpoint of normal serum levels of
  25(OH)D in the elderly, 203–209
 assessment methods, 204
 assays, 205, 206, 207
 calcium intake and serum PTH,
  206–207
 epidemiological and intervention studies,
  205–206
 stages of deficiency, 207
 combined supplementation with vitamin K,
  86–87
 deficiency, 186–188
 deficiency prevention and treatment,
  194–197
 effect on bone, 205, 405–406

 fractures, 265–268
 optimal intake for osteoporosis, 211–223
  dosage determination, 215–217
  dosage recommendations, 219–220
  supplementation in postmenopausal black
   women, 245–271
 1,25(OH)$_2$D (1,25-dihydroxyvitamin D)
  hormonal nature of, 217–219
  metabolic role, 186, 191, 193
  serum levels, 219
 25(OH)D optimal levels (roundtable
  discussions), 264–266
 antiproliferative properties and
  treatments utilizing D_3 analogs,
  193–194
 calcium absorption efficiencies, 228–231
 calcium adsorption regulation, 183, 186
 chromic diseases, 189–193
 clinical importance, 237
 contributors, 263–264
 deficient *vs.* insufficient, 232
 local production of 1,25(OH)$_2$D, 191,
  193
 metabolic pathways, 183–186
 methods applied, 237–238
 optimal serum level, 232
 oral bone health, 154, 162 (*see also*
  Nutrition and teeth)
 osteoporotic fractures, 231–232
 patient evaluation and risk assessment,
  256–258
 prevention of cancers, type 1 diabetes and
  heart disease, 181–201
 PTH *vs.* BMD in threshold assessment,
  236, 240–241
 recommendations, 258–259
 reference ranges, 227–228, 232
 reference ranges, 240–242
 serum level assessment methods, 204
 supplement D_3 dosages, 266–268
 supplementation in elderly after hip
  fracture, adherence
 VDRs, 186, 189, 191, 193
Vitamin E, 122
Vitamin K, 79–92
 action sites, 81–82
 bone health, 84–85
 cardiovascular health, 85–86
 dietary requirements, 87–88
 inflammatory diseases, 83

Vitamin K (*Continued*)
  insufficiency, 80–81
  intervention, safety and side effects, 86–89
  K_1, K_2 (menaquinones), 80, 87–88
  non-inflammatory calcifications, 83
  vascular calcification, 82–83

W
Warfarin, 82, 88–89
Weight reduction, 64
  See also Anorexia nervosa; Dietary restraint,
    cortisol and bone density
Whey protein, 415